MICROVASCULAR
BONE RECONSTRUCTION

MICROVASCULAR BONE RECONSTRUCTION

Edited by

Michael B Wood, MD
Reconstructive Microsurgery
Mayo Clinic
Rochester, Minnesota
USA

and

Alain Gilbert, MD
Institut de la Main
Clinique Jouvenet
Paris
France

Mosby

St. Louis Baltimore Boston Carlsbad Chicago Naples New York Philadelphia Portland
London Madrid Mexico City Singapore Sydney Tokyo Toronto Wiesbaden

Martin Dunitz

First published in the United Kingdom in 1997
by Martin Dunitz Ltd
The Livery House
7–9 Pratt Street
London NW1 0AE

Mosby
Dedicated to Publishing Excellence

A Times Mirror
Company

Distributed in the U.S.A. and Canada by

Mosby–Year Book	Times Mirror Professional Publishing Ltd.
11830 Westline Industrial Drive	130 Flaska Drive
St. Louis, Missouri 63146	Markham, Ontario L6G 1B8

A CIP record for this book is available from the British Library.

ISBN 0 948269 71 5

Composition by Scribe Design, Gillingham, Kent
Printed and bound in Spain by Grafos, S.A. Arte sobre papel

Contents

List of contributors

Peter J Briggs
Department of Orthopaedics
Royal Victoria Infirmary
Newcastle upon Tyne
United Kingdom

Bruno Coessens
University Department of Plastic Surgery
Free University Brussels
Brugmann Hospital
Brussels
Belgium

Timothy R C Davis
Department of Trauma and Orthopaedic Surgery
Queen's Medical Centre
Nottingham
United Kingdom

Alain Gilbert
Institut de la Main
Clinique Jouvenet
Paris
France

Jamal Gousheh
Plastic and Reconstructive Surgery
Shahd Beheshti University
Tehran
Iran

Alain C Masquelet
Service d'Orthopédie et Traumatologie
Hôpital Avicenne
Bobigny
France

Christopher G Moran
Department of Trauma and Orthopaedic Surgery
Queen's Medical Centre
Nottingham
United Kingdom

Marie Claude Romaña
Service d'Orthopédie Pédiatrique
Hôpital Trousseau
Paris
France

Luc Téot
Laboratory for Surgical Research
Faculty of Medicine
Hôpital Lapeyronie
Montpellier
France

Michael B Wood
Reconstructive Microsurgery
Mayo Clinic
Rochester
Minnesota
USA

Preface

The relationship between preservation or restoration of bone blood flow and bone healing has long been recognized. The introduction and refinement of microvascular surgery, particularly over the past fifteen years, has for the first time permitted the possibility of combining the advantages of pedicle bone grafting with the versatility of free bone grafting. This work attempts to provide the reader with an understanding of the rationale, indications, techniques and expected results of vascularized bone grafting. Although the authors recognize that this is a rapidly evolving field, we do attempt to capture the 'state of the art' in 1997 within this text. Moreover, current concepts of bone blood flow control mechanisms and alternative forms of bone grafting are briefly reviewed. The authors realize that vascularized bone grafting for reconstructive purposes is only one of a number of options for most typical clinical challenges involving either bone loss or refractory nonunion. We are at the same time convinced that the ability to carry out vascularized bone grafting is a substantial advance in the field of bone reconstruction and deserves to hold a place in the armamentarium for bone reconstruction in most modern, sophisticated medical facilities.

MBW
AG
March 1997

To my wife, Marilee, and my children, Michael, Hadley, Benjamin, and Luke.

MBW

I GENERAL CONSIDERATIONS: STRUCTURE AND FUNCTION

1. Anatomy of bone

A clear understanding of the form and function of bone is a necessary requisite for any surgeon dealing with skeletal trauma and reconstruction. However, an intimate understanding of both the structural anatomy and the physiology of bone is particularly important for the surgeon dealing with bone reconstruction in cases of skeletal pathology. The mechanisms of simple fracture healing, bone graft incorporation for both nonunions and skeletal defects, healing of vascularized bone transfers, and the response of bone to its soft tissue milieu often require consideration in the selection of the most appropriate management plan for a specific clinical situation. This chapter will attempt to summarize the general morphologic considerations of bone structural anatomy and physiologic response in both health and disease.

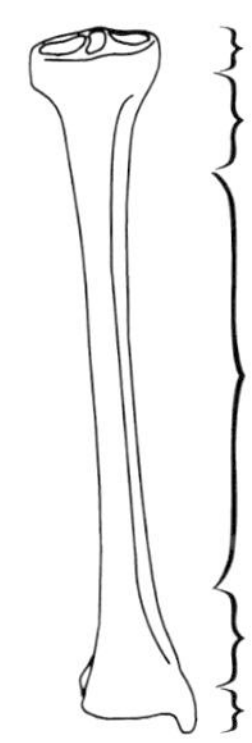

Fig. 1 *Structure of typical long bone.*

Gross structural anatomy

Bone in general can be structurally classified as either flat or tubular. Flat bones develop from connective tissue which differentiates into bone, and include the pelvis (ilium) and scapula. Tubular bones develop from cartilage, and include all the long bones (humerus, radius, ulna, metacarpals and metatarsals, phalanges, femur, tibia and fibula). Tubular bones are in general topographically subdivided into an epiphysis at either end, a central linear diaphyseal portion, and a flared metaphysis at either end, between epiphysis and diaphysis (Fig. 1). All named bones are composed of both cortical (compact) and cancellous (spongy) bone tissue. The relative distribution of cortical or cancellous bone, distribution of marrow, and specific blood flow will vary greatly between bones and regionally within the bone. In general, flat bones and the epiphyses and metaphyses of the tubular bones contain a large proportion of cancellous bone. The diaphyses of long bones are chiefly of cortical composition.

Microscopic anatomy

The cellular components of bone (excluding marrow elements) include osteoblasts, osteocytes, and osteoclasts (Robinson 1965). Osteoblasts are small,

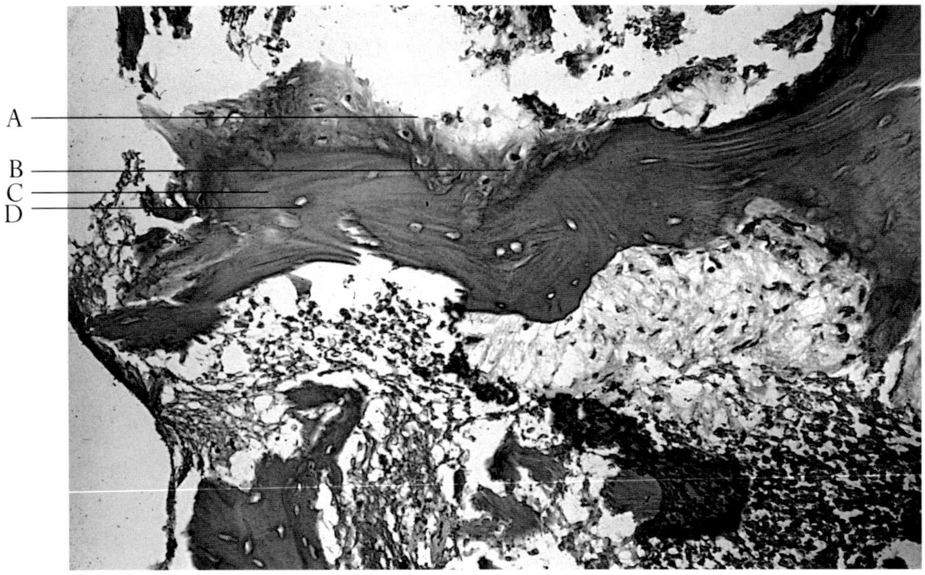

Fig. 2 *Photomicrograph – new bone formation. Note osteoblasts (A), layer of newly elaborated osteoid (B), mineralized bone (C) with contained osteocytes (D).*

cuboidal cells with a single nucleus and are primarily concerned with bone formation. These cells are thought to be derived from undifferentiated circulating osteoprogenitor cells. The factors that signal osteoprogenitor cells and induce their differentiation into osteoblasts at a specific location are not well defined. However, the role of growth factors from a variety of sources is increasingly recognized as important. Fracture, osteotomy, sepsis and the presence of bone marrow grafts appear to be associated with cellular differentiation into bone forming elements. The sequence of events involved in bone formation begins initially with the elaboration by osteoblasts of unmineralized matrix called osteoid (Fig. 2). Osteoid is composed primarily of densely woven collagen and a mucopolysaccharide ground substance. As osteoid is formed the osteoblast itself becomes surrounded and incorporated within the newly formed material. After a delay of approximately 15 days, the osteoid begins to calcify by deposition of hydroxyapatite crystals. The events surrounding the calcification processes are not well understood, but do not appear to be directly cell mediated. When calcification of the osteoid is completed the substance is known as bone and the contained osteoblasts lying within specific spaces termed lacunae become known as osteocytes. Osteocytes, though apparently trapped within a calcified matrix, are interconnected and connected with the extracellular fluid space by small, cytoplasmic processes known as canaliculi. These cells are metabolically active and appear chiefly concerned with calcium homeostasis (Baud and Biovin 1978). Under the influence of parathyroid hormone, osteocytes are capable of directly resorbing surrounding bone. The third cellular components of bone are osteoclasts (Hancox and Boothroyd 1963). These are large, multinucleated cells derived from hematopoietic progenitor cells. The function of osteoclasts is that of bone resorption, which is an integral part of bone remodeling. The mechanism of resorption involves proteolytic enzymatic digestion and phagocytosis. Incompletely mineralized osteoid is resistant to osteoclastic resorption. The processes of bone resorption by osteoclasts and bone formation by osteoblasts are ongoing throughout life and continuously remodel bone. The balance of these two processes determines whether there is a net gain or a net loss of bone mass. In health these two processes should be equal. However, under certain conditions (for example, disuse or senile osteoporosis, hyperparathyroidism, Cushing's disease) resorption may outpace formation. Conversely, under some conditions (osteopetrosis) formation may outpace resorption. Fracture healing and remodeling will exhibit both accelerated bone formation and accelerated resorption, but with a net increase in bone mass. The

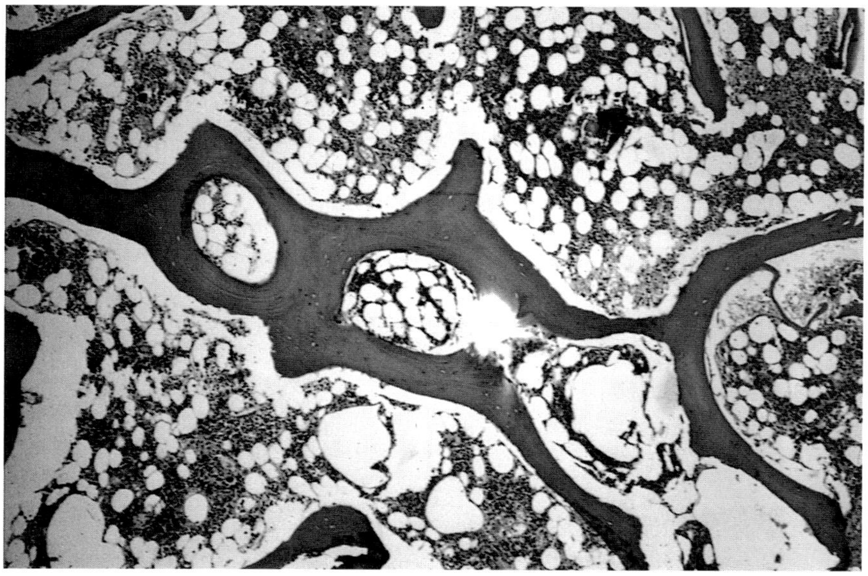

Fig. 3 *Photomicrograph – woven bone (note haphazard arrangement).*

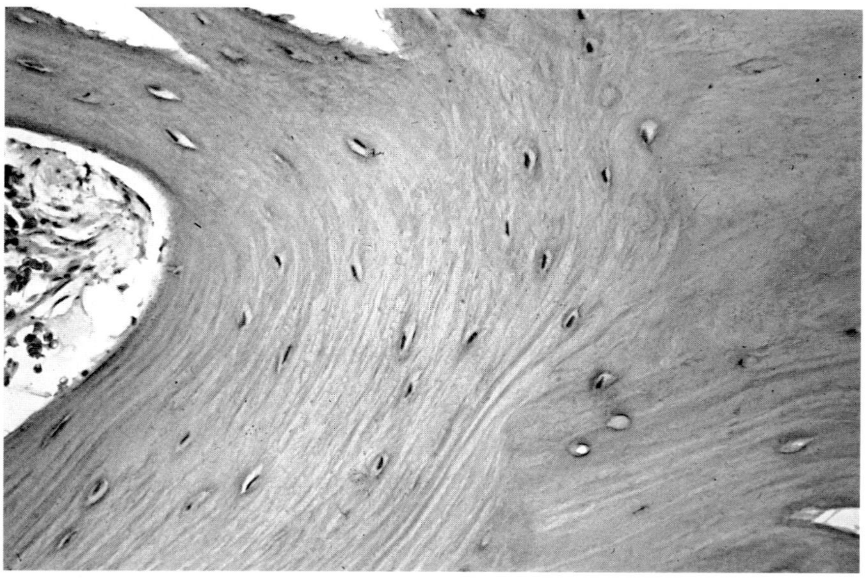

Fig. 4 *Photomicrograph – haversian bone (note dense concentric ringed structure).*

processes of bone formation and resorption involve less than 5% of the total bone surface at any one time in the normal adult. Thus, the majority of bone at any instant is inactive. At the microscopic level bone may be either of woven or compact structure. Woven bone appears haphazardly arranged and is characteristic of immature or newly elaborated bone (Fig. 3). Compact bone is characteristic of mature bone and may be either haversian or nonhaversian. Nonhaversian compact bone is usually periosteal or endosteal lamellar bone. Haversian bone is concentrically arranged about a central vascular channel and appears in a cross-section as multiple concentric rings of dense, well-organized bone (Fig. 4). Each ring unit is called an osteone and extends for a variable distance generally oriented along the longitudinal axis of the bone (Glimcher 1968). Osteones are continuously being breached by osteoclastic resorption activity, with subsequent formation of new (secondary, tertiary, quaternary, etc) osteones directed along axes responsive to imposed loading stresses. In this way bone may adapt to the mechanical demands placed on it in such a way as to attain maximal strength characteristics.

2. Epiphyseal plate: anatomy and growth

Luc Téot

Introduction

The growth plate represents the only temporary structure of the human body that subsequently disappears. This narrow white line of cartilage located deep inside the bone is covered peripherally by the perichondrial ring. Several researchers attempted to transfer the epiphysis experimentally for over a century, but results were unreliable. At the beginning of the 1980s, the development of microsurgical techniques enhanced the hopes of success after pedicled epiphyseal transfer. Most researchers considered that preservation of the epiphyseal vessels was mandatory to keep intact the possibilities of cell development and multiplication in the proliferative layer of the growth plate. Several pioneering attempts were made, the epiphysis being pedicled on the epiphyseal vessels. These vascular sources were not anatomically perfectly defined, and more experiments were necessary before more precise experimental models could be established.

These researchers concluded that reposition in the same location resulted in normal growth possibilities when the epiphysis was well vascularized. In the case of heterotopic transfer, many difficulties were noted concerning the biomechanical conditions that tissue from the donor site was subjected to after transfer into another location. In children, suitable donor sites are not numerous. Three sites of harvesting can be defined: the iliac crest, the upper fibula, and the lower scapula. Two of these are not true epiphyses and are not covered by articular cartilage, and their growth is determined by the traction of the strong muscles that are inserted on these apophyses.

On the basis of this, preliminary clinical series were cautiously initiated and, after being observed for more than 5 years, published. Indications were limited to patients where no other surgical technique had proved its efficacy. Limits to these techniques clearly appeared, comprising a lack of correspondence in size and volume between the possible donor sites and the recipient areas.

The utility of the techniques was, however, confirmed in procedures that used the iliac crest placed into an appositional situation parallel to a bone extremity not large enough to sustain its joint counterpart (radial club hand).

Recent experimental work is more orientated towards research on cryoconservation and preservation of growth plate development after bone banking. Vascularized epiphyseal cryoconserved transfers are a new challenge. If some difficulties now appear to have been solved, the penetration of the protecting agent inside the growth plate itself still remains to be tested.

Beside the clinical problems that are now solved by other techniques (limb lengthening), knowledge of the mechanical, immunological, and vascular requirements of the growth plate has improved and benefited from this surgical enthusiasm for epiphyseal transplantation.

Fundamental aspects of growth plate transplantation

Anatomy of the growth plate

Strictly speaking, the term 'growth plate' suggests a single plane structure. In fact, several anatomical studies have demonstrated that the growth plate presents a shape grossly corresponding to that of the bone extremity inside which it is located. More or less rounded, more or less curved in different directions, the growth structure is globally parallel to the joint cartilage located above or below it. The lower femoral epiphysis is rounded and irregular, and the corresponding growth plate presents a comparable shape. Speer (1982), following Lacroix (1949), Policard and Ranvier (see Trueta 1963), had pursued this line of research, determining the irregular shape of the growth plate and the existence of the mamillary processes, whose role in mechanical resistance has not yet been totally determined.

The epiphysis is initially a homogeneous structure, formed by hyaline cartilage. Progressively, under the combined action of mechanical forces and vascular changes, the secondary nucleus of ossification will appear, determining a zone where the growth plate itself and the articular cartilage will develop. Wilsman and Van Sickle (1970) showed that, from the 21st day of intrauterine life, the hyaline structure is perforated by cartilage canals, each of them including an arteriole, vein, and nerve. The distal ends of the vessels are dilated, and this primitive vascular system provides nutrition to a certain amount of hyaline tissue. These vascular enlargements (glomerulae) are located on the junction site of the first zone of calcification and ossification. Appearance of the nucleus of ossification is initially located near the center of the epiphysis. The growth of the epiphyseal bone will be concentric for some weeks. Later, the growth plate itself will be formed between the epiphysis and the diaphysis, and will be progressively covered on its epiphyseal side by a transverse bone barrier. The cartilaginous growth results from three simultaneous events: cellular hyperplasia (increasing cell multiplication), cell hypertrophy (increasing the size of the cells), and hyperproduction of the ground substance.

Anatomy of the epiphyseal vessels

Epiphyseal vessels can be grouped in three to four main sources, two of them being lateral and one of them penetrating the structure in its central portion.

In some epiphyses, the nucleus of ossification will develop from these central vessels. The initially formed cancellous bone presents communicating channels of perfusion, but it has been clearly demonstrated that the cartilage canals will form the definitive vascular pathway, which remains identical from the beginning of formation until the end of life. It has not been proven that a real vascular supply exists between the different parts of the epiphysis.

In time the peripheral cartilaginous crest becomes progressively thinned, the articular cartilage being penetrated by the synovial fluid. The nucleus of ossification organizes to resist increasing compressive forces.

The end of growth is characterized by the disappearance of the growth plate simultaneously with hormonal changes at puberty.

Few changes occur in the vascular distribution, and the diaphyseal system does not seem to penetrate the epiphysis. The notion of a communicating system existing between the epiphysis and the metaphysis has not been clearly demonstrated, which may explain the fragility of the epiphyseal vascularization. Each epiphyseal portion is vascularized by a specific vascular system which is unique and not biologically capable of supplying a nearby deficiency.

This system can be surgically grouped into three main pedicles:

— the medial epiphyseal vessels;
— the central epiphyseal vessels; and
— the lateral epiphyseal vessels.

All these sources must be harvested and pedicled on one or two principal pedicles, bearing in mind the difficulties of the microsurgical procedure.

Physiology of the growth plate

Bone formation results from a chain of transformations commencing with the cartilage, which is progressively converted to a calcified matrix preliminary to the ossification itself. Cellular chemotactism, proliferation of the mesenchymatous cells, differentiation and hypertrophy of the cartilaginous cells, matrix calcification, vascular invasion, cartilaginous resorption, bone matrix formation and mineralization, and finally bone remodeling are the successive steps that lead to an increase in bone volume.

At present, an understanding of the biochemical events seems more important than studies concerning the function of the growth plate. The main role of the growth plate is to prevent a premature calcification, to multiply and thus to maintain a cartilaginous interposition between two ossified areas.

Amongst the different theories of calcification, those most commonly maintained are:

— proteoglycans inhibit crystal formation by the capture of minerals;
— pyrophosphates directly inhibit the calcification phenomenon; and
— mitochondria act as regulators in crystal formation.

The growth plate that promotes endochondral ossification is a very organized structure, formed by several specialized zones:

- *The reserve zone:* chondrocytes in the reserve zone are usually small in size, and irregularly spread in the matrix. This zone is generally considered a storage zone. Proteoglycans and lipids are found in smaller quantities in this zone than anywhere else in the growth plate. Glycosaminoglycans are identical to those found in the joint cartilage. Initially, some authors considered this zone as playing a fundamental role in cell division. In fact, very few cell division aspects are found here, and the metabolic level of this zone is very low, as indicated by the low pO_2 level.
- *The proliferative zone* is more organized. Chondrocytes are arranged in columns parallel to the long axis of the bone; this columnal organization is found all along the growth plate. The cells present signs of activity, with a discoid shape, and are superimposed one over the other. The surrounding extracellular matrix presents its own characteristics. Inside each cell we can observe mitochondria, a rugous endoplasmic reticulum, and an elongated nucleus. This is the cell division zone. Inhibition of mineralization is maximal in this zone. Pyrophosphates and proteoglycan levels are more important than anywhere else, and it is well known that their role is to inhibit and stop hydroxyapatite formation and development. Epiphyseal vessels end at this level. The pO_2 level is more than 7.5%, explaining the high level of enzymatic activity and the important production of ATP by the mitochondria.
- At the bottom of this proliferative zone, some authors would identify the *zone of matrix synthesis*: cells are elongated and present a larger Golgi system, and numerous dilated cisternae are found in the endoplasmic reticulum. Each cell is separated from the next by a freshly formed cartilaginous matrix, composed of fine fibrils trapped in an amorphous fundamental substance. Inside this matrix, several matrix vesicles inhibiting calcification are observed. Type X collagen seems to play a role in the cartilaginous matrix calcification. It combines with the collagenic fibrils (Type II). When the cartilage undergoes calcification, the mineral formation is very localized to the association between these fibrils and the Type II collagen. Type X collagen seems to have the role of preventing bone crystallization without preventing mineralization. The kinetic modifications are very localized to this zone, and at a lower level at the level of the hypertrophic zone. Hormonal control of the cells in this zone has been clearly demonstrated.
- *The hypertrophic zone* presents larger lacunae, and the longitudinal fibrils are more compressed. The cells show signs of metabolic activity. The most distal cells present an important amount of precipitated calcium, localized outside the cell. In this zone the level of pO_2 is lower (3.2%). The mitochondria bind calcium in the upper part, and deposit calcium in the lower part. Alkaline phosphates are found in the matrix vesicles, facilitating mineralization. The level of neutral proteases is important, enhancing the mineralizing process. The contribution of this zone to the total growth is appreciable. The volume of the cells is directly related to the growth potential of the epiphysis. Several chondrodystrophies can be attributed to pathological changes in the hypertrophy of the growth plate cells, which seem locally modulated by biomechanical and vascular effects. In the lower part of the hypertrophic zone, calcification is induced in the longitudinal septa, between the chondrocyte columns. Penetration of the endothelial cells coming from the metaphyseal vessels is localized in the noncalcified area and the pericellular matrix. The speed of

growth of the hypertrophic cells is about 200 microns per day, and the turnover rate is 9 cells per day. After chondrocyte death, each lacuna is totally empty for about 8 minutes before being filled by the endothelial cells.

Role of the epiphyseal vessel

Toynbee in 1841 suspected the role of the epiphyseal vessels on the growth plate. Flourens (see Trueta 1963) and Ollier (1867) demonstrated at the same time that bone growth occurred at the bone ends. Haas in 1917 induced metacarpal and metatarsal devascularizations in dogs, leading to a constant decrease of growth, but not to a total arrest. In 1923 Nusbaum (see Trueta 1963) obtained an arrest of growth after ligating the epiphyseal vessels. In 1966, Holdsworth thought that epiphyseal ischemia induced only a temporary effect on the growth plate. He first demonstrated that a rapid revascularization takes place after ischemia, and that the loss of growth can be merely transitory when the ischemia is not too drastic.

Trueta in 1960 (Trueta 1963) demonstrated the role of the epiphyseal vascularization in the maintenance of the proliferative layer.

In fact, some authors explain the arrest of growth by some vascular communications between the epiphyseal and the metaphyseal parts, inducing an epiphysiodesis. Brashear (1963) created an experimental model in rats where the lower femoral epiphysis, located above a disarticulated knee, was excised at the periosteal level circularly. An arrest of growth, with an epiphysiodesis, regularly appeared. In fact, the existence of vascular system communication has been a controversial topic, with most authors confirming the important role this can play.

Young in 1956 (see Trueta 1963) induced a devascularization by excision of the capsular insertions on the rat metatarsal, with a rapid revascularization. The growth plate was thinned, owing to a discrepancy between the arrest of growth of germinal cell proliferation on the epiphyseal side, and continuous ossification on the metaphyseal side. This author also developed the interesting theory of a self-regulation of the amount of growth according to the volume of epiphyseal blood flow. This point was more recently confirmed by several studies using microsphere techniques.

These facts tend to lend support to the notion of a minimal break point of ischemia at which the germinal cells are definitively destroyed, leading to an epiphyseo-metaphyseal communication and the formation of an epiphysiodesis.

Experimental models using microsphere techniques were developed, showing that metaphyseal bone blood flow was comparable to epiphyseal bone blood flow. The flow is mainly proportional to the location of the epiphysis in the limb (more distal, less blood flow). No relationship seems to exist between production of new bone and the location of the epiphysis in the human body.

There have been several studies of selective metaphyseal or epiphyseal devascularizations. With regard to the metaphyseal side, all authors agree in observing an enlargment of the hypertrophic layers of the growth plate.

Trueta, Wray (Wray et al 1981), and Goodman induced stimulation of metaphyseal blood flow, mainly by using models involving metaphyseal fracture and periosteal stripping.

Immunology of the growth plate

The immunologic properties of the growth plate remain relatively unknown. The articular cartilage is better understood from the large studies of Friedlander (1983), Mankin et al (1983) and others. The relative resistance of articular cartilage rejection is due to its lack of blood supply and thus is not identical in the growth plate.

The growth plate is formed by a complex spatial arrangement of collagenic fibers (Speer 1982), some of them permeable to the fluid in the upper layers, others totally hermetic, as in the proliferative layer.

Experimental allografts pedicled on the epiphyseal vessels (Weiland et al 1984b; Téot 1983a) have demonstrated the constant development of rejection after transplantation. In a recent study we could observe some growth progression after cryoconservation in a −180°C liquid.

Yaremchuk et al (1985) observed, after an acute rejection, an increase in thickness in the hypertrophic layer.

Experimental studies on epiphyseal transplantation

In recent years, numerous experiments have utilized microsurgical techniques to transplant part or all of an epiphysis for the purpose of developing new surgical methods for traumatic, congenital or infectious sequelae of epiphyseal plate lesions. Donski and O'Brien published their pioneering study of the medullary and cortical vascularization in fibular transplantation in dogs in 1980. Zaleske et al in 1982 published a study involving articular replantation of the knee in rabbits. Growth was found to be practically normal in the vascularized group. The conclusions of this work are comparable to those of a previous work by Judet et al (1981). They indicate that all the structures, the epiphyseal plate, and the secondary ossification center undergo a slight trauma during transplantation or reposition, but keep their structure and function.

Brown et al (1983) studied the development of the proximal end of the fibula after repositioning or transplantation in 48 immature dogs. Conclusions were identical.

In a study of 48 immature dogs, Téot et al (1983a) transferred grafts from the iliac crest after resection of the epiphyseal plate of the distal end of the femur. The good blood supply provided by the revascularized graft appeared to contribute to a remodeling of the epiphyseal plate from the remaining edges of the growth plate.

Taken together, these recent experimental studies show that growth can reasonably be expected from vascularized bone transfers containing a proliferating zone. They also show the limits of this type of transfer, which are essentially imposed by biomechanical considerations. Epiphyses are not interchangeable, even though it has been demonstrated that total preservation of their vascularization is the *sine qua non* for growth.

Grafts coming from all possible zones of growth must be experimentally applied to situations comparable to those found in human pediatric pathology. It is essential that a maximum of guarantees for the reliability of these techniques be acquired by performing further experimentation in animals with long term follow-up of their growth until completion of growth.

There are two crucial zones to be studied in these transfers, and they correspond to the two cartilaginous zones transplanted: the epiphyseal plate and articular cartilage. The latter generally has a higher resistance to traumatic degeneration than the former, but our experience has confirmed the possibility of late arthrotic transformation of the cartilaginous surface of epiphyseal grafts that had previously been considered healthy. These techniques offer attractive solutions to many pathological situations, but their indications and limits must first be defined in animal models.

3. Bone blood flow

Timothy R C Davis and Michael B Wood

In man, skeletal blood flow accounts for 16% of the cardiac output, a figure which is comparable with renal blood flow (Charkes 1980). In comparison to the wealth of knowledge concerning the blood flow to organs such as the kidney, brain, and heart, our understanding of the anatomy and physiology of bone blood flow is sparse. This is partly due to lack of interest in bone blood flow, but is also due to the great difficulties encountered in its study. Study of blood flow is relatively straightforward in organs whose arterial and venous systems are easily isolated and have a reasonably high flow rate. However, in organs such as bone, which have a relatively low blood flow and multiple arterial inputs and venous outlets, it is fraught with problems. This chapter provides an overview of the present concepts of bone blood flow, and first discusses rates of bone blood flow and then describes the anatomy of bone blood circulation.

Rates of bone blood flow

Owing to the difficulty in measuring bone blood flow with noninvasive techniques, the blood flow rates quoted are for laboratory animals. Flow rates in mature mammalian long bones are in the range 5–20 ml/min per 100 g (Charkes 1980; Morris and Kelly 1980), and may be higher in immature bone. Within a long bone, regional differences in flow rates are found, with diaphyseal cortex having the lowest flow rate and red hemopoietic marrow the highest. In general, the ranges of blood flow for cortical bone, cancellous bone, and bone marrow are 5–15, 10–20, and 22–50 ml/min per 100 g respectively (Brookes 1987). Cortical and marrow blood flow are proportional to metabolic activity (McInnis et al 1980). Thus blood flow in metaphyseal cortex is greater than in diaphyseal cortex and flow in red marrow is higher than in yellow (fatty) marrow.

Circulation within a long bone

For many years the arrangement of blood vessels within bone has been disputed and many aspects remain controversial. This description reports the most widely accepted pattern of intraosseous circulation, which was popularized by Brookes (1971).

Arterial supply

All long bones have four arterial inputs, which are the nutrient, periosteal, metaphyseal, and epiphyseal arteries (Fig. 1). Even though this has been recognized for many years (Langer 1876; Lexer et al 1904), the relative importance of these four systems is not fully resolved.

The nutrient artery is the largest artery of a long bone, and for the fibula is usually a branch of the peroneal artery. Most long bones have only one nutrient artery, but the femur has two. The nutrient artery enters the medullary canal through an oblique nutrient foramen in the diaphyseal cortex. The location of each bone's nutrient foramen is relatively constant and, for the fibula, is usually in its middle third (96%) and on or posterior to its medial crest (89%) (Mysorekar 1967). For most (95%) fibulae, the nutrient foramen runs from the periosteal to endosteal surfaces in an

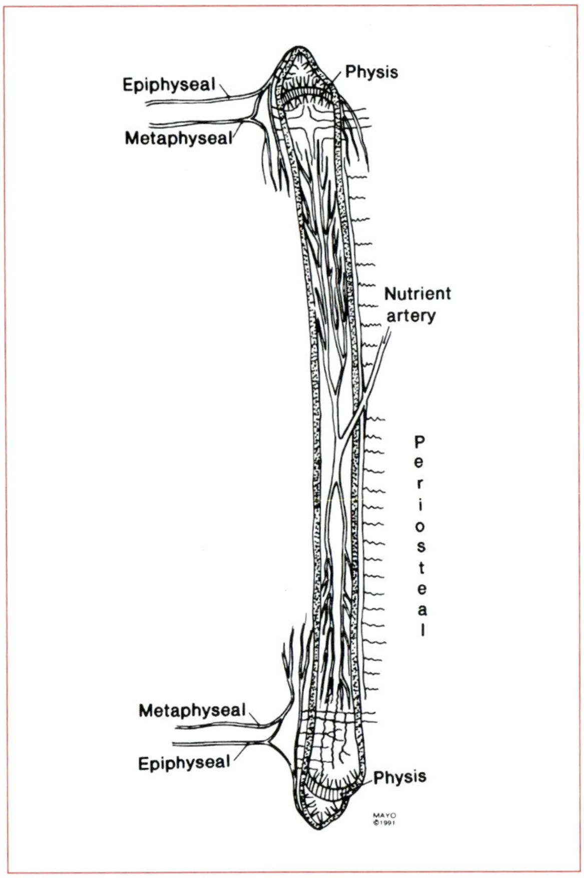

Fig. 1a *Schematic illustrating the arterial circulation within a long bone.*

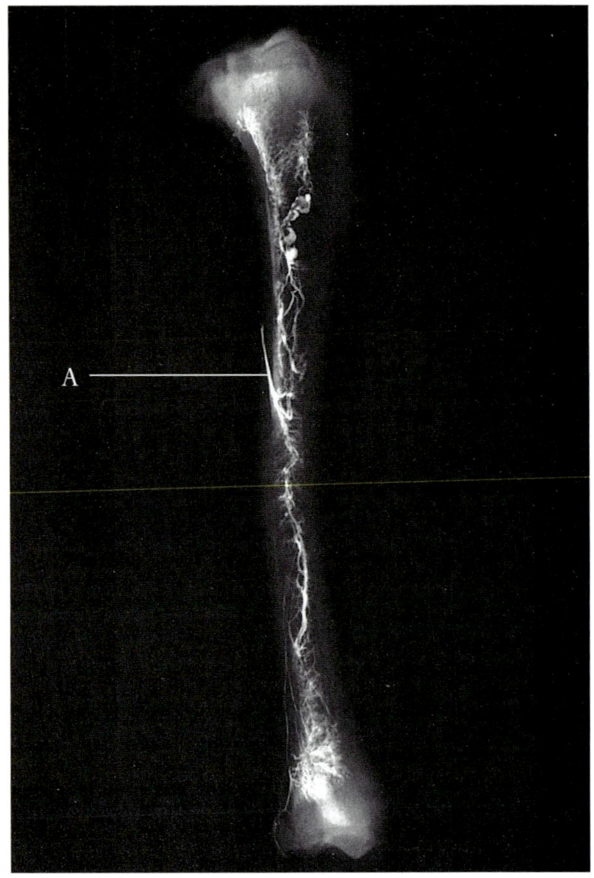

Fig. 1b *Venogram showing the central venous sinus running throughout the length of the medullary canal and draining into a nutrient vein (A).*

oblique distal direction (Mysorekar 1967). Before entering the nutrient foramen, the nutrient artery may send small branches to the periosteum and adjacent muscles, but it does not branch within the nutrient foramen. Once within the medullary cavity, the nutrient artery divides into ascending and descending branches. These repeatedly divide into smaller branches, which pass towards the metaphyses (see Fig. 1). The branches of the nutrient artery tend to lie adjacent to the endosteal cortex, at the periphery of the medullary cavity cross-section. Throughout their length, the arteries of the nutrient system give off radially orientated branches; those running centrifugally feed the capillaries of the cortex, while those running centripetally supply the marrow sinusoids (Fig. 2).

A plexus of small arteries, the circulosus articuli vasculosus (Hunter 1743), surrounds the periosteal surface of the metaphysis. This plexus is fed by articular branches of the major limb vessels and supplies numerous small metaphyseal arteries. These enter the bone in some of the many small foramina that characterize the metaphyseal cortex. Within the marrow cavity, the metaphyseal arteries run towards the center of the metaphysis and supply the metaphyseal cortex and medullary contents.

Extraosseous branches of the circulosus articuli vasculosus run across the surface of the physis and feed the epiphyseal arteries. The epiphyseal arteries pierce the epiphysis in small foramina on its extra-articular surfaces.

Small periosteal arteries lie on, and supply, the periosteum of all long bones. Arteries in the overlying soft tissues feed these vessels and the vascularity of the soft tissues determines the vascularity of the underlying periosteum. For instance, the periosteum on the antero-lateral cortex of the tibia (covered with skeletal muscle) is more vascular than that of the subcutaneous antero-medial cortex. Very small branches of the periosteal arteries enter the underlying cortex in minute foramina, but do not penetrate its complete thickness.

The nutrient artery supplies blood to the diaphyseal cortex and marrow, the metaphyseal arteries supply the metaphyseal cortex and marrow, and the epiphyseal arteries supply the epiphysis. Perfusion studies suggest that in normal circumstances the periosteal arteries are not a significant arterial input of long bones (Brookes 1971), although ablation studies suggest that they are capable of perfusing at least the outer third of the cortex (Johnson 1927). Chronic ablation studies also demonstrate that large anastomoses can develop between the metaphyseal, nutrient, and periosteal arteries; but in normal circumstances few anastomoses exist, and interruption of either the nutrient or metaphyseal arteries will result in regions of marrow necrosis (Brookes 1986). In growing bones the avascular physis prevents intraosseous anastomoses between the epiphyseal and metaphyseal circulations. After physeal closure a few anastomoses may develop between the two circulations, but they tend to remain distinct entities.

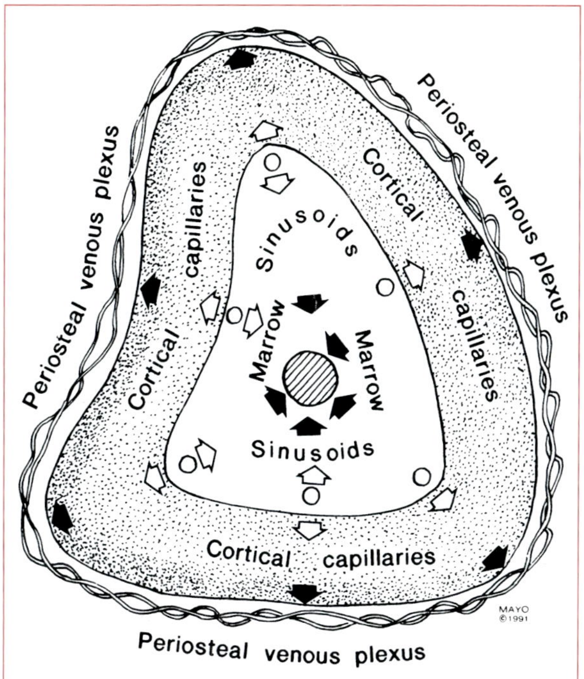

Fig. 2 *Diagram of the blood flow within a cross-section of a long bone. The cortical circulation flows from the endosteal to the periosteal cortices while the marrow circulation passes centripetally from the periphery of the medullary cavity to the central venous sinus (▨). (White arrows = arterial blood; Black arrows = venous blood) (○ = branches of the nutrient artery).*

The microcirculation of bone

Long bones contain two microcirculations whose interrelationship is unresolved. Some consider that the marrow and cortical microcirculations are arranged as a portal system, in which arterial blood first passes through the medullary sinusoids and then perfuses the cortical capillaries (DeBruyn et al 1970). The more widely accepted concept, which is described below, is that the two microcirculations are distinct and separate (Lopez-Curto et al 1980). In physiological conditions both circulations are principally fed by the intramedullary branches of the nutrient, metaphyseal, and epiphyseal systems.

Marrow microcirculation

In the diaphysis the nutrient artery system, which lies at the periphery of the marrow cavity, sends radially orientated branches towards the center of the medullary canal. These branches feed the medullary sinusoids, which are the exchange vessels of the marrow. Medullary sinusoids have a complete endothelial wall but no basal lamina, and are only partially covered by adventitia. The medullary sinusoids of the diaphysis drain through radially oriented venous collecting ducts into the central venous sinus.

In the metaphysis and epiphysis the medullary sinusoids are fed by branches of the respective arterial systems, and blood flow is not centripetal. Cancellous bone is found in the medullary canal of the metaphyses and epiphyses, and consists of a honeycomb of bony trabeculae. Large trabeculae contain blood vessels, whereas small trabeculae do not, and obtain nutrition by diffusion from the adjacent marrow.

Microcirculation of the cortex

In normal situations the cortex is supplied with arterial blood by intramedullary branches of the nutrient, metaphyseal, and epiphyseal arteries. In the diaphysis, branches of the nutrient artery circulation run centrifugally towards the endosteal cortex and feed the cortical capillaries, which lie in the central canals of Haversian systems. These capillaries are abnormally long (up to 2 cm), and run in a longitudinal and outward direction, traversing from the endosteal to the periosteal cortex, where they drain into the periosteal venous plexus.

Venous drainage

The epiphyseal, metaphyseal, and nutrient veins are the main drainage pathways of the marrow cavity. Epiphyseal and metaphyseal veins are more numerous than their arterial counterparts, and exit the bone in the small foramina within the overlying cortices. In the diaphysis, the marrow sinusoids drain through collecting ducts into the central venous sinus. This structure is found at the center of the marrow cavity cross-section (Fig. 2), and runs the whole length of the diaphysis and metaphyses (see Fig. 1b). The central venous sinus empties into the nutrient veins that accompany the nutrient artery in the nutrient foramen. Additional emissary veins pierce the cortex and also drain the central venous sinus. The venous drainage of the cortex is by the periosteal plexus of veins.

Interstitial fluid flow within cortical bone

In common with other organs, bone has an interstitial fluid space in which nutrients are transferred from cortical capillaries to osteocytes. Interstitial fluid is not stagnant but circulates within bone matrix. A recent study has demonstrated the kinetics of interstitial fluid flow (Montgomery et al 1988). At the arterial end of cortical capillaries, plasma is filtered by the capillary wall to produce protein-free interstitial fluid. This filtration is driven by the outward hydrostatic pressure gradient across the capillary wall. Once formed, interstitial fluid flows through the bone matrix until it reaches the venous end of a cortical capillary. Here the inward hydrostatic pressure gradient causes interstitial fluid to re-enter the intravascular space. Alternatively the interstitial fluid can exit the bone matrix in the lymphatic system. It is of interest that, as with cortical bone blood flow, the net direction of interstitial fluid flow is centrifugal.

Lymph flow in bone

Recent evidence suggests that cortical bone has a lymphatic system (Montgomery et al 1988). Prelymphatic matrix vessels are present within bone matrix, and drain into perivascular prelymphatic vessels, which lie alongside cortical capillaries within the central canal of the Haversian systems. These prelymphatic vessels are similar to those of the bone marrow, the brain, and the retina, and do not have an endothelial lining.

In summary, the arterial blood supply of a long bone in normal conditions is provided by the nutrient, metaphyseal, and epiphyseal arteries. All these enter the medullary cavity before supplying both the marrow and cortical microcirculations. Flow in the diaphyseal marrow is centripetal (into the central venous sinus), whereas that of the diaphyseal cortex is centrifugal (into the periosteal venous plexus).

Effects of fracture and fracture fixation on bone blood flow

Fracture initially reduces blood flow in the adjacent cortex and disrupts the normal pattern of bone blood flow (Rhinelander 1968; Smith et al 1990). With displaced fractures, the periosteal blood supply of bone becomes prominent at the fracture site, and, as healing and remodeling progress, blood flow at the fracture site is increased. As these processes reach completion, fracture site blood flow returns to normal over a period of months. Operative fracture fixation can further disrupt fracture blood flow, and consequently can delay fracture union. Plating of an osteotomy/fracture results in damage to the periosteum directly under the plate. Thus the venous drainage of the cortex under the plate is destroyed, and blood flow to this region is reduced (Rhinelander 1968). Intramedullary nailing may damage the intramedullary nutrient and metaphyseal arterial networks, and can cause necrosis within the adjacent endosteal cortex (Rhinelander 1968; Smith et al 1990). However, if the normal intramedullary cortical arterial supply is destroyed, the ischemic cortex can obtain a circulation from the periosteal arteries: this circulation may not prevent necrosis of the endosteal cortex, but allows the outer cortex to remain viable. Recruitment of the periosteal arterial circulation explains how cortical bone remains viable following intramedullary reaming. Studies show that intramedullary reaming causes a dramatic decline of blood flow to the endosteal cortex (and concurrent bone infarction), whereas blood flow in the periosteal cortex is preserved (Smith et al 1990: Trueta and Cavadias 1955). Fracture fixation by an external fixator does not necessitate exposure of or further damage to the fracture site. It is therefore not surprising that peri-fracture blood flow is damaged least by this form of fracture fixation.

Bone blood flow in a flat bone

Periosteal vessels feed and drain areas of thin bone such as the scapula. In general, flat bones, such as the innominate, have one main nutrient artery, which is found near the center of the bone. This is reinforced in the peripheral regions by branches of extraosseous arteries such as the deep lateral circumflex iliac artery, whose branches pierce the iliac crest and anastomose with the terminations of the central nutrient artery (Taylor et al 1979). Venous drainage is by veins that accompany the arteries. This arrangement is not markedly different from the situation in a long bone.

Capillary recruitment

There is evidence that suggests that cortical capillaries are not always perfused, and may at times be closed (Charkes 1980; McInnis et al 1980; Montgomery et al 1988). If this is correct then it is possible that, as with skeletal and cardiac muscle, the rate of uptake of nutrients can be increased by increasing the density of open capillaries (recruitment). Presumably mechanisms that act on precapillary sphincters control the density of open capillaries; but these have not yet been identified.

4. The control of bone blood flow

Peter J Briggs

The rate of blood flow to bone, as to other organs and tissues, is controlled by systemic and local control mechanisms. Systemic arterial pressure, cardiac output, and circulating blood volume affect bone blood flow, with, as expected, flow declining with decreased blood pressure (Shim and Patterson 1967). This is, in part at least, mediated by baroreceptor reflexes, stimulation of which increases flow, with denervation decreasing flow (Gross et al 1979).

This chapter will review our understanding of the major local mechanisms underlying the control of blood flow in bone. These mechanisms can be considered under the following headings:

1. Autoregulation
2. Neural control
3. Humoral factors
4. Metabolic factors
5. Endothelial cell mechanisms.

Autoregulation

Autoregulation can be defined as the ability of a vascular bed to maintain a constant blood flow despite changes in arterial pressure (Ganong 1989). The precise mechanism for this phenomenon is uncertain, but a number of hypotheses have been proposed to explain it. The myogenic hypothesis proposes that the vascular smooth muscle responds to changes in distension pressure. The metabolic hypothesis suggests that accumulation and dispersion of metabolic products influences vascular tone to maintain them at a constant level. The tissue pressure hypothesis is not generally favored as an explanation, but essentially suggests that an increase in flow causes the accumulation of interstitial fluid, which leads to a rise in extrinsic pressure on the vasculature. It is possible that autoregulation may be explained in part by the function of the vascular endothelium in the control of blood flow.

The ability to autoregulate varies between vascular beds. Using intramedullary pressure as an indicator of bone blood flow Tøndevold et al (1979a) found that medullary pressure was maintained constant if the systemic pressure was above 81 mmHg. Below this the medullary pressure falls, which has been interpreted as indicating reduced arterial flow. Medullary pressure is, however, an unreliable indicator of bone blood flow, and at best only gives a qualitative estimate of changes in flow (Azuma 1964; Shim et al 1972). It remains uncertain whether the osseous vascular bed has the ability to autoregulate its blood flow.

Neural control

Sympathetic nerve fibers have been identified entering the nutrient foramen with the nutrient artery (Sherman 1963; Duncan and Shim 1977). They divide with the branching of the nutrient artery, and ultimately end as multiple varicosities in a rich plexus on the adventitial surface of the small arterioles supplying the marrow and the bone.

A number of studies have shown the importance of the sympathetic innervation in the control of bone blood flow. Sympathetic stimulation causes a decrease in bone blood flow and a rise in perfusion pressure (Shim and Patterson 1967; Azuma 1964; Drinker and Drinker 1916; Herzig and Root 1959; Driessens and Vanhoutte 1979; Tran 1980), and sympathectomy is associated with an increase in flow (Trotman and Kelly 1963). In other vessels, however, chronic sympathectomy, which necessarily occurs with free tissue transfer, is associated with an increase in vascular smooth muscle tone (Mangiarua et al 1986). Impaired production of relaxing factors by the endothelial cells has also been observed (Mangiarua and Bevan 1986).

Sympathetic nerve fibers act primarily via α_1-adrenergic receptors (Driessens and Vanhoutte 1979), which in bone appear to be extremely sensitive to stimulation (Brinker et al 1990). The sympathetic innervation of bone is therefore likely to contribute to the redistribution of the cardiac output during exercise or hypovolemic shock, causing a reduction in bone blood flow (Gross et al 1979).

Neuropeptide Y is found in sympathetic perivascular nerve terminals, and has recently been identified in bone vasculature (Bjurholm et al 1988a). In many tissues it appears to potentiate the action of other vasoconstrictor agents, and in others it has a direct action on vascular smooth muscle, which may explain the inability of α-adrenergic antagonists to completely inhibit the constrictor effect of sympathetic nerve stimulation (Neild and Brayden 1991). Exogenous neuropeptide Y has a potent vasoconstrictor action in bone vasculature, but its physiological importance in the regulation of bone blood flow is unknown (Lindblad et al 1993).

There is as yet no definite evidence for a neural vasodilator mechanism in bone vasculature. Vipergic nerve fibers (containing vasoactive intestinal peptide – VIP) have been identified in periosteum and possibly bone, particularly in the epiphyses; but the nerve endings do not appear to be associated with blood vessels (Bjurholm et al 1988a; Hohmann et al 1986). VIP is a vasodilator in most vascular beds, and has been found to cause relaxation of arterioles isolated from cancellous bone (Lundgaard et al 1993); but a physiological role in the regulation of bone blood flow has not been established.

VIP is often found in conjunction with acetylcholine in parasympathetic nerve endings (Lincoln and Burnstock 1990), but cholinergic nerve fibers have not been identified in bone. Muscarinic cholinergic receptors are present in bone vasculature, and exogenous acetylcholine causes attenuation of the responses to noradrenaline, which can be inhibited by atropine (Driessens and Vanhoutte 1979; Woodhouse 1963). High doses of acetylcholine will also cause vasodilatation (Brinker et al 1990). The purpose of these acetylcholine receptors in the control of bone blood flow is uncertain, but is likely to be related to the role of the endothelial cells in the regulation of blood flow.

Agents such as substance P, dopamine, and calcitonin gene-related protein (CGRP) have been identified as possible neurotransmitters with potent vasodilator actions (Neild and Brayden 1991). Substance P- and CGRP-containing nerves have been demonstrated in bone, marrow, and periosteum (Bjurholm et al 1988b). Some of the nerve endings have varicosities adjacent to blood vessels. Their role in the control of bone blood flow is unknown. In other tissues substance P and CGRP have been found in sensory nerves, and CGRP may modulate osteoclast activity.

Humoral factors

Circulating catecholamines such as adrenaline and noradrenaline increase bone vascular resistance and reduce bone blood flow (Drinker and Drinker 1916; Woodhouse 1963), an effect mediated by both α_1- and α_2-adrenergic receptors (Dean et al 1992; Moran et al 1993). α_1 receptors are thought to be primarily postsynaptic and associated with sympathetic nerve endings (Van Zwieten 1988), whereas α_2 receptors are noninnervated and regarded as hormone receptors for circulating adrenaline and noradrenaline. α_2 receptors are found on the luminal aspect of smooth muscle cells, where they mediate vasoconstriction, and presynaptically, where they inhibit noradrenalin release (Langer and Hicks 1984).

β-adrenergic receptors have been identified in bone, but their role in the control of bone blood flow remains uncertain. Shim et al (1972) and Brinker et al (1990) showed that isoproterenol (nonspecific β agonist) caused vasoconstriction in bone, in contrast to vasodilation in most other vascular beds. Propranolol (nonspecific β antagonist) causes a reduction in the constrictor responses to exogenous noradrenalin (Dean et al 1992).

This effect may possibly be explained by the presence of presynaptic β_2 receptors that mediate noradrenalin release from sympathetic nerve endings (Van Zwieten 1988) and the absence of postsynaptic β receptors. Lack of a postsynaptic β-mediated dilator mechanism may contribute to the observed marked constrictor responsiveness in bone vasculature to sympathetic stimulation (Brinker et al 1990).

Calcitonin has a direct action on bone vascular smooth muscle, causing vasoconstriction, but parathyroid hormone does not appear to have any effect on bone vascular resistance (Driessens and Vanhoutte 1981). This action of calcitonin may be part of its physiological mechanism of action. Glucocorticoids modify the responses to exogenous noradrenalin probably by changing the sensitivity of the β-adrenergic receptors (Driessens and Vanhoutte 1981).

The platelet products adenosine, serotonin, and thrombin have dilator effects on vascular smooth muscle in other organ systems (Vanhoutte 1991). In bone adenosine causes vasodilatation (Gross et al 1979), but the responses to serotonin and thrombin have not been determined. Thromboxane A_2 causes vasoconstriction in the vasculature of bone, which can be inhibited by a specific PGH_2/TXA_2 receptor antagonist (Brinker et al 1990). The hormones angiotensin and vasopressin are primarily concerned with the systemic regulation of the circulating blood volume and blood pressure. They probably have a vasoconstrictor action in bone (Stein et al 1958), as in other tissues.

Metabolic factors

Metabolic factors are important in the control of bone blood flow (Shim 1968). The hydrogen ion concentration has a modulating effect on the baseline vascular resistance and also modulates the responses to exogenous noradrenalin (Davis and Wood 1993). In vivo experiments in bone show that CO_2 retention and acidosis causes vasodilation (Shim and Patterson 1967; Gross et al 1979; Woodhouse 1963). Cumming (Cumming and Nutt 1962) in cross-perfusion studies in the rabbit also showed that bone blood flow is affected by systemic metabolic manipulations, which appear to be mediated by neural reflexes. This complicates interpretation of in vivo studies with regard to the study of local blood flow control mechanisms.

Increased H^+ concentration may affect the contractile ability of vascular smooth muscle by a variety of mechanisms. It may affect intracellular mechanisms or membrane ion transport (Kwan et al 1988; Wray 1988). It also reduces the α adrenoreceptor responsiveness (Korstanje et al 1985), and may possibly inhibit endothelial-cell-derived relaxing factors (Wray 1988; Furchgott 1988).

Hypoxia has been found to cause an increase in bone blood flow (Shim and Patterson 1967), and also a decrease in flow (Gross et al 1979). The reason for this contradiction in results is not apparent. Hypoxia may cause vasodilation at a local level by changes in the cell membrane permeability to Ca^{2+}, causing hyperpolarization, but alterations in other ion transport mechanisms, as well as by interference with electromechanical coupling and ATP production in smooth muscle (Lombard et al 1988). In vascular smooth muscle 50% to 80% of glucose is metabolized by the glycolytic pathway to lactate under aerobic conditions, but 50% to 60% of the ATP production is dependent on oxygen via the tricarboxylic acid cycle and hexosemonophosphate shunt (Lundholm et al 1977).

Tøndevold et al (1979b) found that bone intramedullary pressure falls during hypoxia, but hyperoxia and manipulations of pH and pCO_2 did not have any effect. Why they did not observe any changes with pH and pCO_2 in contrast to other studies is uncertain. It may possibly relate to combined systemic and local effects in the in vivo situation, anesthesia, or the indirect method of estimating changes in bone blood flow.

Endothelial cell mechanisms

The importance of the vascular endothelium in the local control of blood flow in the microcirculation has been recognized over the last 10 years. Endothelial cells are able to produce a number of vasodilator and vasoconstrictor agents.

The most important of the vasodilators appear to be endothelium-derived relaxing factor, which is probably nitric oxide, and vasodilator prostaglandins, most likely prostacyclin and PGE_2. The production of these agents has been demonstrated in the bone microvasculature (Davis and Wood 1992). Amongst the endothelium-derived vasoconstricting agents the family of endothelin peptides is the only one that has been positively identified; and it has a potent action in bone vasculature (Brinker et al 1990).

The vascular endothelium, rather than being an inert lining to the cardiovascular system, has been shown to have many functions apart from a role in the control of vascular tone. It is able to synthesize connective tissue components; it has procoagulant, anticoagulant, antiplatelet, and fibrinolytic properties; it can activate and inactivate angiotensin; it is involved in the metabolism of lipoproteins; it interacts with activated, and may activate, neutrophils; and it is responsible for an unidentified smooth muscle growth factor (Jaffe 1985; Ryan 1986).

Vasodilator prostaglandins

Prostacyclin (PGI_2) is probably the most important and potent of the vasodilator prostaglandins (Moncada et al 1977; Gerritsen and Cheli 1983). Its production can be stimulated by thrombin and trypsin (Weksler et al 1978). Prostaglandin E_2 is also an important vasodilator, which can be stimulated by bradykinin and noradrenalin (Vane and McGiff 1975).

Vasodilator prostaglandins have been found to attenuate vasoconstrictor responses (Davis and Wood 1992; Messina et al 1976), and are important in mediating autoregulation and postischemic reactive hyperemia (Vane and McGiff 1975). Prostacyclin is also a potent inhibitor of platelet adhesion and aggregation (Weksler et al 1977; Moncada et al 1978).

Endothelium-derived relaxing factor

Furchgott and Zawadzki (1980) discovered the importance of the endothelium in the vasodilator response to acetylcholine, and demonstrated the presence of a factor that could be transmitted from the endothelial cells to the smooth muscle. The substance was named endothelium-derived relaxing factor (EDRF). The similarity of the vascular responses to nitrovasodilators (GTN) and EDRF led to the speculation that EDRF was nitric oxide (Furchgott 1983). The biological behaviour of exogenous nitric oxide (NO) and EDRF appears to be identical (Palmer et al 1987).

Endothelium-dependent vasodilator responses have been demonstrated in response to a variety of stimuli such as serotonin, adenine nucleotides, bradykinin, substance P, adrenaline, vasopressin, thrombin, and increased flow rate (Rapoport et al 1984; Rubanyi et al 1986; Vanhoutte 1988). Increases in intraluminal pressure induce vascular smooth muscle contraction, which may in part be related to inhibition of EDRF production (Rubanyi 1988a). The ability of the endothelial cells to cause vasodilation is also impaired after chronic sympathetic denervation (Mangiarua and Bevan 1986).

EDRF is an important modulator of vascular tone. It mediates the vasodilator function of bradykinin and serotonin, which would otherwise cause vasoconstriction by a direct smooth muscle action (Vanhoutte 1991; Lüscher et al 1990). The role of the vascular endothelial cell muscarinic receptors and others may be explained by the finding that endothelial cells can themselves produce acetylcholine, and also contain substance P and serotonin. These agents are released from endothelial cells in response to hypoxia (Parnavelas et al 1985; Burnstock et al 1988; Milner et al 1989), suggesting a further possible mechanism for hypoxic vasodilatation. Serotonin and adenine nucleotides may also arise from platelets.

In addition to its vasoactive role, EDRF acts synergistically with prostacyclin to inhibit platelet adhesion and aggregation (Radomski et al 1987).

EDRF and vasodilator prostaglandins are produced widely by vascular endothelial cells, but major differences are seen between species and between different vascular beds, as well as between arteries and veins (Messina et al 1976; DeMey and Vanhoutte 1982). EDRF is the main endothelial-cell-derived relaxing factor produced by the microvasculature of bone in response to acetylcholine (Davis and Wood 1992), where it can attenuate the contractile response to noradrenalin.

Endothelin

Endothelin is a 21-amino-acid peptide initially defined in the supernatant of cultured bovine aortic endothelial cells (Hickey et al 1985; O'Brien and McMurtry 1984), and later isolated and purified (Yanagisawa et al 1988). In vitro it produces a long-lasting contraction of vascular smooth muscle that is resistant to antagonism of known vasoconstrictor

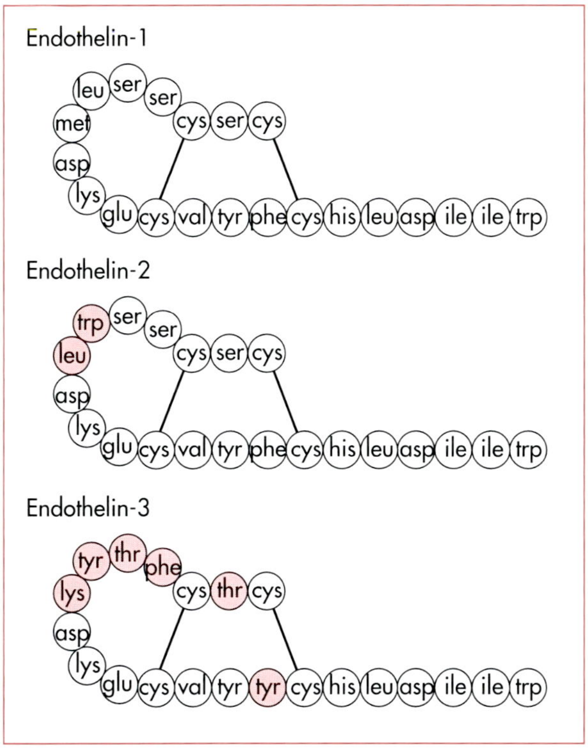

***Fig. 1** Endothelin peptide structure: 21 amino acids with two disulfide linkages between cysteine residues.*

mechanisms (e.g. α and β adrenergic, muscarinic, serotonergic and histaminergic). As a vasconstrictor it is the most potent known, being ten times more potent than angiotensin II, vasopressin or neuropeptide Y (Yanagisawa et al 1988).

In vivo endothelin produces a prolonged rise in mean arterial pressure and total peripheral resistance, often with an initial transient vasodilator response (Yanagisawa et al 1988; Wright and Fozard 1988; Inoue et al 1989; Eglen et al 1989).

Induction of endothelin synthesis by endothelial cells above basal levels takes 2 to 5 hours, and involves new gene transcription, with increase in mRNA synthesis (Zoja et al 1991). It may be stimulated by thrombin, transforming growth factor β, interleukin-1, endotoxin, high glucose, fluid mechanical shear stress, vasopressin, and in some cells by endothelin itself (Yanagisawa et al 1988; Zoja et al 1991; Sugiura et al 1989; Yamauchi et al 1990; Bakris et al 1991). It may also be stimulated by hypoxia (Rubanyi 1988b), and adrenaline (Yanagisawa et al 1988). Secretion of endothelin is inhibited by atrial natriuretic factor (Saijonmaa et al 1990), and by EDRF (Boulanger and Lüscher 1990). Endothelin is formed from a 203 amino acid precursor peptide called preproendothelin (Yanagisawa et al 1988). The 21-amino-acid peptide is produced by the action of specific endopeptidases (McMahon et al 1991).

Genomes for three different endothelins have been identified in the human (Inoue et al 1989). They have very similar peptide structures, consisting of 21 amino acids with two disulfide linkages between cysteine residues (Fig. 1). Endothelin-1 can be obtained from cultured endothelial cells. No tissue has yet been identified as a source of endothelin-2, and endothelin-3 has been isolated in brain tissue, suggesting its role may be that of a neurotransmitter (Yanagisawa and Masaki 1989).

The mechanism of action of the endothelins appears to be complex, and differences are seen between different species and different vascular beds (Eglen et al 1989). At least two, and possibly more, endothelin receptors are known to exist in the peripheral vascular system. The ET_A receptor was the first described (Arai et al 1990); this has a high specificity for endothelin-1. These receptors have been found on vascular smooth muscle cells, and mediate the contractile responses (Hirata et al 1988a,b; Lin et al 1991). They stimulate calcium ion entry into smooth muscle cells, as well as the release of stored intracellular calcium (Simonson and Dunn 1992).

Another receptor, ET_B, has been identified (Sakurai et al 1990), which has been localized to vascular endothelial cells (Takayanagi et al 1991) and has not been found in smooth muscle (Sakurai et al 1990). It has equal affinity for the different endothelins, and is thought to mediate the vasodilator actions of endothelin, possibly via prostaglandins and EDRF (Sakurai et al 1992).

Calcium channel blockers such as nifedipine are effective in many but not all vascular beds in antagonizing the contractile responses to endothelin (Yanagisawa et al 1988; Eglen et al 1989; Auguet et al 1988). In some tissues the contractile response to endothelin is in part mediated by constrictor prostaglandins, which can be inhibited with indomethacin (Macquin-Mavier et al 1989; Reynolds and Mok 1990).

Low concentrations of endothelin may have a vasodilator action. The mechanism for this remains uncertain, but may involve the stimulation of the release of vasodilator prostaglandins or EDRF depending on the animal species and the tissue vascular bed (Tabuchi et al 1989; Warner et al 1989). Receptor antagonists for endothelin have been developed and are under evaluation (Ihara et al 1991; Ihara et al 1992; Fukuroda et al 1992). These may help clarify the mechanisms of action of endothelin.

Endothelin may interact with other constrictor mechanisms. It appears to inhibit the contractile response to sympathetic nerve stimulation, either by reducing noradrenalin release from nerve endings (Tabuchi et al 1989; Wiklund et al 1988) or by a postjunctional effect (Reid et al 1989). In contrast it is also able to potentiate the action of other agonists on vascular smooth muscle (Inoue et al 1989; Goto et al 1989; Yang et al 1990).

The physiological importance of endothelin is not yet clearly understood. Although detectable in the plasma at levels of 0.5–5.0 pmol/l in the human (Ando et al 1989; Cernacek and Stewart 1989; Heublein et al 1989a; Pittet et al 1991) and in the dog (Heublein et al 1989b), these levels are generally below concentrations required to activate ET_A receptors. This suggests that endothelin derived from endothelial cells primarily acts at a local level rather than as a circulating hormone. Delay between stimulus and *de novo* synthesis of endothelin suggests that it may be involved in long-term homeostasis.

In contrast endothelin has been implicated as an important factor in a number of pathological situations such as acute myocardial ischemia (Miyauchi et al 1989) and septic shock (Pittet et al 1991). Plasma levels are raised, and in septic shock appear to correlate with the severity of the condition. Tissue ischemia is associated with increased release of endothelin on reperfusion in the lungs (Vemulapalli et al 1992) and the heart (Watanabe et al 1991; Maulik et al 1992), and numerous studies have shown that there is an increase in the endothelin receptor density or increased affinity for endothelin after ischemia to the heart or the kidneys (Liu et al 1990; Clozel et al 1991; Neubauer et al 1991; Watts et al 1992). These findings suggest that endothelin may be important in ischemia–reperfusion injury. This conclusion is further supported by the finding that calcium channel blockers and endothelin antibodies are effective in reducing infarct size and restoring normal vascular resistances in experimental ischemia of the myocardium and the kidney (Watanabe et al 1991; Kon et al 1989).

Brinker et al (1990) have demonstrated that endothelin-1 is a potent vasoconstrictor in bone microvasculature. The other endothelins also cause vasoconstriction in bone and the pattern of their potencies suggests that the receptor is similar to that found in other tissues (Briggs 1994). The action of endothelin in bone can be modulated by changes in the metabolic environment, but is not affected by calcium channel blockers or by EDRF.

Other endothelium-derived vasoactive factors

A number of other as yet unidentified endothelium-derived vasoactive agents have been demonstrated in organ-bath studies. Until their precise nature is known their presence and role in the control of the microvasculature of bone would be difficult to determine.

Endothelium-derived contracting factor-1 ($EDCF_1$) is a product of arachidonic acid metabolism (Rubanyi 1988b), which in most vascular beds appears to be a cyclo-oxygenase metabolite (Miller and Vanhoutte 1985; Lüscher and Vanhoutte 1986). The active agent is probably a prostaglandin (Katusic et al 1988a), but in some vascular beds thromboxane A_2 or leukotrienes are possibilities (Miller and Vanhoutte 1985; Altierre et al 1986; Katusic et al 1988b). Anoxia is known to facilitate contractile responses by an endothelium-dependent mechanism that is not entirely explained by the inhibition of EDRF production during anoxia (Rubanyi 1988b; DeMey and Vanhoutte 1983; Katusic and Vanhoutte 1986). A diffusible factor – termed $EDCF_3$ – has been demonstrated (Rubanyi and Vanhoutte 1985), but its identity is unknown.

Acetylcholine, bradykinin and histamine, as well as stimulating EDRF production, stimulate a transient hyperpolarization in vascular smooth muscle cells that is dependent on the presence of endothelial cells (Feletou and Vanhoutte 1988; Komori and Vanhoutte 1990). Methylene blue, which inhibits the effects of EDRF, fails to inhibit the hyperpolarization, which is also not inhibited by indomethacin (Chen et al 1988).

This substance has been called endothelium-derived hyperpolarizing factor. The hyperpolarization is transient and much shorter in duration than the relaxation induced by EDRF. Its role in the local regulation of blood flow is probably minimal.

Conclusions

Appreciation of the normal mechanisms involved in the regulation of bone blood flow, and how these may be affected in certain situations such as transplantation, fracture nonunion, aseptic necrosis, and bone tumors, may ultimately allow predictable therapeutic manipulation of blood flow. Recent advances have been made in our understanding of the normal bone blood flow control mechanisms (Driessens and Vanhoutte 1979; Brinker et al 1990; Lindblad et al 1993; Dean et al 1992; Driessens and Vanhoutte 1981; Davis and Wood 1992, 1993).

Sympathetic mechanisms are mediated by α_1, α_2, and β adrenoreceptors (Fig. 2), and these can be modulated by the metabolic environment. The vascular endothelium produces smooth-muscle-relaxing factors, in particular EDRF and to a lesser extent prostaglandins, in response to acetylcholine. Vasoconstrictor responses to thromboxane A_2 via the PGH_2/TXA_2 receptor, endothelin, neuropeptide Y, and vasopressin have also been demonstrated.

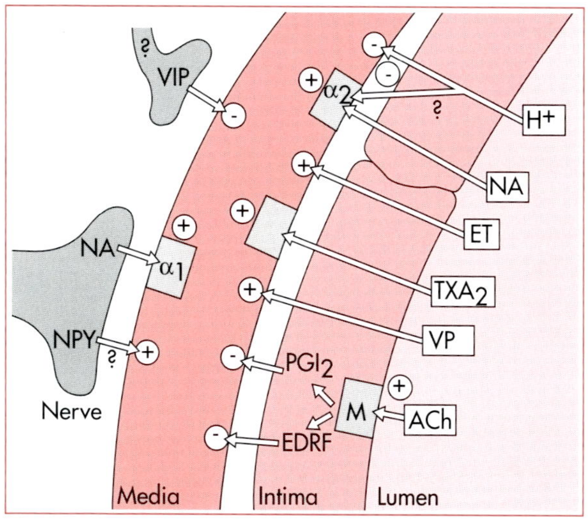

Fig. 2 *Schematic illustrating proposed neurohumoral mechanisms involved in the local control of bone blood flow.*

II NORMAL BONE HEALING MECHANISMS

5. Fracture union

The course of fracture healing will depend upon a number of variables, including the degree of vascular insult to the fractured bone ends, the degree of injury to the surrounding soft tissues, the intimacy of coaptation of the fractured bone ends, the adequacy of fracture immobilization, and the presence or absence of infection or surgical intervention. The typical process, however, for a closed, long-bone fracture with adequate reduction and immobilization involves the following sequence of events (Ham 1930; Ham and Harris 1956; McMinn and Pritchard 1969; Brand 1983; Bieber and Wood 1986). At the moment of fracture, intraosseous blood vessels coursing over the long axis of the bone are disrupted, and surrounding soft tissue, including periosteum, is stripped for a variable distance over one or both bone ends. As a consequence of this, the fractured bone ends are rendered avascular or ischemic to a variable degree, depending upon the amount of fracture displacement, comminution, and topographical location within the bone. Proportionally to the extent of vascular insult, bone cellular elements will undergo necrosis (McKibbin 1978).

As early as 48 hours following fracture the process of repair may begin with the initial steps towards formation of an external callus. Osteogenic cells derived from the deep (cambium) layer of the viable periosteum begin proliferating, tending to form a thickened cellular cuff, which advances the cell multiplication towards the fracture site from either bone end (Cruess 1984). Concurrently with the periosteal cellular activity, capillary buds appear within the cellular mass, particularly along the deepest aspects adjacent to the bone. Those cells closest to the capillary buds tend then to differentiate into osteoblasts, which then elaborate osteoid trabeculations along the surface of the fractured bone ends. More peripherally over the cuff of advancing cells capillary buds are less plentiful, and the cell line here tends to differentiate into chondroblasts and fibroblasts. In the absence of interposed soft tissue, sepsis, excessive fracture motion, extreme ischemia, and other conditions, the cellular cuffs (external callus) surrounding both fractured bone ends will grow toward each other and eventually unite. The initial union achieved by external callus is based on woven bone haphazardly elaborated about the periphery of the fracture. Therefore, although this will splint the fracture well, it is mechanically a tenuous union.

Concurrently with the healing events involving the external callus, cells of the endosteum and possibly osteogenic cells of marrow origin begin proliferating and elaborating woven bone trabeculations on the endosteal bone surface. As union through the external callus rigidly splints the two bone ends, endosteal new bone formation (internal callus) progresses from each bone end, eventually to meet and unite (Fig. 1). Union of the medullary callus appears to require rigid immobilization of the fracture. It is therefore seen following union by external callus or rigid surgical internal fixation or in cases of inherently very stable fractures. Moreover, internal callus is not seen in the absence of a second bone end (for example, in the case of an amputation). This suggests that it must be dependent on some mechanical or humoral stimulus. Union of

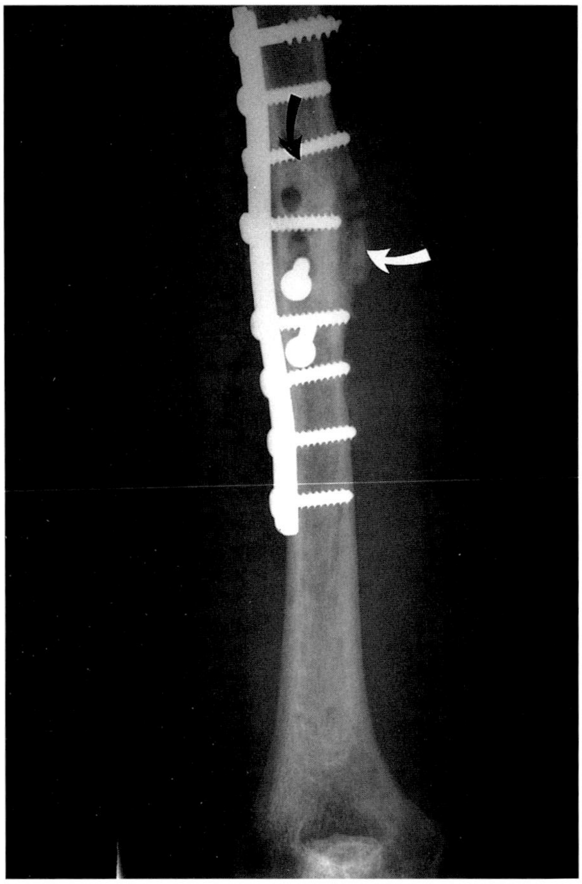

Fig. 1 *Fracture union by external callus (white arrow) and internal callus (black arrow).*

the internal callus substantially contributes to the strength of the healing fracture. From this point on the process of osteoclastic resorption of the necrotic bone ends and remodeling of the woven bone of both the internal and external callus into compact lamellar bone progressively occurs. Thus the structure and the strength of the original bone may be gradually restored.

The actual course of fracture union may be modified by a number of factors. Rigid immobilization by internal fixation with precise fracture reduction appears to impair the formation of an external callus (Fig. 2). Indeed, with such cases an external callus may in fact be unnecessary. With rigid internal fixation the course of union may be that of internal (medullary) callus formation alone. Furthermore, in instances of rigid internal fixation and perfect reduction, some authors have demonstrated primary cortical union with an absence of both internal and external callus. If the latter situation does occur in the clinical situation, it is relatively infrequent.

Electromagnetic fields may be internally generated by a fracture, and when applied externally to a fracture may influence the course of bone healing. Electronegativity appears to be associated with osteoblastic (bone formation) activity, and electropositivity with osteoclastic (bone resorption) activity

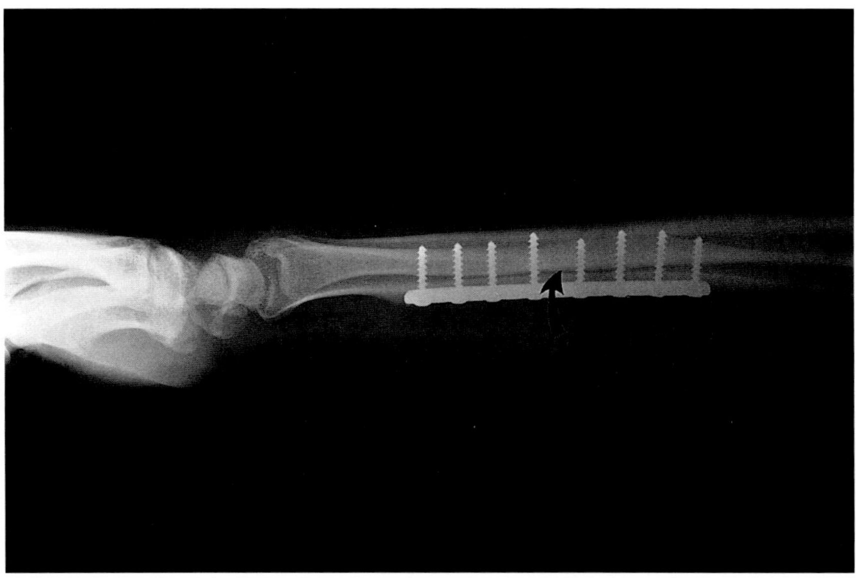

Fig. 2 *Fracture union by internal callus (arrow) without initial external callus, as a result of rigid immobilization afforded by a compression plate.*

(Bassett 1972). Cyclic fracture loading by either weightbearing (Sarmiento et al 1977) or active muscle activity appears to enhance fracture union. The mechanism of this enhancement may depend on piezoelectric effects or other undefined mechanisms. Although the stimulus to fracture union remains obscure, a possible and intriguing theory is that of a humoral agent. Increasing evidence is available to support the existence of growth factors that initiate the events that lead to fracture union (Urist et al 1972; Bolander 1991). To the present time, however, no mechanical or pharmacologic agent has been convincingly documented to accelerate or enhance the incidence of union with a typical fracture in the clinical setting.

6. Bone autograft incorporation

Christopher G Moran and Michael B Wood

Bone autografting is a well-established and common clinical procedure. The chief indications for bone autografting are to promote healing of an ununited fracture, to reconstruct bony defects, and to provide skeletal structural support for a variety of situations (Bost 1947; Phemister 1947; Chase and Hemdon 1955; Heiple et al 1963; Zuchman et al 1968; Piotrowski 1975; Burchardt et al 1975; Bonfiglio 1983; Burchardt 1983; Heppenstall 1983; Mankin et al 1983). Common to the success of any bone grafting technique is adequate revascularization from the host bed (Ray and Sabet 1963). Any circumstance that significantly reduce the potential for graft revascularization, including an ischemic host bed from prior surgery, trauma, radiation, infection, or excessive fracture site motion, will diminish the chances for successful graft incorporation. However, in the presence of an ideal soft tissue bed, the revascularization process of bone is impressively rapid (Ray 1972; Wood 1983). In general, bone autografts may be classified by structure as cancellous, cortical, or corticocancellous. The clinical indications and healing mechanisms for cancellous and cortical bone autografts differ somewhat.

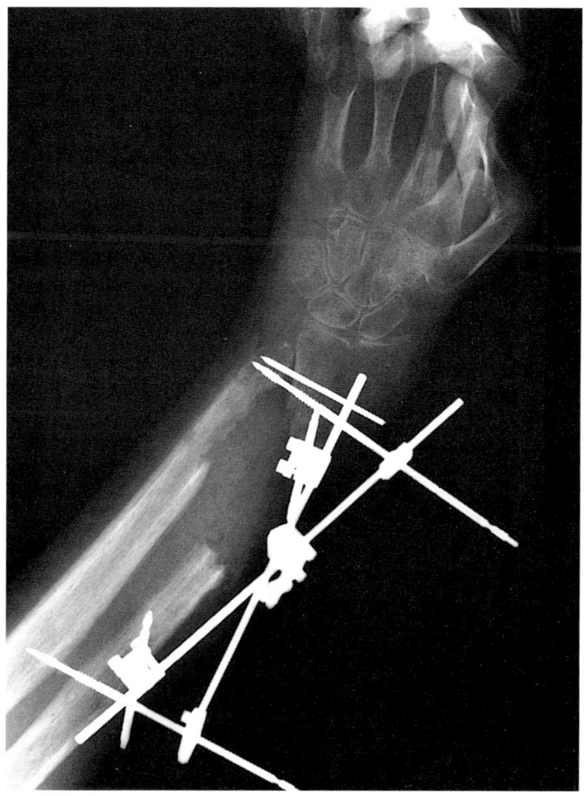

Fig. 1 *Cancellous bone graft impacted in a defect of the radius resulting from osteomyelitis and subsequent debridement.*

Cancellous bone autografts are chiefly of value for promoting bone union of unhealed fracture or for providing bone mass in situations not requiring immediate skeletal support. Cancellous bone grafts are particularly well suited for obliteration of relatively small cavities left by pseudarthrosis excision or fracture comminution, because this material can be firmly impacted, much like grouting material (Figs 1 and 2). By virtue of their structure, cancellous bone grafts have a large number of

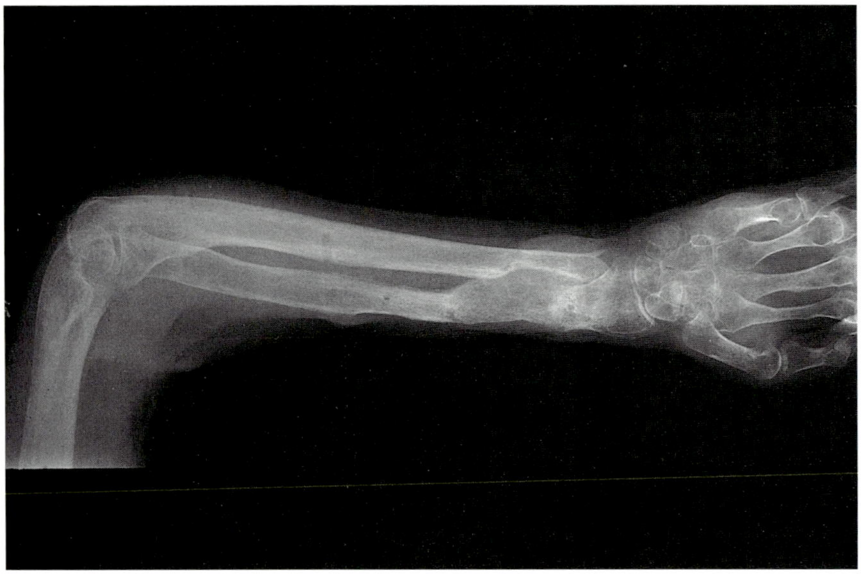

Fig. 2 *Note the mature incorporation of cancellous graft material 6 months after surgery.*

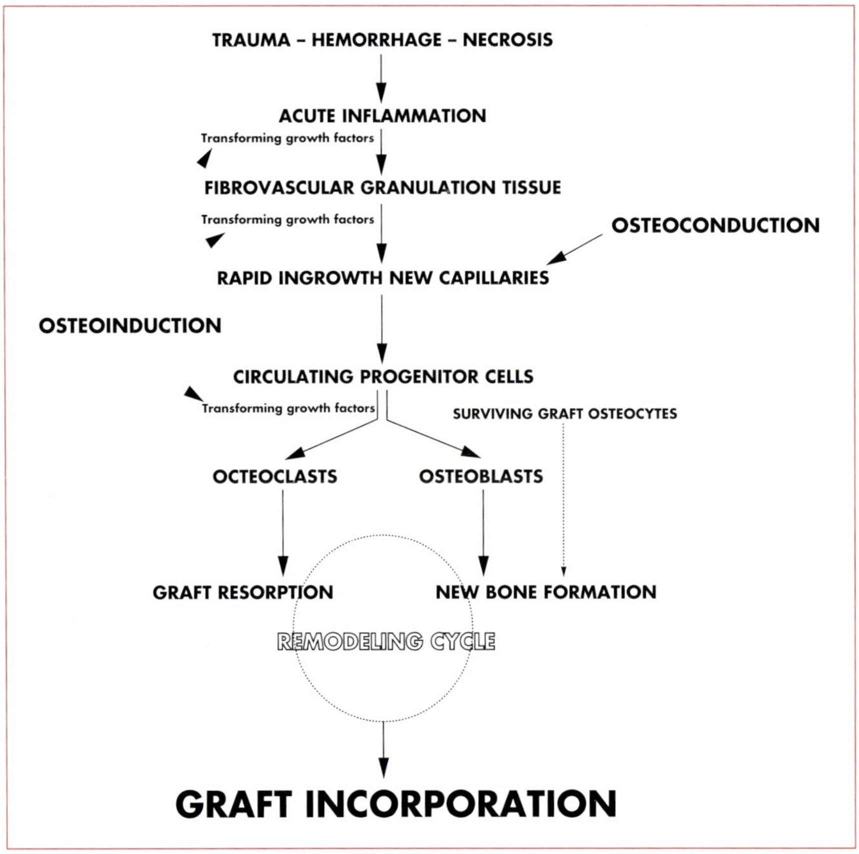

Fig. 3 *The incorporation of bone grafts. Osteoinduction is an active process: the graft releases transforming growth factors, such as the bone morphogenic proteins, which stimulate the migration and transformation of precursor cells. Osteoconduction is a passive process whereby the graft provides a scaffold for the ingrowth of blood vessels and the laying down of new bone.*

exposed bony trabeculae. Thus, a massive bone surface is presented to the host bed with a limited mechanical barrier to the diffusion of nutrients or the ingrowth of blood vessels and osteoprogenitor cells. The process of incorporation for cancellous grafts, therefore, involves direct vascular ingrowth and elaboration of osteoid followed by new bone formation on existing bony trabeculae.

The initial events during the incorporation of fresh, nonvascularized, autogenous cortical and

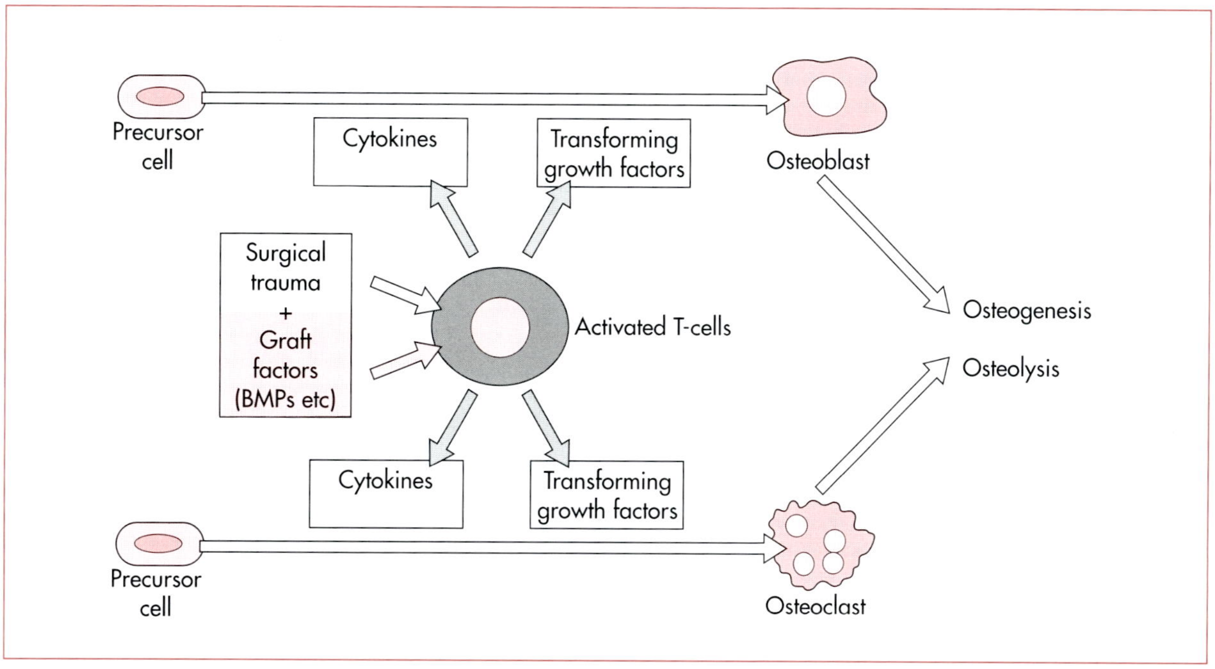

Fig. 4 *T-cells play a central role in the incorporation of bone grafts. Helper T-cells (CD4+) and cytotoxic T-cells (CD8+) produce cytokines and growth factors. Precursor cells transform into osteoblasts and osteocytes and commence bone remodeling.*

cancellous bone grafts are identical. A few endosteal and periosteal (cambium) graft-derived cells remain viable by diffusion (Arora and Laskin 1964; Heslop et al 1960a), but the majority die. Graft necrosis and surgical trauma stimulate a local inflammatory response to produce host granulation tissue. This connective tissue transports blood vessels, and osteogenic precursor cells, to the graft. The contributions of the graft to this process are termed osteoinduction and osteoconduction (Urist and Strates 1971; Fig. 3). Osteoconduction is a passive process whereby the graft provides a trellis on which new bone is deposited. Osteoinduction is an active process: the graft produces several chemical messengers, including osteogenin and bone morphogenic proteins, which act on mesodermal progenitor cells in the host tissue (Sampath and Reddi 1981). These differentiate into chondrocytes and osteoblasts, which line the edges of dead trabeculae and deposit osteoid (Luyten et al 1989; Wozney et al 1988). An important source of these mediators is necrotic cells and bone matrix (Bolander 1991). It is likely that activated cells of the immune system play a major role in modulating, if not controlling, these changes (Friedlaender 1991; Horowitz and Friedlaender 1991; Stevenson and Horowitz 1992; Fig. 4). The role of surviving graft cells in osteoinduction remains uncertain.

In the presence of a healthy soft tissue bed the incorporation of cancellous autografts may be well under way as early as 2 weeks after surgery (Shaffer et al 1987; Siegert and Wood 1990). With time osteoclastic activity will remove necrotic trabeculae and remodel the woven bone into more mature lamellar bone. This lengthy process has been termed, rather descriptively, as 'creeping substitution' by Phemister (1914). The remodeling of the graft may be incomplete: even years later remnants of necrotic bone trabeculae, from the original graft, covered by new lamellar bone may be noted. In terms of mechanical strength, the cancellous graft is weakest initially. Thereafter, it progressively increases in strength because bone is elaborated about it prior to the osteoclastic removal of necrotic trabeculae.

Cortical bone grafts are mainly of value for spanning lengthy bone defects, or for providing

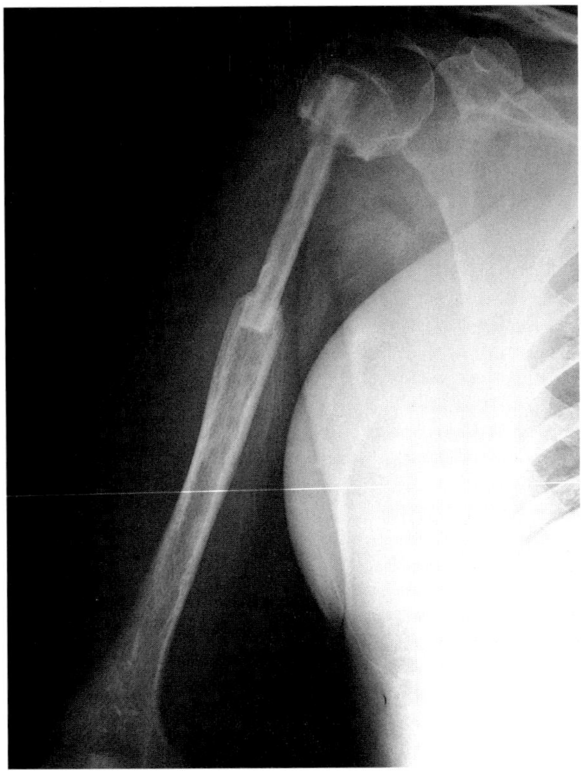

Fig. *5 Cortical bone autograft. Note the stress fracture and the atrophic appearance.*

immediate mechanical strength. Because of the dense composition of cortical bone, these grafts provide a more limited bony surface to the host bed and present a formidable mechanical barrier to the diffusion of nutrients and the ingrowth of vascular buds. Therefore, in contrast to cancellous bone, a cortical graft must first undergo osteoclastic resorption to create pores and channels. Very few, if any, graft cells are thought to remain viable in cortical bone. Following the formation of resorption spaces, vascular invasion can occur. This brings with it osteoprogenitor cells that elaborate osteoid and new bone on the surfaces of such resorption cavities. Once under way, vascular invasion can advance through pre-existing haversian or Volkmann canals. The overall 'creeping substitution' process with cortical grafts is more protracted than with cancellous bone. Significant volumes of nonviable interstitial lamellae may persist, and incorporation of the graft may be incomplete (Weiland et al 1984b). Because cortical grafts require resorption before new bone elaboration, they tend to lose mechanical strength following implantation, and exhibit their greatest weakness at 6–12 months after surgery (Enneking et al 1980). Cortical grafts regain strength only late, when the balance of the bone turnover process is shifting towards mature bone remodeling. Thus, although union of cortical grafts is not a major problem, late complications of stress fracture are frequent (Fig. 5). Depending on the specific site of implantation and length of bony defect, some form of protection of cortical grafts may be required for as long as 2–3 years after surgery.

There are no fixed guidelines regarding the length of a bony defect amenable to reliable reconstruction by conventional bone autografts. It is generally agreed that, in the presence of a reasonably healthy soft tissue bed, bony defects up to 6 cm in length can be very effectively reconstructed using cancellous autografts (Shaffer et al 1985). This is also true in the presence of infection, provided debridement of devitalized bone and soft tissue has been adequate and granulation tissue completely covers the bony defect. Defects exceeding 6 cm in length can also be effectively managed by conventional autografts, provided the surrounding tissue bed is well vascularized and protection from excessive mechanical stress can be ensured. For the longer defects, cortical autografts are usually preferable to cancellous grafts. Enneking has successfully managed skeletal defects of up to 25 cm in length using single or dual fibular strut grafts (Enneking et al 1980). For defects of 7.5–12.0 cm he has reported a union rate of 67%, with a fatigue fracture complication rate of 17%. For defects of 12–25 cm in length the union rate is 68%, but fatigue fracture complications have occurred in 58%. This latter figure should underscore the need for late, long-term protection.

7. Vascularized autograft healing

Christopher G Moran and Michael B Wood

Vascularized bone grafts may either be employed as pedicled bone segments or as free microvascular bone transfers. A pedicle bone graft will retain a degree of cellular viability proportionate to the adequacy of its vascular pedicle (Blair 1917; Baadsgaard and Medgyesi 1965; Medgyesi 1965, 1973). In general, pedicle bone grafts based on either a major nutrient arteriovenous pedicle or on a generous muscle cuff retain an appreciable degree of viability. Those based on skin, tendon, or ligament, without a defined accompanying vessel, may receive only scant volumes of blood flow (Medgyesi 1965). Clinical experience as well as animal laboratory data support the superiority of pedicle bone grafts over free, nonvascularized bone grafts in terms of cell viability, the speed of union and graft hypertrophy. It is likely that a pedicle bone graft can itself participate in the healing process by the mechanism of fracture union (Medgyesi 1973). Depending upon the quantity of retained vascular supply, however, it is likely that some portion of the bone will be rendered ischemic and may thus require incorporation by 'creeping substitution' (earlier discussed in Chapter 6).

A number of pedicle bone donor sites have been effectively used clinically. The fibula, on the basis of its nutrient arteriovenous pedicle as well as its attached muscles, was perhaps the earliest described (Huntington 1905), and still enjoys popularity for management of tibial defects and nonunions (Harmon 1945; Chacha et al 1981; Figs 1 and 2). Judet has employed this technique widely, both regionally adjacent to nonunions, and also about the hip (Judet and Patel 1972). Meyers has utilized a portion of ischium based on a muscle pedicle for femoral neck fractures (Meyers et al 1973). Davis et al have based

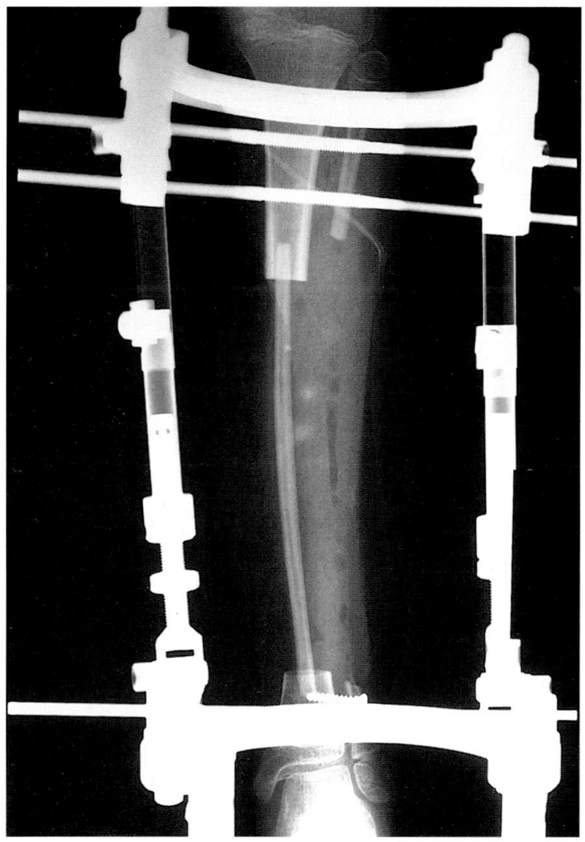

Fig. 1 *AP radiograph taken immediately after surgery of a pedicle fibula bone graft for reconstruction of a post-traumatic tibial defect.*

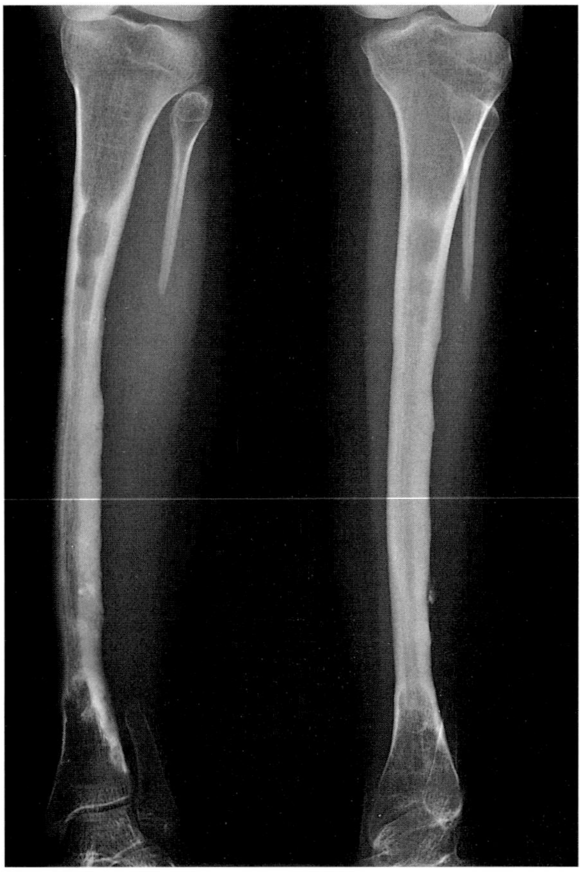

Fig. 2 *AP radiograph of the same pedicle fibula bone graft depicted in Fig. 1 in its healed state 8 months postoperatively.*

iliac crest on the tensor fasciae femoris to augment hip fusion (Davis and Taylor 1952). Iliac crest, based on the superficial circumflex iliac artery via a conventional groin flap, may be utilized for osteocutaneous reconstruction, particularly to the upper limb (Finseth et al 1976). Other described donor sites include clavicle based on a skin flap, rib based on intercostal vessels or muscle, radius based on radial artery or muscle, pisiform based on flexor carpi ulnaris, and metacarpal based on dorsal metacarpal vessels (Snyder et al 1970; Strauch et al 1971). The clinical applications of pedicle bone grafts are to some extent limited, owing to constraints related to the length and adequacy of the vascular pedicle. These constraints, however, are for the most part obviated by free microvascular autogenous bone transfer.

The major objective of a vascularized bone transfer is the immediate restoration of a physiological blood supply so that the cellular elements of the graft can survive (Arata et al 1984; Doi et al 1977). Although conventional bone grafts may be rapidly revascularized, most osteogenic elements are unable to survive this period of normothermic hypoxia. Immediate surgical restoration of the blood supply to a bone graft minimizes bone necrosis and allows graft osteogenic cells to initiate bone remodeling and healing. Incorporation of large vascularized cortical grafts thus should be rapid and complete. This process

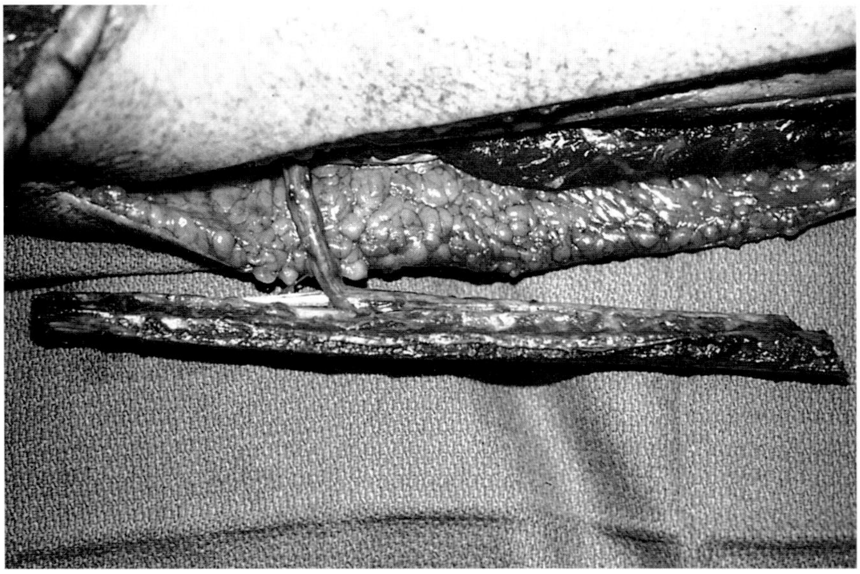

Fig. 3 *Photograph of a prepared fibula segment isolated on the peroneal arteriovenous pedicle.*

requires a patent vascular anastomosis and an adequate capillary blood flow (Siegert and Wood) 1987).

Numerous clinical (DeBoer and Wood 1989; Minami et al 1989; Weiland 1981, 1991) and experimental (Arata et al 1984; Doi et al 1977; Berggren et al 1982a; Goldberg et al 1987; Haw et al 1978; Shaffer et al 1985) studies have demonstrated that microarterial patency is maintained after vascularized bone graft. Remodeling progresses rapidly along the haversian canals, with an increase in bone porosity. However, the architecture of the cortex is preserved, and there is a rapid increase in the number of osteons (Schwarzenbach et al 1989). Histomorphometric studies have confirmed that vascularized grafts maintain a greater cross-sectional area of cortical bone (Goldberg et al 1987), and peripheral new bone deposition is much less marked than in avascular autografts, where cortical bone is replace by woven reactive bone. Experimental and clinical studies have confirmed that the rate of callus formation and union are significantly higher in vascularized bone grafts (DeBoer and Wood 1989; Haw et al 1978; Shaffer et al 1985; Zdeblick et al 1988). Thus most of the evidence suggests that vascularized cortical bone grafts enjoy a biological advantage over non-vascularized cortical bone grafts.

A variety of donor bones are available for free microvascular bone transfer. The two most commonly used, the fibula based on the peroneal arteriovenous pedicle (Taylor et al 1975; Gilbert 1979; Fig. 3) and the iliac crest based on the deep circumflex iliac vessels (Taylor et al 1979), were both originally described and clinically utilized by Taylor. Other potential donor sites include the rib, the scapula, a portion of the radius or humerus, the metatarsal, and bone from damaged or useless parts.

8. Bone allografts

Christopher G Moran and Michael B Wood

Advances in the management of musculoskeletal tumors, and the need to reconstruct failed joint replacements, have increased the use of bone allografts. The incorporation of these grafts will be influenced by two major factors: immunogenicity of the grafts and the effect of long-term preservation on the graft (Friedlaender 1987, 1991).

The majority of grafts used at the present time have been stored in a bone bank. Deep freezing (to less than –70°C) results in a loss of activity of proteolytic enzymes (Ehrlich et al 1983) and a reduction in immunogenicity (Friedlaender 1983). Incorporation of the graft starts with the formation of a hematoma rich in cytokines (Bolander 1991; Stevenson and Horowitz 1992). Surgery, and the presence of the graft, stimulate an acute inflammatory response. This is associated with infiltration of large numbers of lymphocytes. The majority of these lymphocytes are T-cells, and their activation may be the first step in graft rejection (Von Boehmer and Kisielow 1990). The graft is rapidly surrounded by fibrovascular (granulation) tissue, with the invasion of vascular buds and osteogenic precursor cells into the bone. In cortical bone this usually occurs through pre-existing haversian or Volkmann canals (osteoconduction). The interface between invading host fibrovascular tissue and allograft bone is the site of osteoclastic activity and the resorption of bone. This activity may be greater in fresh allografts, which present a greater antigenic load to the host's immune system.

The delicate balance between osteolysis and osteogenesis must be maintained for the graft to be revascularized and substituted without appreciable loss of strength. In many experimental animals there is a substantial uncoupling of these events: the immune stimulus for bone resorption is greater than for bone formation, resulting in weakening of the graft (Friedlaender 1983). Clinical experience would suggest that the immune response is less active in humans: it may abate or there may be a chronic immune response with slow resorption of the graft (Friedlaender et al 1984; Fig. 1) and an increased susceptibility to infection (Enneking and Mindell 1991). Activated T-cells appear to play an important

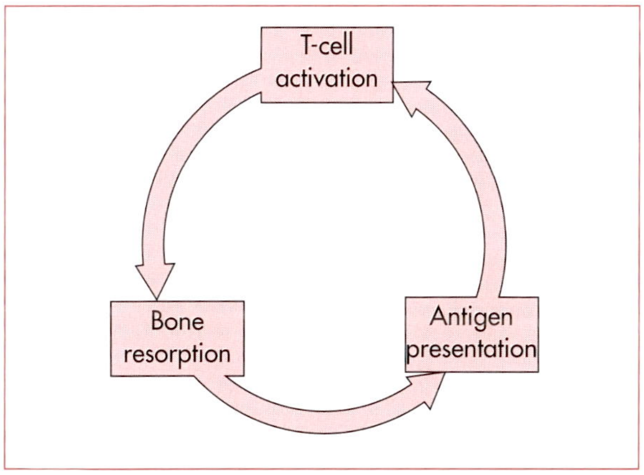

Fig. 1 *Progressive and indolent resorption of bone allografts as a result of ongoing rejection response.*

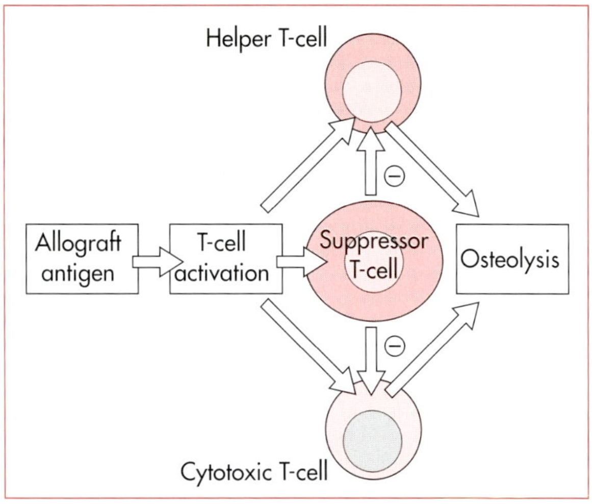

Fig. 2 *The balance between osteogenesis and osteolysis may depend upon the relative number and action of different subsets of T-cells. Successful incorporation of an allograft may require suppressor T-cells to inhibit the immune response.*

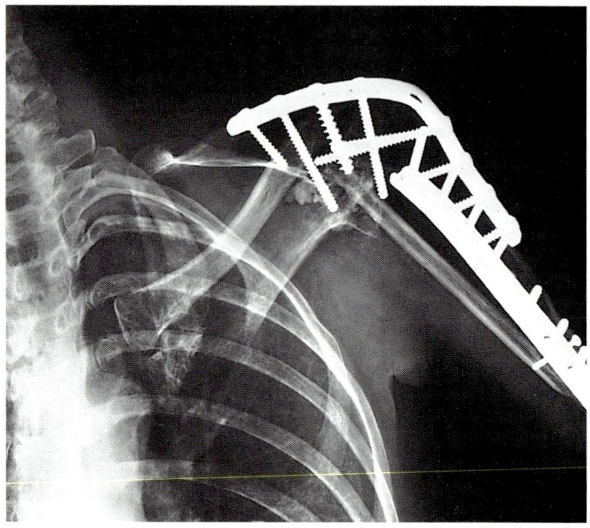

Fig. 3 *Combined proximal humerus allograft and vascularized fibula autograft for scapulohumeral arthrodesis following humeral resection.*

role in controlling this process (Friedlaender 1991; Horowitz and Friedlaender 1991; Stevenson and Horowitz 1992), and the biological response to an allograft may depend upon the specific types of T-cells that are activated. Large numbers of suppressor T-cells, which reduce the immune response, may be related to the success of bone allografts (Stevenson and Horowitz 1992; Fig. 2). Presumably on the basis of variations in host–donor histocompatibility, three patterns of allograft repair have been observed experimentally in animals (Burchardt et al 1975; Burchardt 1983; Heslop et al 1960a). Type I repair, essentially identical to autograft incorporation, may be seen in 20%. Type II repair exhibits delayed and incomplete revascularization and new bone formation, with concomitant accelerated osteoclastic resorption. This pattern occurs in as many as 60% of cases, and is associated with a higher incidence of nonunion and late loss of mechanical strength, with fatigue fracture. The Type III pattern occurs in 20% of cases, and involves a marked rejection response with allograft resorption. When the allograft has revascularized, remodeling can commence. There is evidence that revascularization only occurs to a depth of a few millimeters into the graft (Enneking and Mindell 1991; Burwell 1969). This is sufficient to allow union to the host bone, and for soft tissues to attach to the allograft surface biologically. A large volume of the allograft remains avascular and is not incorporated. However, this bone may continue to function as a structural graft for many years (Enneking and Mindell 1991). Thus the majority of massive nonvascularized allografts are successful in clinical practice. Because incorporation is not complete, allografts are not as strong as a similar-sized autograft. Adaptive remodeling to changes in stress patterns is limited, and stress fractures are likely to be a recurrent problem.

The combination of nonvascularized allograft and vascularized autograft for certain bone reconstructions about the knee and shoulder has been reported to show encouraging results (Zinberg et al 1985; Wood 1986; Fig. 3). Such an approach may permit the combined benefits of immediate structural support with the allograft and late structural support as a result of union and hypertrophy of the vascularized autograft.

Vascularized bone allografts

Vascularized bone allografts may have great potential for reconstructive surgery. Vascularization offers the possibility of complete incorporation of the graft, allowing adaptive changes to the biomechanical environment. However, the direct consequence of revascularization is the immediate exposure of the host to a far greater antigenic mass of tissue. Experimental studies have shown that fresh vascularized bone allografts, transplanted across major histocompatibility barriers, undergo rejection and necrosis between 3 and 7 days after transplantation (Garnet et al 1991; Gotfried et al 1987). The primary site of damage appears to be the vascular endothelium, resulting in secondary ischemic damage to the osteocytes. The primary effect of the host immune response on allograft osteocytes is not known. The immunological response to vascularized allograft bone is reduced by genetic matching, and suppressed by cyclosporin A. In this situation, early incorporation appears to be similar to vascularized isograft (and, presumably, autograft) (Innis et al 1991). Long-term survival studies need to be performed before the ultimate fate of these grafts can be evaluated. However, cessation of immunotherapy is consistently followed by a rejection response. Because of the risk of serious complications related to presently available systemic immunosuppression, vascularized bone allografts cannot be justified in the usual clinical setting.

III MICROVASCULAR BONE TRANSFER: EXPERIMENTAL

9. Laboratory basis

Christopher G Moran and Michael B Wood

Bone grafting is one of the most frequently performed procedures in orthopedic surgery, and is used in a variety of clinical situations. Conventional techniques of bone grafting can be used in the vast majority of cases, but their efficacy in treating large, segmental bone defects is often limited. Advances in microvascular surgery have made it possible to reconstitute these defects with autogenous bone grafts on a vascular pedicle. With the nutrient blood supply preserved, osteoblasts and osteocytes in the graft can survive and allow union to the recipient bone. The optimum application of this technique requires a thorough understanding of the biological and mechanical characteristics of transplanted bone.

History

The first bone graft procedure was described, in 1668, by the Dutch surgeon Job van Meekeren. This graft, taken from a dog's skull, was used for a successful repair of a traumatic defect in a soldier's cranium (DeBoer 1988). Bone autografts were first used in clinical practice in the early part of the nineteenth century (Von Walter 1821). However, it was not until the early twentieth century that Albee (1915) popularized this procedure.

The first scientific investigations into the problem of osteogenesis were undertaken by DeHeyde (1684). Ollier (1867) was interested in bone grafts, and demonstrated that bone and periosteum remain viable when transplanted. Ollier thought that a bone graft contributed directly to new bone formation, and did not recognize any contribution by the mesenchymal cells of the host bed. Barth (1894) challenged this theory, and suggested that the transplanted bone, marrow, and periosteum were necrotic. He believed that the viable cells for bone production were derived from the host-bed tissue. Barth wrote about *schleichenden ersatz*, absorption of dead tissue in a bone graft and then formation of new bone which grew into the graft. This process was later termed 'creeping substitution' by Phemister (1914). More recently, Urist and Strates (1971) have suggested that this process is stimulated by chemical mediators released from bone grafts. This process is termed osteoinduction, and a number of such mediators have now been isolated (Sampath and Reddi 1981).

The development of vascularized bone grafts

The earliest record of autogenous pedicled grafts is in a Sanskrit text from India, the *Sushrista Shamita* (Flye 1989). These grafts were used to repair mutilations of the face in the second century BC. The modern concept of transplanting a vascularized, living bone was proposed by Phelps (1891) and Curtis and Morrey (1893), and the first pedicle transfer, of the ipsilateral fibula on to the tibia, was described by Huntington (1905). However, the use of these grafts is limited by the length of the vascular pedicle. In most anatomical sites, vascular bone transplantation did not become practical until the operating microscope, and improved microsurgical instrumentation, became available (Östrup and

Frederickson 1974). The first report of a free vascularized fibular graft was by Taylor (Taylor et al 1975), and this new technique has been successfully applied in a large number of clinical situations (DeBoer 1988; Weiland and Daniel 1979; Wood and Cooney 1984).

Biology

Bone heals by regeneration and replacement, producing additional bone rather than scar tissue. Thus the final common pathway of bone homeostasis, fracture repair, and graft incorporation is the remodeling cycle.

The remodeling cycle

The remodeling cycle has three phases: activation, resorption, and new bone formation. The activation of bone remodeling remains poorly understood, but it appears that both local and systemic factors can initiate this process (Friedlaender 1987). In addition to these biological factors, physical modalities, such as mechanical stress and electrical signals, may induce the same activity (Canalis 1985).

Bone resorption is characterized by the appearance of osteoclasts on the trabecular surfaces. These are multinucleate giant cells that probably originate from hemopoietic, stem-cell precursors of macrophage lineage (Felix et al 1990; Wiktor-Jedrzejczak et al 1990). The osteoclasts remove mineral and matrix, an action which may be stimulated by a number of cytokines and growth factors released from activated reticuloendothelial cells (Stevenson and Horowitz 1992). Formation of new bone generally follows resorption, and occurs when osteoblasts deposit osteoid on bone surfaces. This matrix is subsequently mineralized, with the bone-forming cells persisting as osteocytes. Regulation of bone resorption is complex, and it is likely that bone morphogenic proteins and transforming growth factors play a central role in the control mechanisms (Bolander 1991).

When resorption and formation are synchronous, bone mass remains constant. Repair and incorporation of bone grafts are characterized by a substantial uncoupling of these events, and there are significant differences between vascularized and nonvascularized bone grafts.

Preservation of the blood supply to a bone graft should prevent bone necrosis and allow graft osteogenic cells to initiate bone remodeling and healing. Thus incorporation of these large, cortical grafts should be rapid and complete. This process obviously requires that an adequate capillary blood flow be maintained, so that the osteogenic cells can remain viable.

Blood flow in vascularized bone grafts

The viability and circulatory status of bone grafts has been assessed by a number of techniques. In experimental models arteriography and microangiography have been used to judge arterial patency (Doi et al 1977; Shaffer et al 1985), but provide no information on the bone blood flow. Scintigraphy can measure quantitative differences in blood flow, and has been used to demonstrate normal or increased blood flow 4 days after revascularization of a canine rib graft (Berggren et al 1982b). At this time, there is no uptake of the radionuclide in nonvascularized bone. However, by 1 week nonvascularized cortical bone may have a positive scintillation scan, and histological studies demonstrate that this is due to neovascularization around the cortical bone (Bos 1979; Shaffer et al 1987).

Hydrogen washout has also been used to measure blood flow to bone grafts. Using a canine tibia model, based entirely on its nutrient artery, Zdbelick et al (1988) observed that the bone blood flow increased threefold. These authors also demonstrated that the blood supply to nonvascularized segments was significantly reduced throughout this period, and did not gain parity with the vascularized segments until 3 months postoperatively. However, it should be noted that no microvascular anastomosis was performed in this experiment. Thus the effect of ischemia, local endothelial damage, and the no-reflow phenomenon were not evaluated.

Quantitative evaluation of blood flow in vascularized bone segments has also been performed using the radiolabeled microsphere method (Siegert and Wood 1990). In this study a segment of canine tibia, based upon the nutrient artery, was revascularized by arterial and venous anastomosis in a heterotopic site. At 2 days the vascularized bone transfers exhibited intermediate levels of cortical blood flow (1.4 ± 0.4 ml/min per 100 g) compared with undisturbed

Dog	Specimen,[a] blood flow[b] CV	CC	V	C
8	3.2	4.1	2.1	5.7
9	2.9	1.9	6.9	2.0
10	1.7	0.7	6.5	1.7
11	2.9	2.4	2.6	4.9
12	1.0	1.2	6.6	4.0
13	1.2	0.9	1.9	1.2
14	1.3	1.9	0.7	1.1
15	3.7	3.6	4.0	4.4
Mean[c]	2.2	2.1	3.9	3.1
SD	1.0	1.1	2.3	1.7
SEM	0.3	0.4	0.8	0.6

[a] C, conventional graft; CC, control for conventional graft; CV, control for vascularized graft; V, vascularized graft.
[b] Expressed in ml/100 g of bone/min.
[c] With paired Student's t test: CC:C, $p < 0.05$.

Fig. 1 *Blood flow as measured by microsphere technique to microsurgically revascularized canine tibia segment compared to nonrevascularized canine tibia over a 2-week period (from Siegert and Wood 1990).*

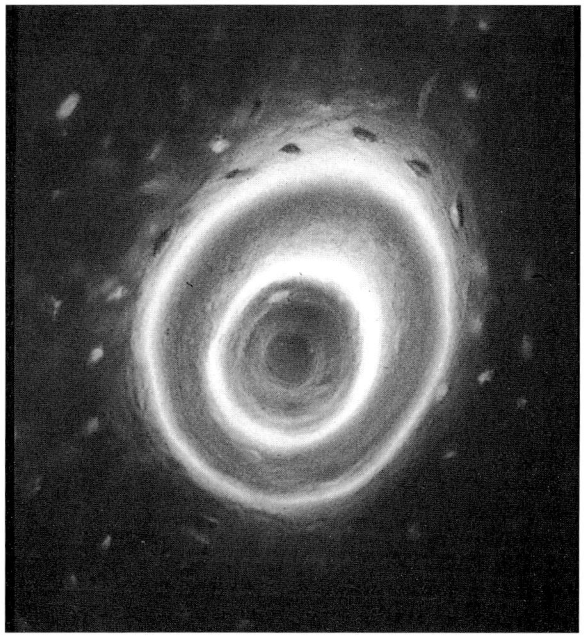

Fig. 2 *Photomicrograph of vascularized bone graft following two labels of fluorochrome (tetracycline) given 5 weeks apart, illustrating active osteones taking up label. Note that the distance between tetracycline labels illustrates the amount of osteoid elaborated over this period.*

control bone (2.7±0.5 ml/min per 100 g) and nonrevascularized conventional cortical bone grafts (0.0±0.0 ml/min per 100 g). At 1 week all conventional grafts demonstrated some blood flow (0.2±0.1 ml/min per 100 g) and, by 2 weeks, the blood flow values in both types of bone graft were significantly greater than in normal bone (Fig. 1).

These results demonstrate the rapidity (and the extent) of neovascularization in cortical bone grafts, and may be analogous to the hyperemia seen after fracture or osteotomy (Trueta 1957; Rhinelander 1974). In this experiment the bone grafts were placed in subcutaneous fat and not subject to internal fixation or mechanical stress. There was marked osteopenia of the grafts and, because of this change in bone mass, the serial microsphere method could not be used to estimate changes in bone blood flow. The blood flow changes observed may not accurately reflect those seen in the clinical situation. An additional problem was that only 76% of vascular anastomoses were confirmed to be patent at sacrifice. This is similar to other studies in the dog (Shaffer et al 1985; Berggren et al 1982a,b), but lower than that reported in most clinical series of free tissue transfer (DeBoer and Wood 1989; Weiland 1991). This difference probably reflects surgical expertise, but may also be due to false positive bone scans in the clinical group.

Viability of osteogenic cells in vascularized bone grafts

The major objective of a vascularized bone transfer is the immediate restoration of a physiological blood supply so that the cellular elements of the graft can remain viable. Although conventional bone grafts are rapidly revascularized, most osteogenic elements are unable to survive this period of normothermic hypoxia (Heslop et al 1960b; Arora and Laskin 1964). A number of studies have investigated the viability of cells within a vascularized bone graft. This may be estimated by the morphologic appearance of osteocytes on light microscopy; or the number of viable cells may be studied by fluorochrome analysis. Fluorochrome dyes are only taken up by osteons that are actively involved in the process of bone formation (Milch et al 1958; Harris 1960; Fig. 2). Because this process is variable (Tam et al 1974) the quantity of fluorochrome uptake may not be a direct measure of the quantity of viable cells within a bone specimen.

Doi et al (1977) utilized morphologic osteocyte counts 7 days after transplantation of a vascularized canine rib autograft. The percentage of cells judged viable was 94%, compared with 8% in nonrevascularized bone. However, it is likely that this is an overestimate of the viability of the graft, since it has been shown that osteocytes appearing relatively normal to light microscopy may be present in the lacunae for 2 weeks after cell death (Usui et al 1989). Arata et al (1984) assessed the osteocyte viability in a revascularized canine tibia 6 weeks after surgery. The percentage of viable osteocytes was 52%, compared with 69% in normal bone and 28% in nonrevascularized bone. Longer-term studies, using the same model (Schwarzenbach et al 1989), have confirmed these results, and demonstrate a more rapid increase in the number of osteons taking up fluorochrome dye in vascularized bone grafts. This observation may reflect an increased rate of remodeling in this type of graft.

The origin of the blood supply may also be important in determining the viability of the graft. Berggren et al (1982a) have demonstrated that canine posterior rib grafts, with an intact medullary and periosteal blood supply, have the same fluorochrome labeling pattern as normal bone. In contrast, posterolateral rib grafts, with only a periosteal blood supply, had fewer viable osteons. Despite this, there was no difference in healing between the two grafts, and the number of graft-derived osteogenic cells needed to ensure rapid graft incorporation is unknown.

Healing and remodeling of vascularized bone grafts

With an intact blood supply and viable osteogenic cells, incorporation of a vascularized bone graft should be rapid and resemble fracture healing. Experimental studies, however, have demonstrated that significant bone resorption still occurs in these grafts (Weiland et al 1984b; Shaffer et al 1985; Goldberg et al 1987). This is due to remodeling, which progresses rapidly along the haversian canals. There is an increase in bone porosity, but the architecture of the cortex is preserved (Schwarzenbach et al 1989). Histomorphometric studies have confirmed that vascularized grafts maintain a greater cross-sectional area of cortical bone (Goldberg et al 1987), and peripheral new bone deposition is much less marked than in avascular autografts, where cortical bone is replaced by woven reactive bone. It should be noted that the type of remodeling depends upon the experimental model. Vascularized canine ulna autografts have a greater volume of periosteal new bone formation than vascularized canine rib or tibial grafts.

Experimental and clinical studies have demonstrated that the rate of callus formation and union are significantly higher in vascularized bone grafts (Weiland et al 1984b; Zdeblick et al 1988; DeBoer and Wood 1989). Haw and O'Brien (Haw et al 1978) replaced segments of dog tibias with immediately vascularized grafts and achieved 100% union, compared with only 50% union when nonvascularized grafts were used. Weiland et al (1984b) reconstructed segmental defects in the canine femur using vascular and avascular rib autografts. There was no difference in the union rates at 6 months, but union occurred more rapidly in the vascular group.

Similar results have been observed in the canine ulna (Shaffer et al 1985) and tibia (Zdeblick et al 1988), where 87% of vascularized segmental osteotomies had healed at 3 months. Thus most experimental evidence suggests that vascularized bone grafts enjoy a biological advantage over nonvascularized cortical bone grafts.

Biomechanics of vascularized bone grafts

Experimental study of vascularized bone grafts is complex, and so there have been few investigations of the biomechanical properties of these grafts. Puckett et al (1979) compared the bone formation resulting from nonvascular grafting techniques with the osteogenesis after vascular rib grafts. At 4 months vascular grafts had a slightly greater tolerance to stress than nonvascular grafts, but quantitative assessment of all grafts was not done. Davis et al (1982) compared the torsional strength of vascularized and nonvascular bone grafts. A rib autograft was used to reconstruct a nonunion of the ulna in nine dogs. There was a wide variation in the torsional strengths of the grafts, but in all dogs the maximum torque sustained by the specimen was greater in the vascularized graft. Using a similar model, Moore et al

(1984) concluded that vascular grafts were 234% stronger in torsion than conventional bone grafts. However, biomechanical testing was reported for only 3 months postoperatively.

Weiland et al (1984b) also report considerable variation in the mechanical strength of various types of bone graft, but vascularized grafts achieved the highest strength. These results were confirmed by Shaffer et al (1985), who demonstrated that vascularized bone grafts have superior torsional strength and stiffness throughout the repair process. However, the biomechanical properties of vascularized bone grafts remain controversial. Dell et al (1985) evaluated a nonweightbearing canine fibula model. The vascularized grafts were transiently stronger than the conventional grafts (at 6 weeks), but thereafter there was no difference. Nather et al (1990) were also unable to demonstrate any difference in mechanical properties between vascularized and nonvascularized cat tibia grafts. It should be noted that the mechanical strength of vascularized bone graft is diminished when compared to normal bone (Goldberg et al 1987; Nather et al 1990). This loss of mechanical properties occurs during incorporation of the vascularized graft, and thus these grafts must be protected during incorporation and remodeling.

IV MICROVASCULAR BONE TRANSFER: CLINICAL

10. Surgical techniques: donor sites

A. ILIAC CREST OSTEOCUTANEOUS FLAP: DEEP CIRCUMFLEX ILIAC ARTERY

The anterior iliac crest based on the deep circumflex iliac vessels is particularly well-suited for reconstructions requiring a broad, somewhat short bone graft (Wood 1990a). It may be readily used for defects up to 12 cm in length. Because of its shape, it is useful for metaphyseal reconstructions (Fig. 1). The anterior iliac crest is chiefly cancellous in composition (Fig. 2). This feature may be an advantage in terms of bone surface contact and rapid union, but is disadvantageous in regard to inherent strength and stable internal fixation. The broad, flat structure and multitude of direct vascular perforating vessels. (Fig. 3) from the overlying iliac muscle allow one or several osteotomies through this segment. Thus it may be shaped to accommodate to the recipient site defect geometry with considerable versatility. Perhaps the most useful characteristic of anterior iliac crest is the fact that it is easily isolated with an accompanying skin flap of large dimensions (Taylor et al 1979). The overlying skin is congruent with the design and dimensions of the well-known groin flap. Thus the iliac crest based on the deep circumflex iliac vessels may provide well-vascularized bone with a large skin flap for one-stage reconstructions of compound defects.

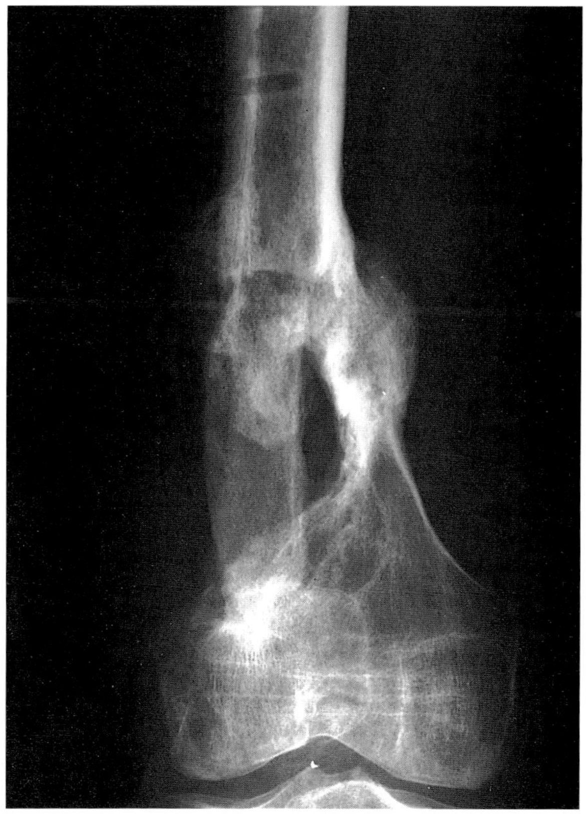

Fig. 1 *AP radiograph illustrating vascularized iliac crest transfer based on deep circumflex iliac vessels to reconstruct a post-traumatic metaphyseal defect of femur.*

The anterior iliac crest is convex when viewed externally. The vascular pedicle enters its anterior margin. Thus the selection of right or left side may be relevant, depending upon the recipient site location, bone defect length, and recipient vessel location. Whenever its use is possible for lower-extremity reconstruction, selection of the ipsilateral iliac crest facilitates postoperative immobilization by avoiding weightbearing on the donor side and it is

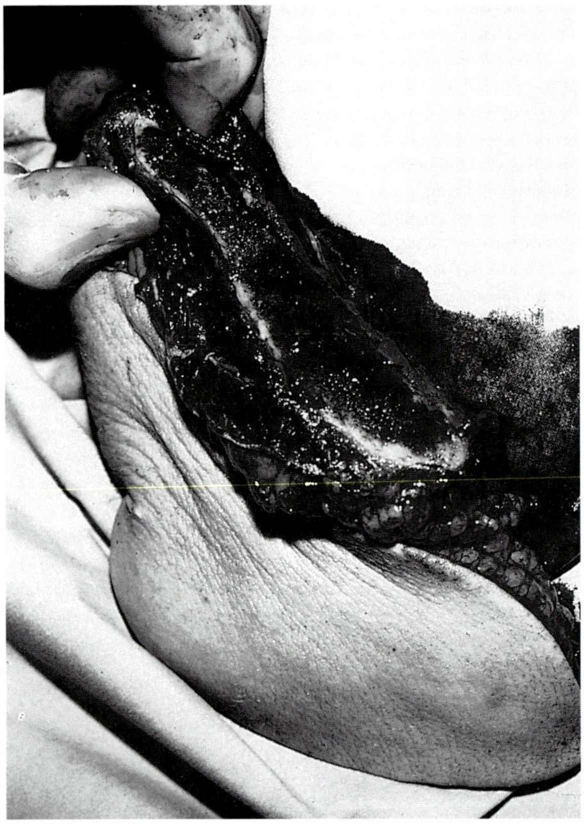

Fig. 2 Photograph illustrating cancellous composition of anterior iliac crest.

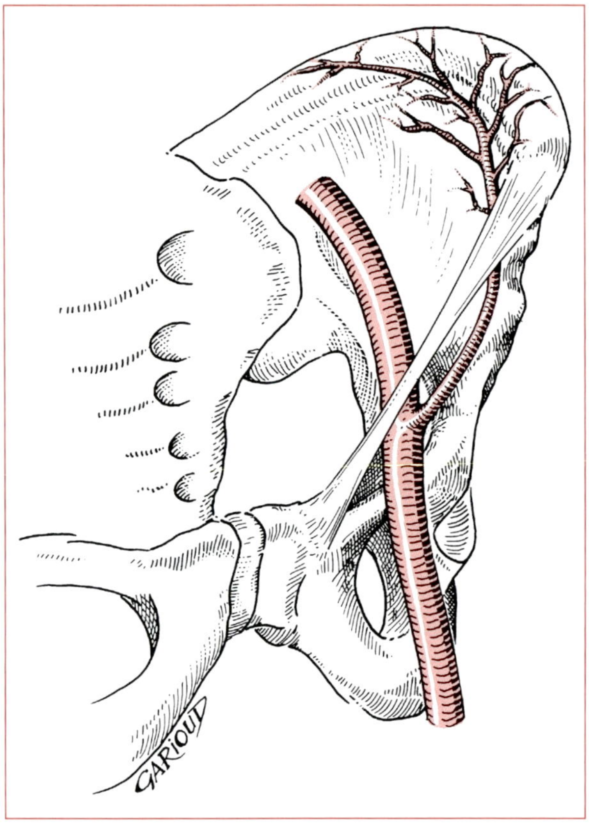

Fig. 3 Schematic illustrating of multiple vascular perforating vessels coursing to inner table of anterior ilium from deep circumflex iliac vessels.

preferred for this reason and for ease of access. However, the contralateral iliac crest should be selected if its curvature will fit better at the recipient site.

Following selection of the more appropriate donor side, the patient is placed on the operating table in a supine position with a soft roll beneath the donor side buttock. The surgical field should be prepared and draped to include the costal margin cephalad, the midline and pubic tubercle medially, and extend as far posterolaterally as is required to meet the dimensions of the skin flap to be included with the bone. Distally the lower extremity should be prepared and draped circumferentially, so that it may be readily positioned with the hip in flexion to facilitate skin closure of the donor defect.

The intended surgical incision is marked to begin medially directly over the femoral artery at a point 3–4 cm distal to the inguinal ligament (Fig. 4). In most patients this point can be accurately localized by palpating the femoral pulse in the groin. The incision passes cephalad over the course of the femoral artery until the level of the inguinal ligament. It is then directed laterally along the course of the inguinal ligament until it engages the outline of the accompanying skin flap. The skin flap design is centered at or slightly lateral to the longitudinal axis of the iliac crest (Fig. 5). The distal margin of the skin flap should overlie the anterior superior iliac spine. The skin is incised along the line thus marked and carried through subcutaneous tissue. The incision is then deepened to expose the fascia overlying the inguinal ligament and the external oblique muscle. Great care is required at this point in order to avoid undermining the skin flap and severing it from its soft tissue connections to the fascia overlying the external oblique muscle and iliac

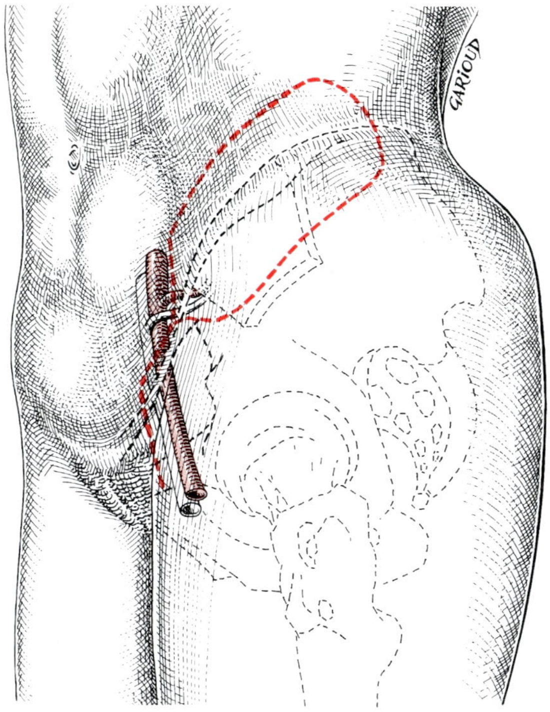

Fig. 4 *Schematic illustration of the surgical incision for the isolation of an iliac osteocutaneous flap based on the deep circumflex iliac vessels.*

crest. The fascia and muscle of the external oblique are then incised parallel and slightly cephalad to the inguinal ligament, exposing the inguinal canal. Medially the spermatic cord in the male or the round ligament in the female is identified and protected. The dissection is then further deepened through the posterior wall of the inguinal canal by incising the conjoined internal oblique aponeurosis and the transversalis fascia. Closely applied to the undersurface of the transversalis fascia is the deep circumflex iliac artery and its accompanying veins (Fig. 6).

The deep circumflex iliac artery arises from the external iliac artery. Its point of origin should be isolated along with the terminations of the deep circumflex iliac veins draining into the external iliac vein. These vessels should then be traced and mobilized in a lateral direction towards the anterior superior iliac spine. Along its course several small arterial branches and venous perforators will require isolation and ligation. A large consistent branch of the deep circumflex iliac artery is its ascending branch, which courses in a cephalad direction in a plane lying between the internal oblique and transversus abdominis muscles (Fig. 7). This branch should be identified and ligated near its point of origin 1–3 cm medial to the anterior superior iliac spine. Lateral to the ascending branch,

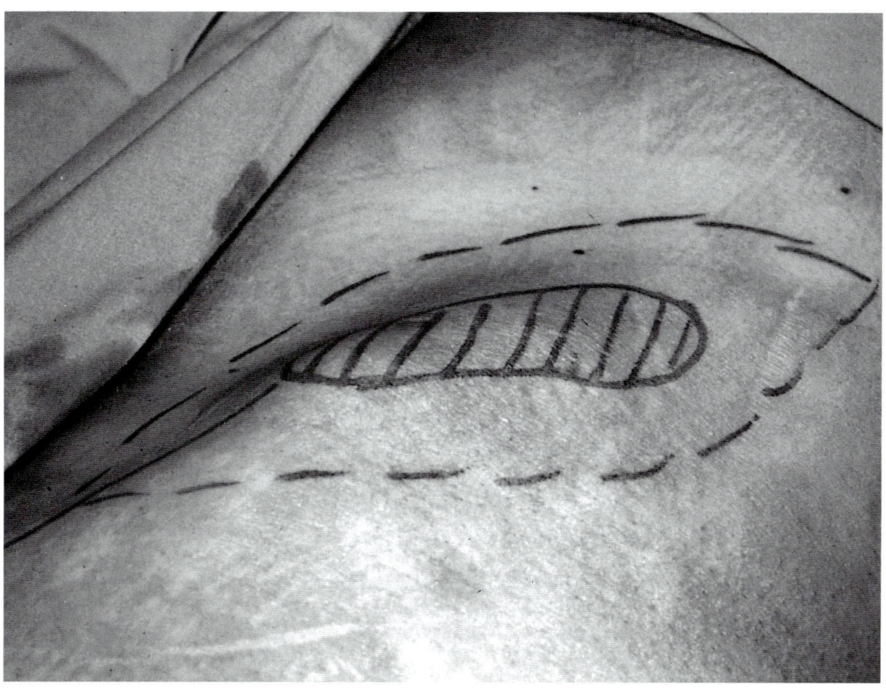

Fig. 5 *Photograph illustrating the design of a groin skin flap overlying the anterior iliac crest.*

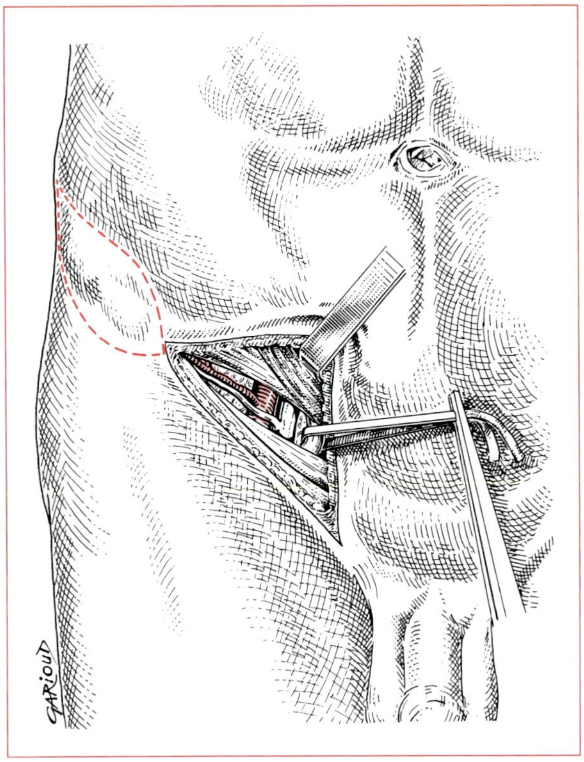

Fig. 6 *Schematic illustration of the relation of the deep circumflex iliac vessels to the abdominal wall musculofascial layers within the inguinal canal.*

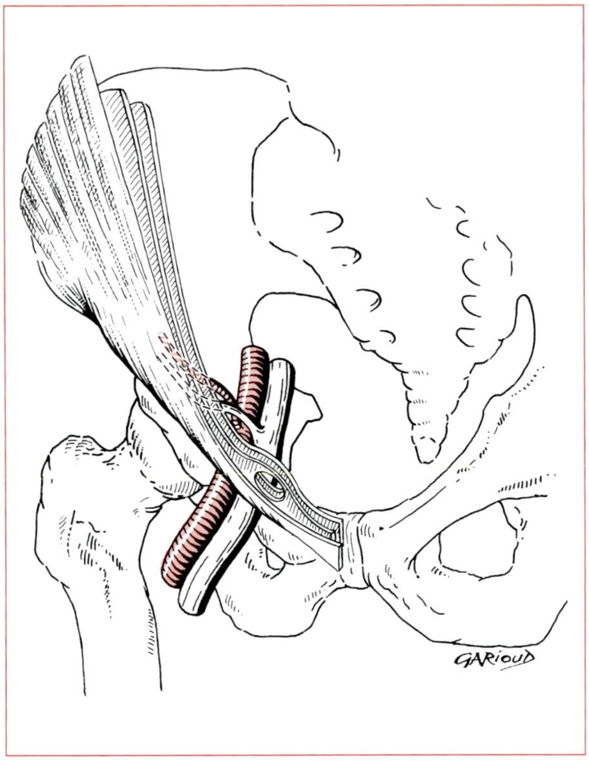

Fig. 7 *Schematic illustration of the ascending branch of the deep circumflex iliac artery between the internal oblique and transversus abdominis muscles.*

the deep circumflex iliac vessels ascend along the inner surface of the anterior ilium or within the iliac muscle, approximately 2 cm caudal to the iliac crest. Multiple perforating vessels course from the deep circumflex iliac vessels through the iliac muscle and the inner table of the anterior ileum (Fig. 3).

Just medial to the anterior superior iliac spine, the lateral femoral cutaneous nerve passes either deep or superficial to the deep circumflex iliac vessels. If superficial, the nerve may require sectioning, but if it courses deeply it can be preserved. The iliac muscle and fascia about the course of the vascular pedicle must be meticulously preserved where it is applied to the inner table of the bone. It may be incised down to the iliac inner table parallel with the course of the deep circumflex iliac vessels along a line lying 1–2 cm caudal to the vessels (Fig. 8). Posteriorly the vessels are ligated and sectioned, and the iliac fascia is incised at the same level as the intended posterior osteotomy of the iliac crest. The abdominal wall muscles, consisting of the external oblique, the internal oblique, and transversus

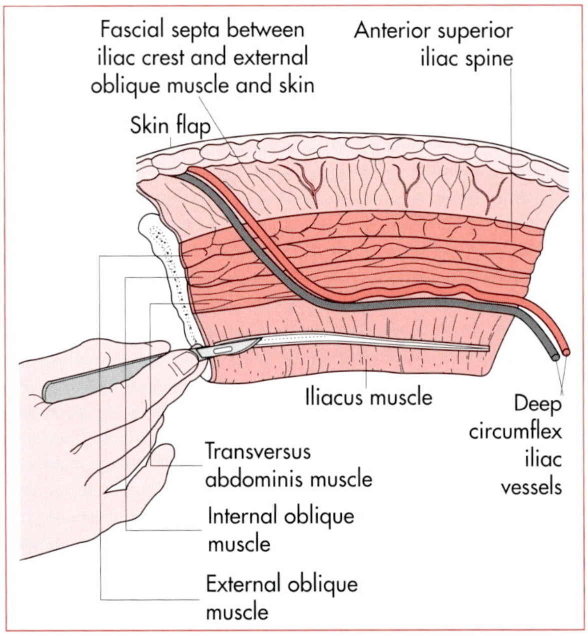

Fig. 8 *Schematic illustration of the incision through the iliacus down to the inner iliac table 1–2 cm caudal to the course of the deep circumflex iliac vessels.*

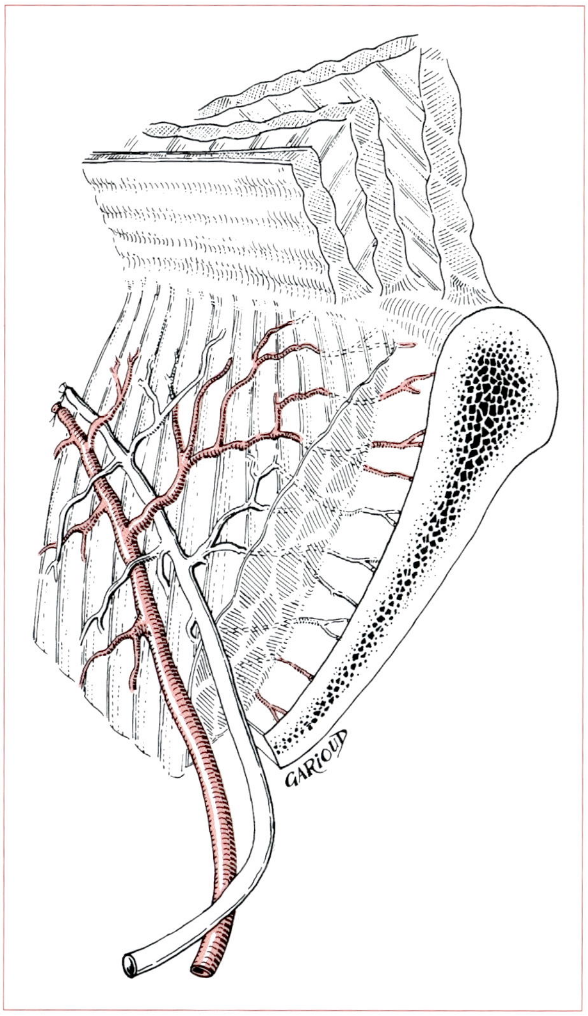

Fig. 9 *Schematic illustration of an iliac bone segment with muscle attachments of the external oblique, internal oblique, and transversus abdominis and back along the inner table.*

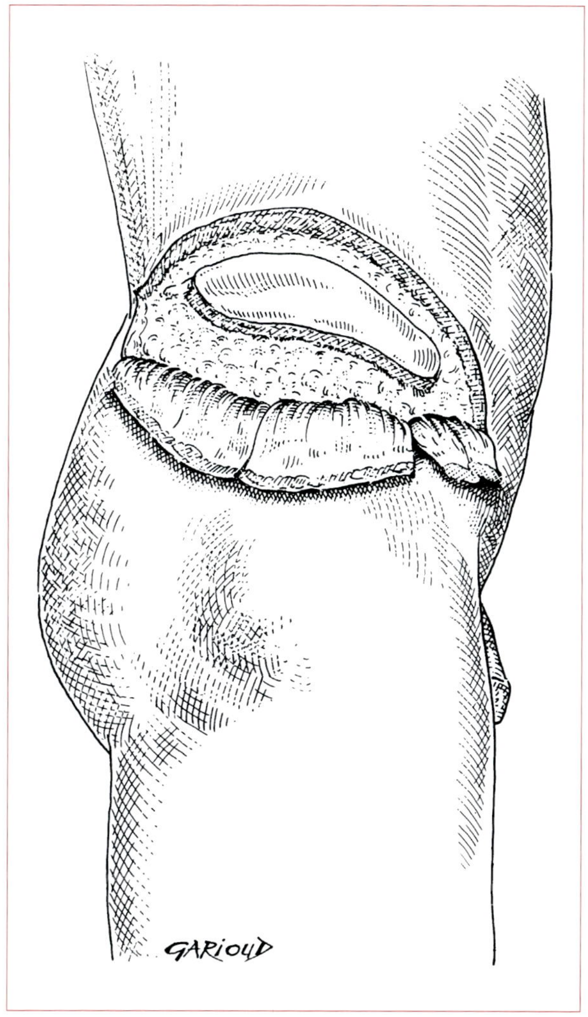

Fig. 10 *Schematic illustration of the lateral incision of the skin flap down to gluteal and tensor fasciae femoris fascia along the outer iliac table.*

abdominis, are released from the anterior iliac crest along the desired bone length, leaving about 1 cm of muscle tissue attached to the crest (Fig. 9).

After completion of vascular pedicle isolation with the attached surrounding iliacus muscle, attention should be turned to the lateral margin of the skin flap. Dissection here is deepened through the subcutaneous tissue down to the fascia overlying the gluteal and tensor fasciae femoris muscles (Fig. 10). As was emphasized for the dissection of the medial portion of the flap, great care should be taken to avoid undermining the skin flap from its soft connections to the underlying fascia. The gluteal and tensor fasciae femoris fascia is incised in line with the lateral margin of the skin flap, and then reflected from the underlying muscle to a point approximately 2 cm caudal to the iliac crest. The dissection is then deepened through muscle to bone, preserving a 1- to 2-cm rim of muscle tissue on the outer side of the iliac crest. The remaining muscles covering the outer iliac table and those attached to the anterior superior iliac spine (sartorius and rectus femoris) are then reflected extraperiosteally in a distal direction until the intended bone segment osteotomy sites are exposed.

Using a reciprocating saw and with great care to avoid injury to the vascular pedicle and the attached

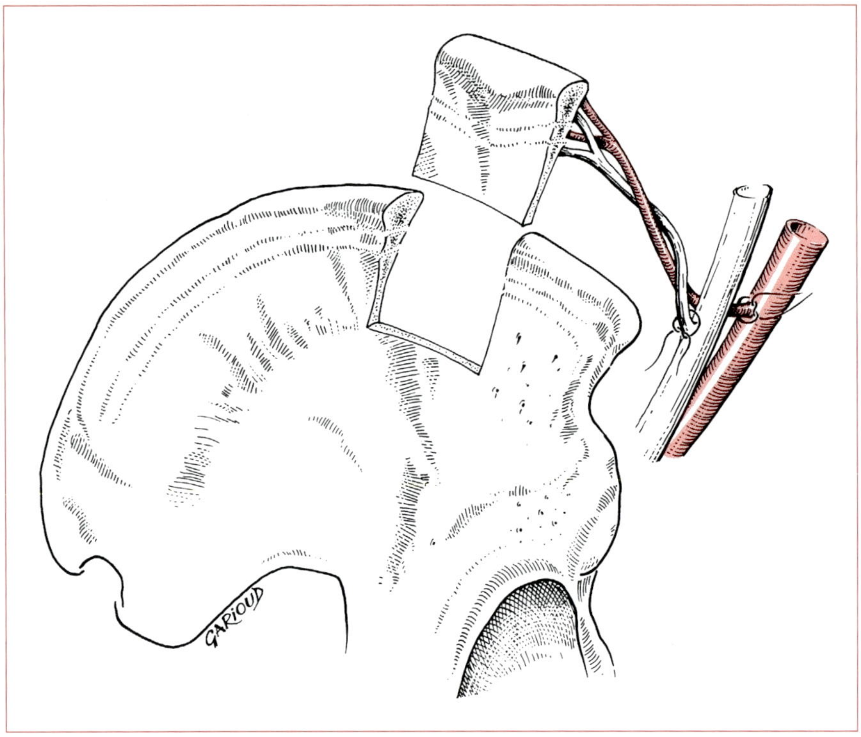

Fig. 11 *Schematic illustration of an isolated iliac bone segment following osteotomy based on the deep circumflex iliac vessels.*

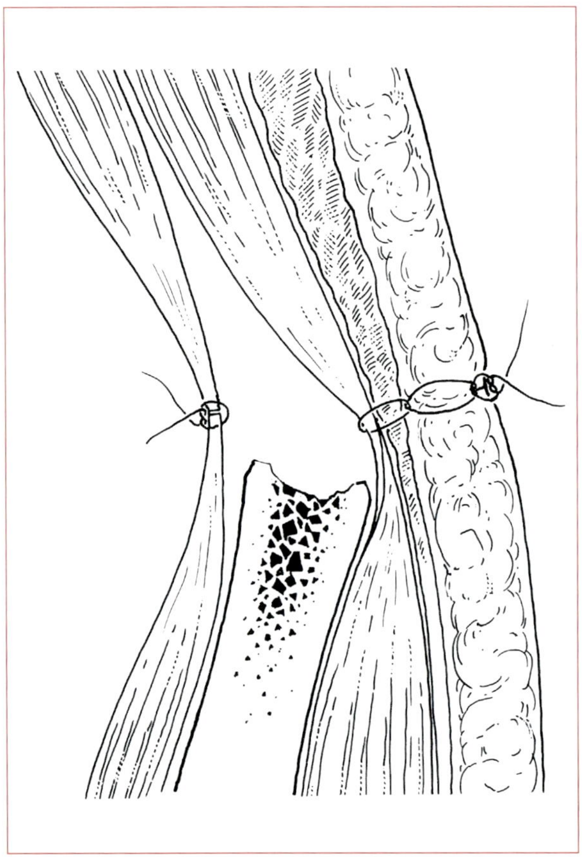

Fig. 12 *Schematic illustration of layered closure of the iliac donor site.*

iliac muscle segment lying along the inner table, an anterior, posterior, and caudal osteotomy of the iliac crest is accomplished from the lateral incision. Following completion of the osteotomies, the iliac bone segment will be completely isolated, with only its vascular pedicle intact (Fig. 11). At this point bleeding from the ends of the isolated bone segment and viability of the attached skin flap should be confirmed. The deep circumflex iliac artery and accompanying deep circumflex iliac vein(s) should then be ligated and sharply sectioned at their juncture with the external iliac vessels. The multiple deep circumflex iliac venae comitantes are usually joined to form a single vein before they terminate into the external iliac vein. Typically a pedicle length of 6–8 cm is possible.

Closure of the donor site defect must be carefully carried out in order to prevent an abdominal wall wound hernia. The transversalis fascia adjacent to the bone must be tightly coapted to the iliac fascia laterally with 2-0 or 3-0 braided polyester interrupted sutures. This is followed by repair of the aponeurosis of the external and internal oblique muscles to the gluteal fascia in a similar manner (Fig. 12). In the medial aspect of the wound, repair of the incision in the posterior wall of the inguinal canal consisting of the conjoined internal oblique aponeurosis and transversalis fascia

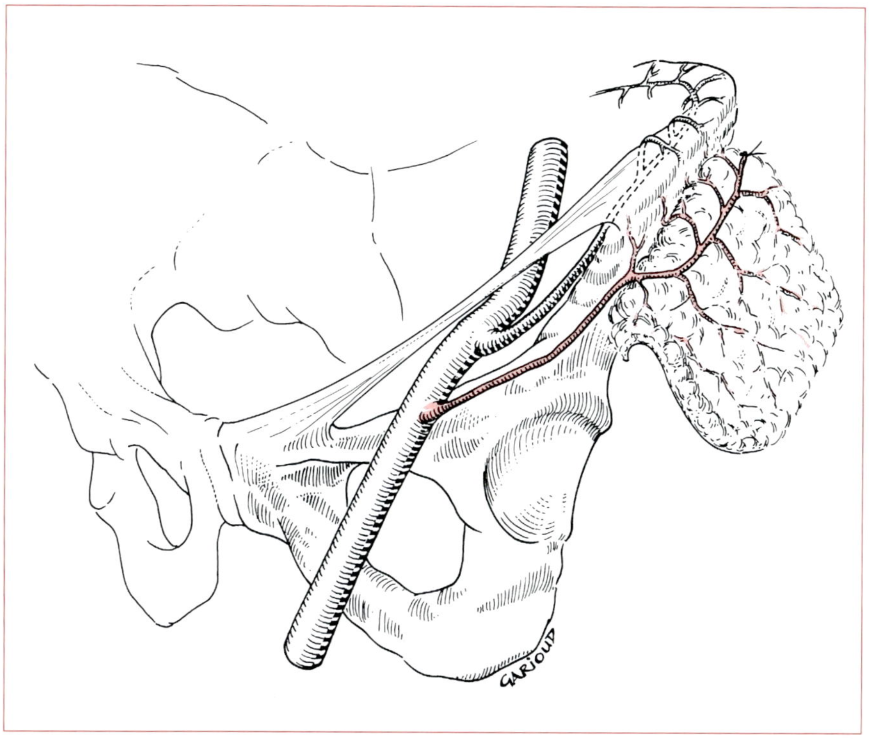

Fig. 13 *Schematic illustration of fasciocutaneous perforators from the skin flap to the underlying ilium from superficial circumflex iliac vessels, by contrast to direct bone-perforating vessels from the deep circumflex iliac vessels.*

with interrupted 3-0 braided polyester suture is necessary. Following this, repair of the anterior wall of the inguinal canal, consisting chiefly of the external oblique aponeurosis, is carried out in a like manner. Care must be taken to avoid injuring the ilioinguinal nerve, the lateral femoral cutaneous nerve, or the spermatic cord with the sutures during the course of closure. Following the deep closure, the subcutaneous tissue and skin should be closed in a layered manner, using the technique of surgeon's preference Temporary deep suction drains are recommended.

Postoperatively the patient should be kept at bedrest, with the hip gently flexed to decrease repair site wound tension, for 3–5 days. Thereafter a progression of activities, with weightbearing on the donor side, is permissible. A strengthening program for the muscles of the abdominal wall and the hip abductor and flexor muscles may be initiated 4–6 weeks postoperatively.

B. ILIAC CREST BONE FLAP: DEEP CIRCUMFLEX ILIAC ARTERY

The iliac crest can be isolated as a bone-only flap based on the deep circumflex iliac vessels when an accompanying soft tissue flap is not required. Such may be the case when a relatively short, broad, flat bone segment is desired, but there is no accompanying soft tissue defect. The technique of bone isolation is identical, with the exception that an elliptical skin flap is not designed, and instead the lateral aspect of the incision courses in a cephalad direction directly over the anterior iliac crest. It is, of course, necessary to preserve the iliac fascia and muscle along the inner table of the isolated bone segment in order to ensure inclusion of the bone-vascular perforators arising from the deep circumflex iliac vessels. However, preservation of a rim of external oblique, internal oblique, gluteal, and tensor fasciae femoris muscle is not necessary, and instead these should be reflected directly off the periosteum of the crest. Thus closure is simplified by virtue of the fact that there is less tension along the muscle aponeurosis suture line.

C. ILIAC CREST OSTEOCUTANEOUS FLAP: SUPERFICIAL CIRCUMFLEX ILIAC ARTERY

The anterior iliac crest may be isolated as a compound flap based on fasciocutaneous perforating vessels from a standard groin flap supplied by the superficial circumflex iliac vessels (Fig. 13) (Finseth et al 1976;

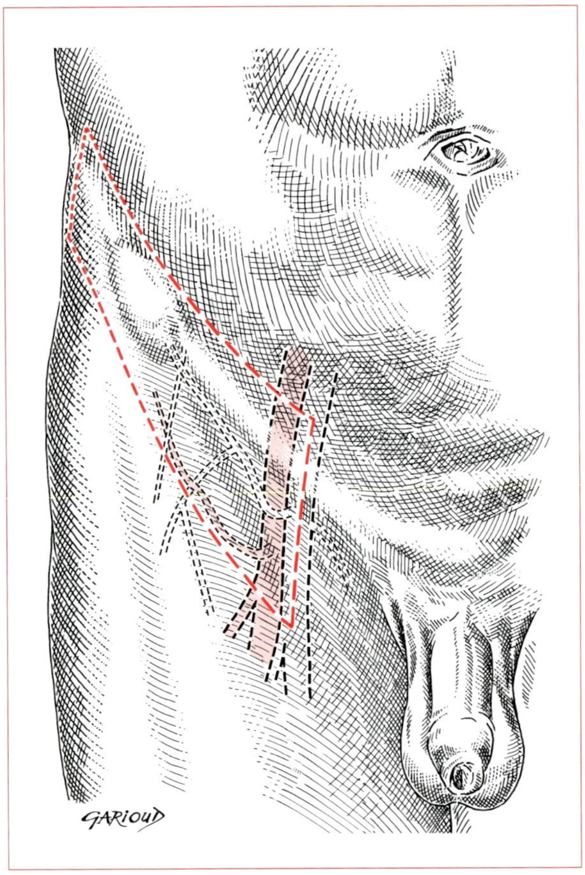

Fig. 14 *Schematic illustration of the central arterial axis of a groin flap. The origin overlies the femoral artery 2.5 cm distal to the inguinal ligament, and then courses laterally and cephalad to the anterior superior iliac spine.*

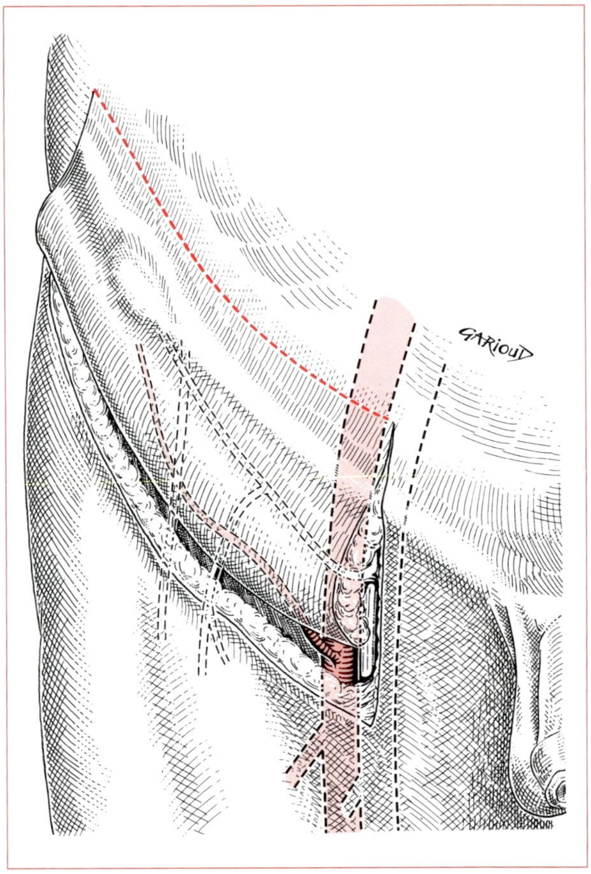

Fig. 15 *Schematic illustration of the elevation of the caudal margin of a groin skin flap.*

Taylor and Watson 1978). Although there is some controversy in regard to the adequacy of bone vascularity, it is likely that the blood supply to the bone with this flap is sparse. Vascular perfusion studies as well as clinical experience have confirmed that some blood flow to the bone may be seen with this compound flap. However, in contrast to the iliac flap based on the deep circumflex iliac system, there are no demonstrable direct vascular perforators from the superficial iliac vessels to bone. Moreover, as a free tissue transfer, the iliac crest osteocutaneous flap based on the superficial circumflex iliac vessels is less desirable, because the length and diameter of the pedicle vessels are smaller than those of the deep vessels. Thus it would seem that the only obvious indication for the use of this flap is a situation requiring an iliac osteocutaneous flap in the absence of the deep circumflex iliac vessels as a result of prior injury. The superficially based compound iliac flap might also be considered when a conventional pedicle groin flap is to be carried out in conjunction with a small iliac bone graft. Such may be the case in patients undergoing osteoplastic thumb reconstruction or in the management of certain distal forearm or wrist compound skin and bone defects. For the most part, the technique of elevation of an iliac crest compound flap based on the superficial circumflex iliac vessels is identical to that of a groin flap elevation (Smith et al 1972).

The patient is positioned supine on the operating table with a soft roll beneath the donor side buttock. The surgical field to be prepared and draped is identical to that described for the iliac crest flap based on

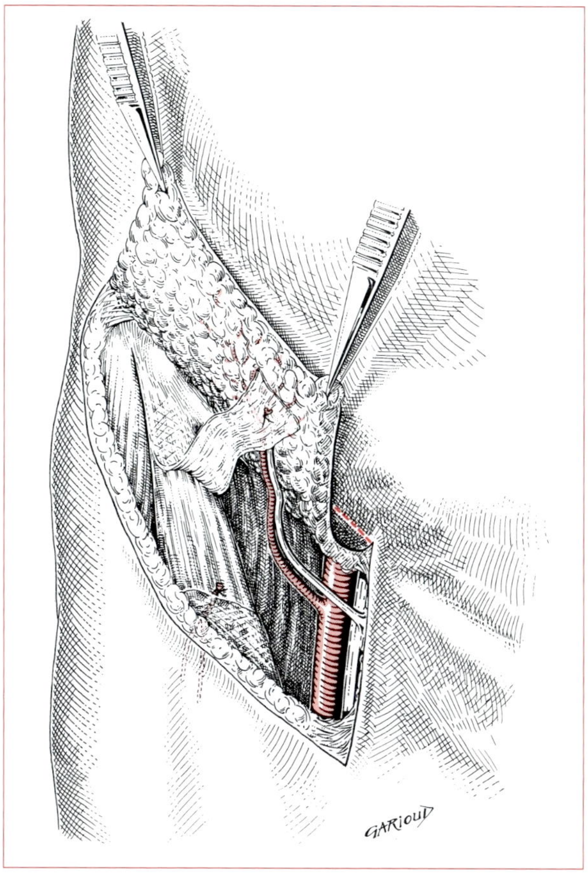

Fig. 16 *Schematic illustration of cephalad elevation of sartorius fascia during the course of groin flap elevation.*

the deep circumflex iliac vessels. The positions of the femoral artery, inguinal ligament, pubic tubercle, and anterior iliac crest are marked with a surgical pen. The central axis of the flap is designed as a line that begins medially at a point 2.5 cm distal to the inguinal ligament over the femoral artery, and then passes laterally to cross the anterior superior iliac spine (Fig. 14). A skin flap of desired dimensions is then outlined over this central axis, with its medial margin overlying or slightly lateral to the course of the femoral artery. The flap should be designed so that the lateral aspect covers the anterior iliac crest.

Once the flap margins are outlined, the actual skin incision begins along the distal margin of the flap (Fig. 15). The dissection is carried down to the fascia overlying the anterior thigh muscles. The fascia overlying the sartorius and tensor fasciae femoris (if overlying the flap dimensions) muscles is incised. Just deep to the sartorius fascia, near the anterior iliac spine, the lateral femoral cutaneous nerve may be encountered. It should be identified and protected. The dissection should then be directed in a cephalad direction along the sartorius muscle; but it must remain deep to the sartorius fascia (Fig. 16). As the medial border of the sartorius is encountered, the superficial circumflex iliac vessels can be visualized through the fascial layer lying on its medial and superficial aspect. At this point a deep branch of the superficial circumflex iliac artery may be seen piercing the fascia and entering the sartorius muscle. This branch should be ligated where it enters the muscle; but all vessels running along the undersurface of the fascia superficial to the muscle should be preserved. Following identification of the medial border of the sartorius and elevation of the sartorius fascia, the medial border of the skin flap is developed. This dissection is carried down through the subcutaneous tissue to the femoral artery and vein.

Using the previously identified superficial circumflex iliac vessels, lying medial and superficial to the sartorius fascia as a guide, dissection proceeds along the medial sartorius fascia in a cephalad direction until the origin of the superficial circumflex iliac artery is seen to arise from the anterior or lateral surface of the femoral artery. The accompanying vein(s) will be seen to terminate in the femoral vein nearby. Following identification and isolation of the superficial circumflex iliac pedicle, the remaining proximal and lateral margin of the skin flap may be incised. The lateral portion of the proximal margin dissection is carried deeply onto the aponeurosis of the external oblique muscle. Medially the flap may be elevated superficial to the external oblique fascia until the sartorius fascia is encountered. The dissection is then carried through the sartorius fascia where it joins the previously developed plane of flap elevation deep to the sartorius fascia (Fig. 17). Extreme care should be taken during this aspect of the dissection to visualize and protect the superficial circumflex iliac vascular pedicle arising from the femoral artery and vein.

Finally, the lateral aspect of the flap is elevated by carrying the dissection through external oblique and gluteal fascia. Care must be taken to avoid flap

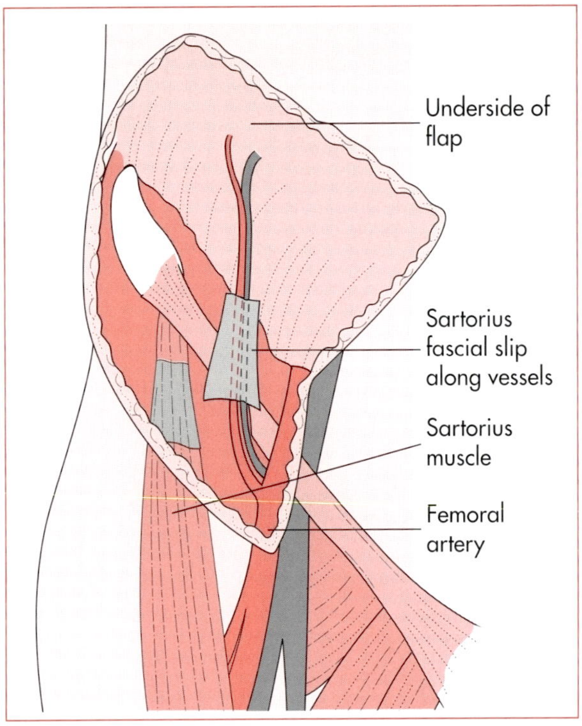

Fig. 17 *Schematic illustration of fully isolated superficial circumflex iliac vessels with an attached island of sartorius fascia.*

separation from the deep fascia where it overlies the iliac crest. The plane of dissection then proceeds deep to the muscle fascia towards the iliac crest on the proximal, distal, and lateral margins. The sartorius, abdominal wall muscles, gluteal muscles, and tensor fasciae femoris muscle are then detached extraperiosteally from the anterior iliac crest sufficiently to expose the required bone segment. The bone is then osteotomized from the lateral aspect in a similar manner to that described in the previous section. All fascia and adipose tissue lying between the skin flap and the osteotomized bone segment must be meticulously preserved in order to maintain the minute fasciocutaneous perforating vessels to the bone. If the compound flap is intended as a free tissue transfer, the origin of the superficial circumflex iliac artery from the femoral artery and the termination of the accompanying veins at the femoral vein are ligated and sectioned, thus fully freeing the flap. If the flap is to be used as a pedicle flap, the vascular pedicle should of course be preserved, with tubulation of the cutaneous base as for a standard groin flap.

Closure of the donor defect should begin with careful approximation of the conjoined external and internal oblique aponeurosis to the lateral aspect of the inguinal ligament and remaining gluteal and tensor fasciae femoris fascia. A layered subcutaneous tissue and skin closure may then be carried out in the manner of the surgeon's preference over suction drains. The postoperative management is identical to that described for the iliac crest flap based on the deep circumflex iliac vessels.

D. FIBULAR TRANSFER

The fibula is now the most common bone donor area. It was used first by Taylor in 1975 (Taylor et al 1975), but the use of a posterior approach was very rapidly abandoned. The lateral approach was described in 1976 and in detail in 1979 (Gilbert).

Choice of donor limb

The choice of the donor limb depends mostly on the recipient area. When we have to deal with a lesion of the femur or femoral neck it is usually better to take the contralateral fibula.

This is, of course, also necessary when we deal with a tibial defect, although it may be possible to use the ipsilateral fibula as a pedicle flap (see below).

Taking the right or left side does not make any difference, as the fibula is a triangular, highly cortical bone, the pedicle being on one of its faces.

Position and draping (Fig. 18)

The patient is supine, and the knee acutely bent, with a tourniquet on the proximal thigh. A small cushion under the ipsilateral buttock will allow some adduction of the thigh and a more comfortable position. The foot and knee may be fixed in this position, as it will not vary during the operation. It is then necessary before fixation to express the blood and inflate the tourniquet. In the case of some recipient areas (those in the other leg), fixation is not possible and the limb must stay free, being merely supported by an assistant. For some occasions (femoral reconstruction) the patient is in a prone position, usually on a fracture table. We then use the other leg as a donor; the knee is slightly flexed (45°) and fixed in that

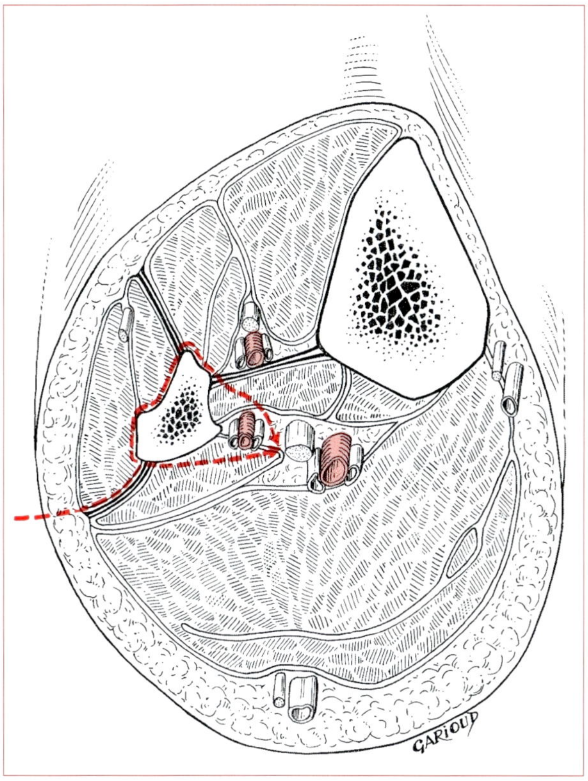

Fig. 18

(a) The approach to the fibula is lateral, including the peroneal vessels.

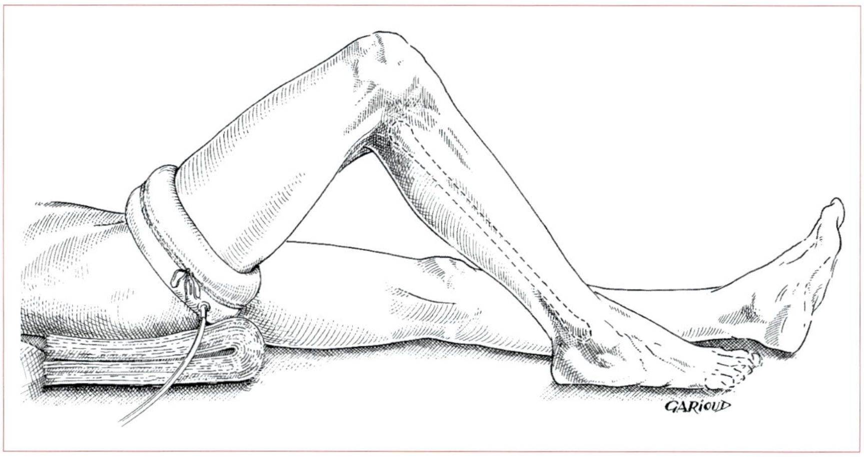

(b) The patient is lying on his back with a cushion under his buttocks.

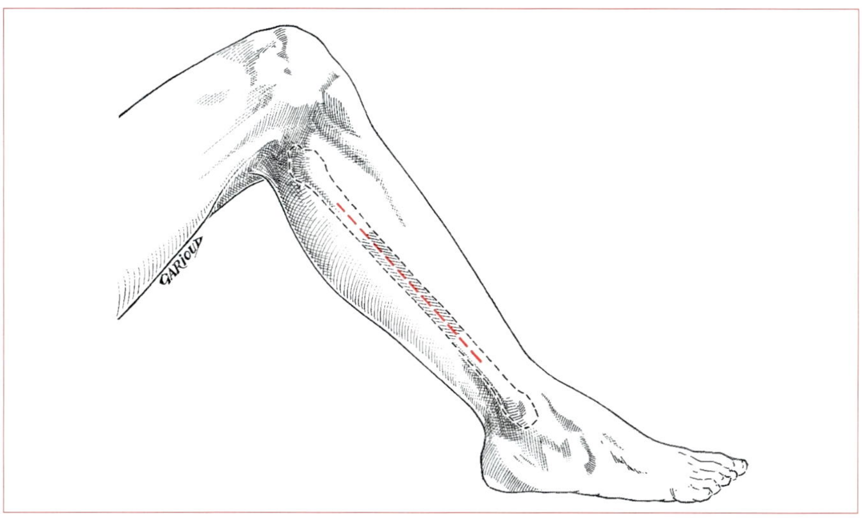

(c) The fibular graft will be taken in the middle part of the bone, where the nutrient artery is usually situated.

Fig. 18 continued

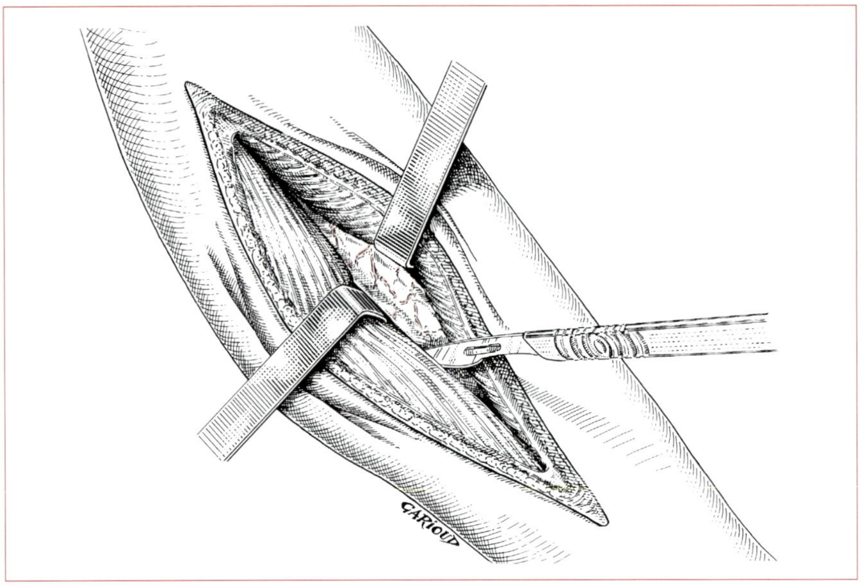

(d) *After skin incision, the soleus and peroneal muscles are separated.*

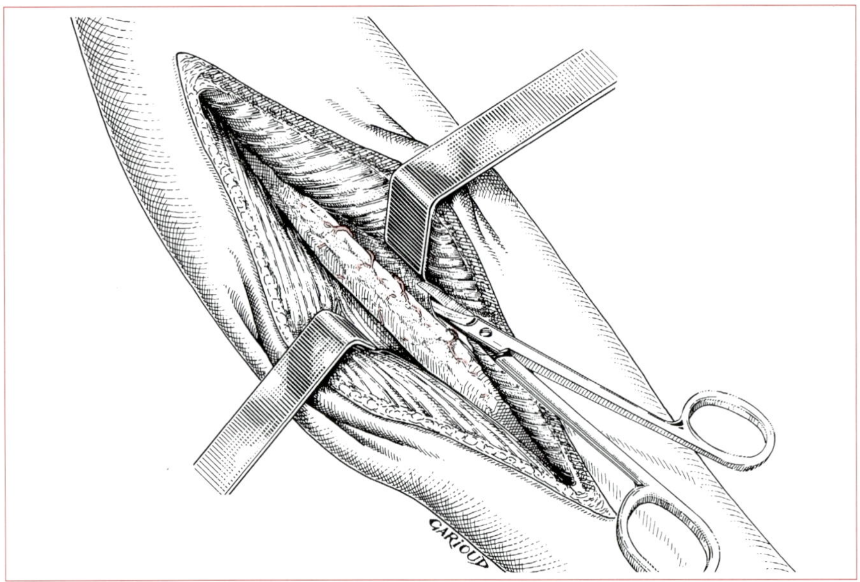

(e) *The muscles are separated from the bone, leaving the periosteal cuff.*

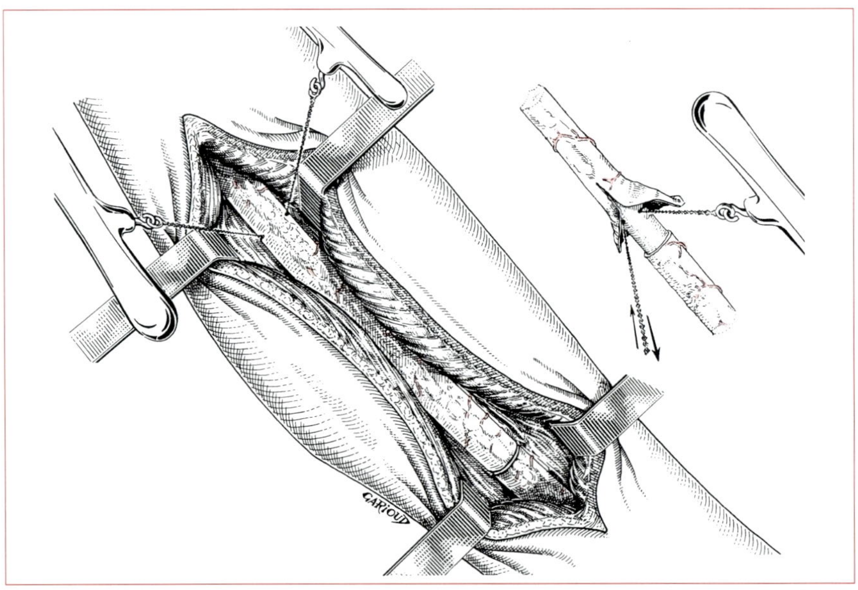

(f) *The bone is cut at each extremity with a Gigli saw. In children, care is exercised to preserve the periosteum.*

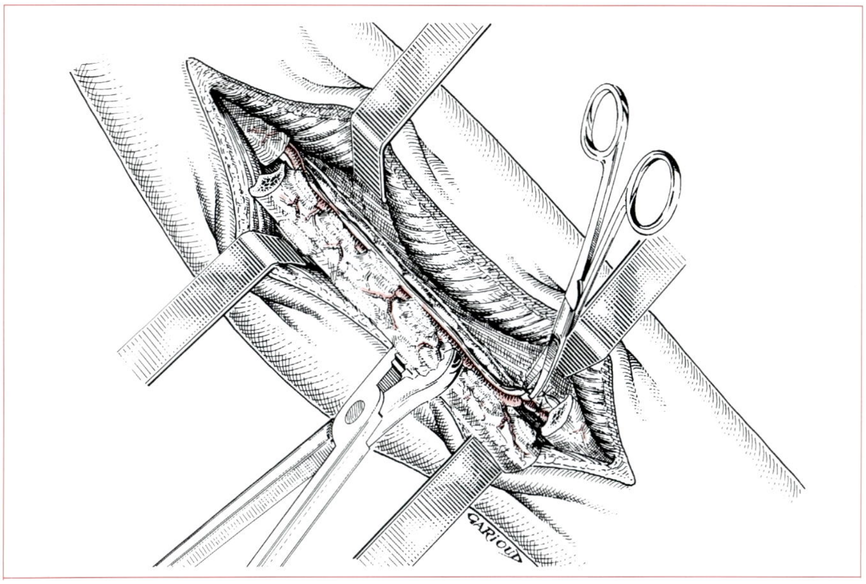

Fig. 18 continued

(g) The distal vessels are ligated and cut.

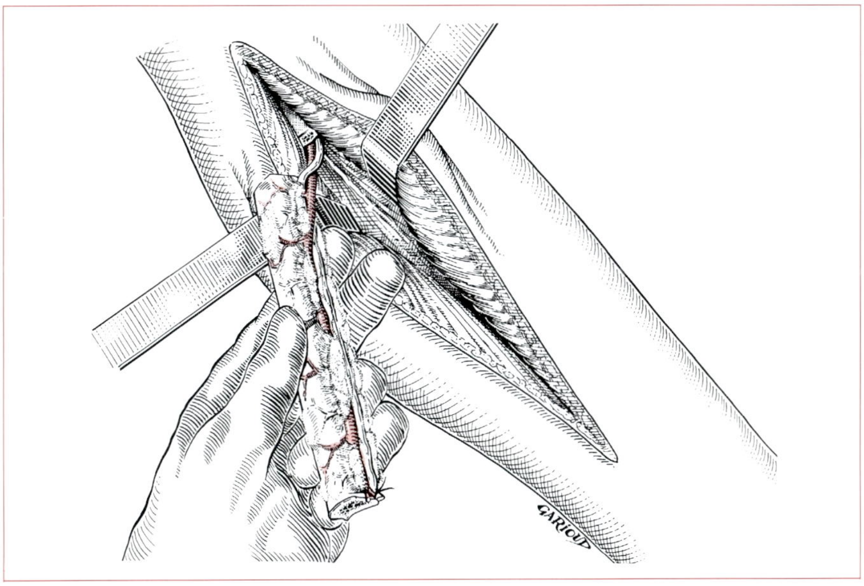

(h) The bone is isolated on its pedicle.

position. The approach will be the same, and is probably even easier in that position, as the muscles do not get in the way.

Incision (Fig. 19)

First the fibula should be outlined on the skin with a dermographic pen. The expected place of the nutrient artery should be marked at the mid-shaft. Then one must draw the approximate length of bone required, centered on the nutrient vessel. Once this is well defined, an incision is made directly over the fibula, extending 5–8 cm proximally and distally than the segment required.

The superficial fascia is opened and the peroneus longus muscle appears. It is retracted anteriorly and progressively detached from the sagittal fascia separating it from the soleus (Fig. 18d). When the peroneus longus muscle is detached and retracted, the fibula appears (Fig. 18e). The peroneus longus and brevis are then detached from the lateral aspect of the bone. It is not necessary to keep a muscle cuff on the bone, but is important to preserve the periosteum and its

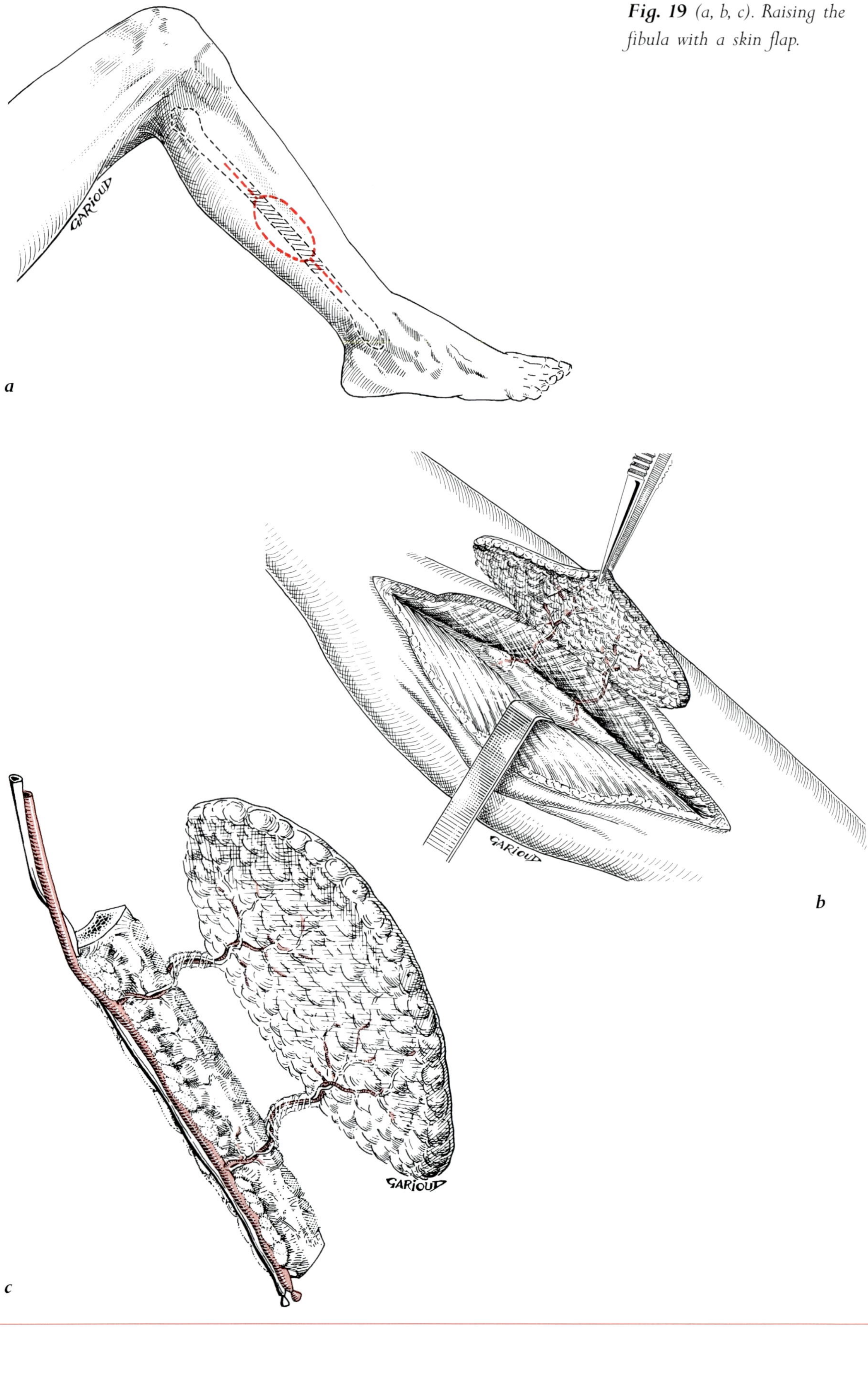

Fig. 19 *(a, b, c). Raising the fibula with a skin flap.*

circulation. The muscles are detached slowly with scissors until one comes to the strong deep fascia separating the anterior and lateral compartments. The anterior compartment is then opened and dissection proceeds, detaching more muscles: extensor digitorum longus and extensor hallucis longus. We have then reached the interosseous membrane, which should be seen for the whole of its length. Deep retractors will allow a good view of the membrane without any risks for the anterior tibial pedicle. The membrane is opened and cut with large scissors.

The dissection returns to the posterolateral part of the fibula. The flexor hallucis longus is slowly and carefully retracted. The peroneal pedicle lies just behind it, and it is better to preserve 5–8 mm of muscle around the pedicle to avoid damage. Once the posterior aspect of the peroneal vessels has been exposed the first part of the dissection is finished.

The bone graft is sectioned to the defined length. The best instrument to cut the bone is the Gigli saw, which can be passed around the shaft with a special curved instrument. It is not dangerous and allows good control (Fig. 18f).

When the bone is cut on both sides, it can be mobilized with a bone holder. The distal part is then retracted laterally, bringing with it the peroneal vessels. The distal pedicle is ligated using vessel clips, and the dissection proceeds gently from distal to proximal, coagulating the small branches and using clips for the larger (Fig. 18g). When we come to the upper third of the fibula, there is usually a very large branch of the peroneal artery going to the lateral soleus. This branch is ligated. The dissection proceeds up to the tibioperoneal division, and should be very cautious, as the posterior tibial nerve and very large veins are adjacent. Once the pedicle is completely dissected, the bone is free. Hemostasis must be very precise, as hematoma is a real danger after such a dissection. The tourniquet is released and bone circulation is checked (Fig. 18h). We should have not only a good periosteal bleeding but also a consistent bleeding from the medulla. It is then time to cut the pedicle, dip it into heparinized saline, and transfer it to the recipient area.

Closure

Skin is closed directly. We should not try to close the fascia. A suction drain is used. Compressive bandaging avoids hematoma.

Postoperative care

This depends mostly on the recipient area. If it is an upper limb reconstruction, the patient is allowed to stand and begin walking at 2 days. The donor area is not very painful, and there are no particular risks in early movement.

Variations

Osteocutaneous flap (Figs. 20–26)

The lateral aspect of the leg is partly vascularized by the perforating branches of the peroneal artery (see above).

It may be of use to employ a cutaneous flap for closure of a small defect or for monitoring the circulation.

At times the fasciocutaneous perforators may be detected with a Doppler and marked. The flap is usually situated in the inferior third of the leg and should be narrow, as closure may otherwise be a problem.

The anterior margin of the flap is dissected first, and then the fascia over the peroneus longus is opened. The perforators are situated between the peroneus longus and the soleus. Most often they are inside the fascia or on the soleus side of the fascia. They can be completely dissected out, but they are long and thin and there is a risk of rupture, so they can also be taken with a part of the fascia to protect them. Once they are dissected, the posterior margin of the flap is dissected. The vessels are, of course, carefully followed towards the peroneal vessels (Fig. 20).

Musculocutaneous flap (Fig. 21)

The use of this flap was proposed by Baudet (1981). The main branch of the peroneal artery is the artery to the lateral soleus.

This muscle can easily be taken, either completely or in part, with this pedicle.

The dissection is not difficult. There is, however, a high risk of hematoma after partial resection of the muscle (Fig. 22).

Osteotomies of the fibula

For some indications (mandible reconstruction, double-barrel fibula), the bone needs to be osteotomized. This is possible, but we are then relying completely on the periosteal vascularization. The osteotomy should be subperiosteal, and the periosteum itself should be protected with care (Figs. 23, 24).

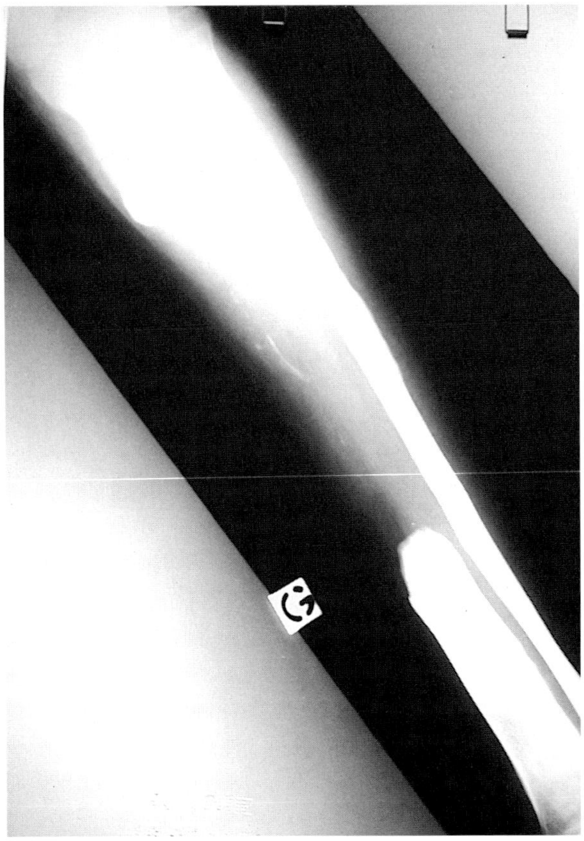

a

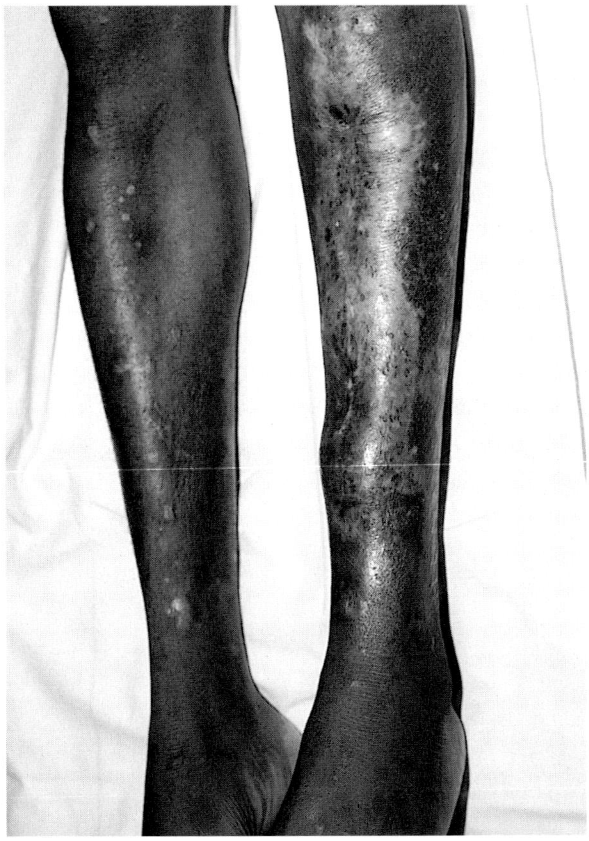

b

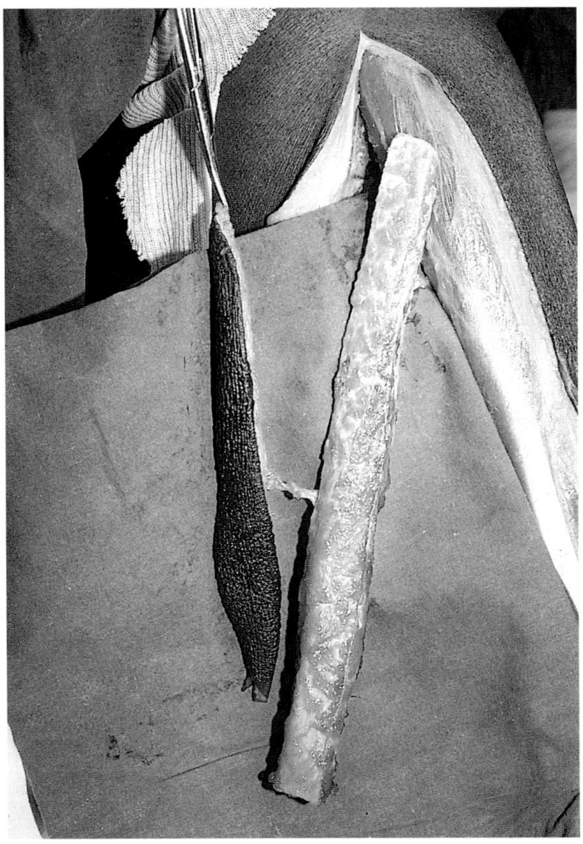

c

Fig. 20 *Osteocutaneous flap.*

(a,b) A 25-year-old patient with osteitis. The bone defect is 16 cm long and the anterior skin is in poor condition.

(c) Harvesting a fibula with the skin flap.

(d) Vascular suture.

(e) The skin flap is in place.

(f,g) Result at 2 years.

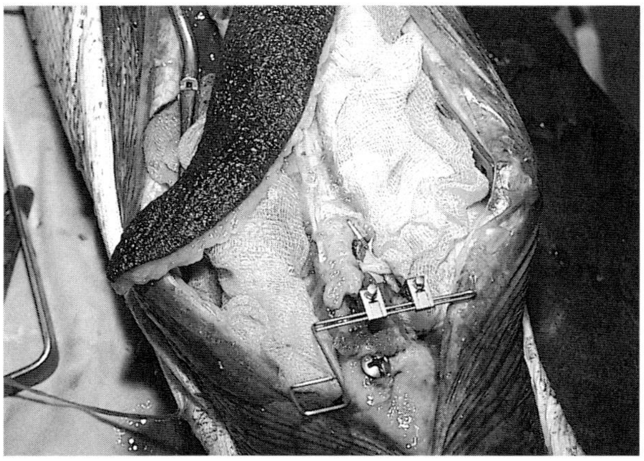

d

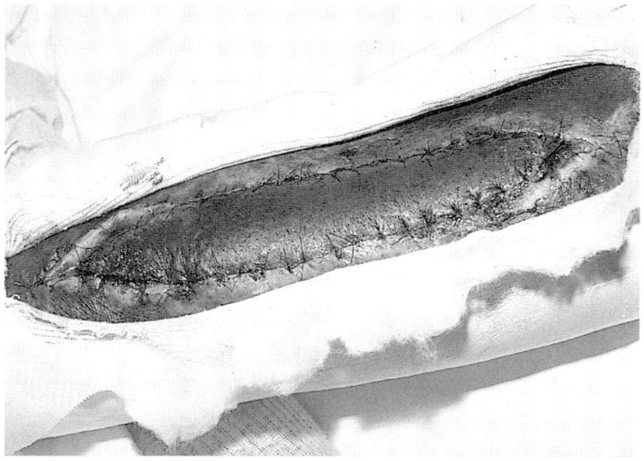

e

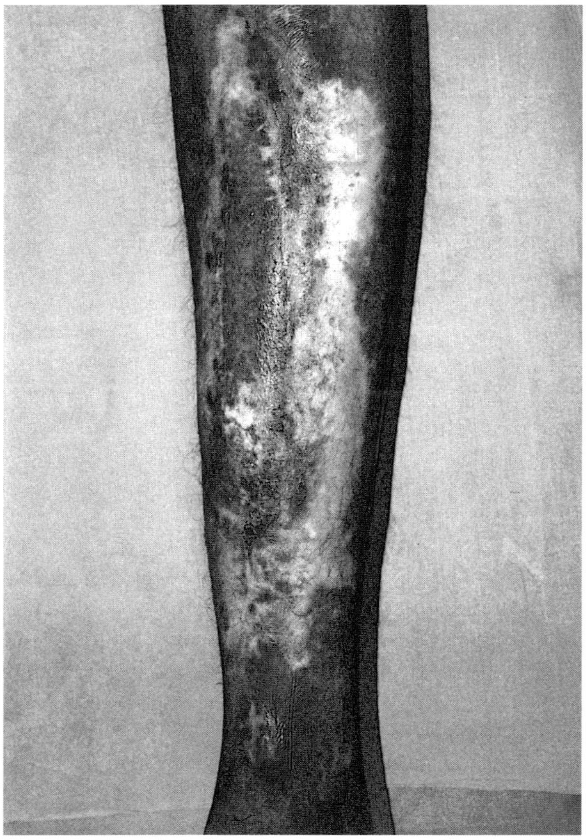

f

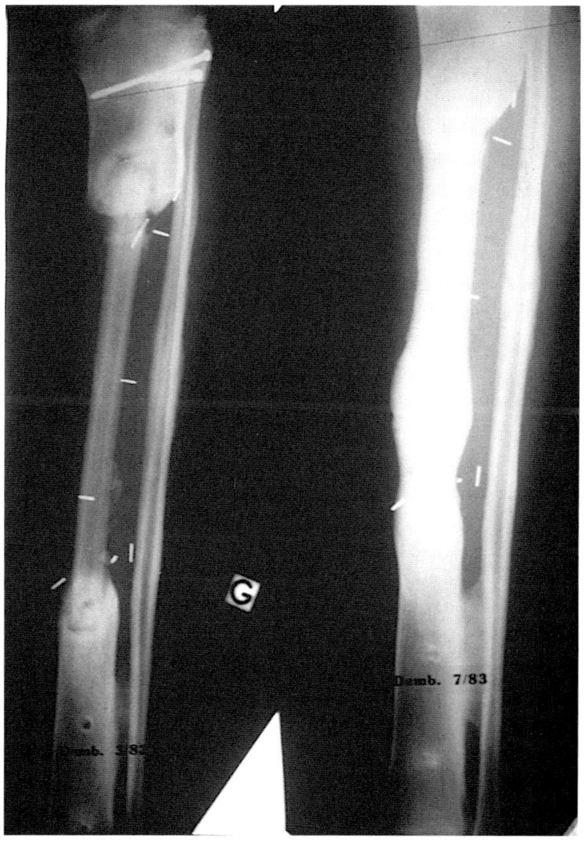

g

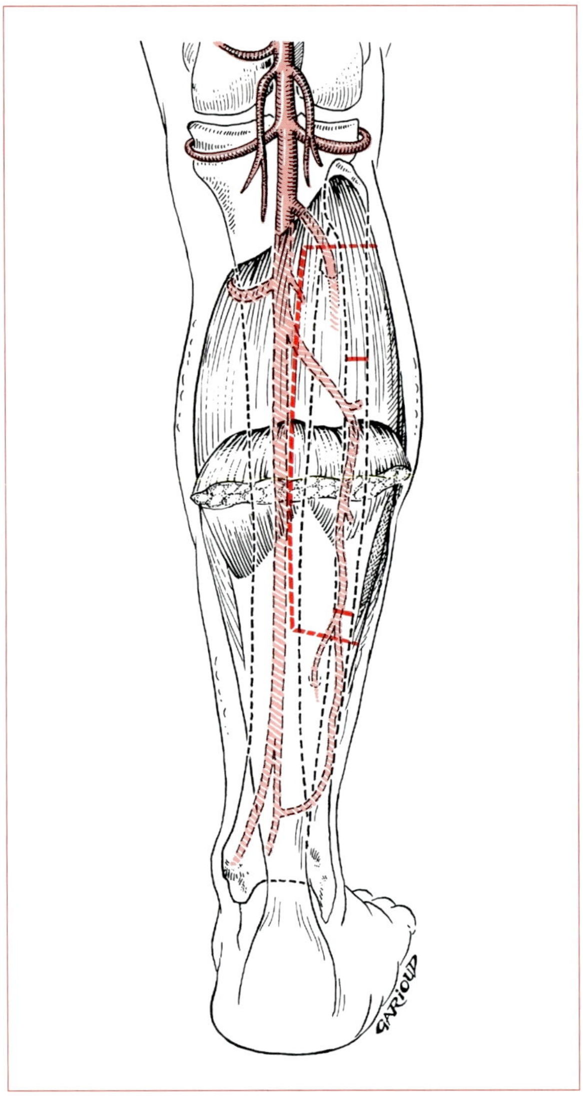

a

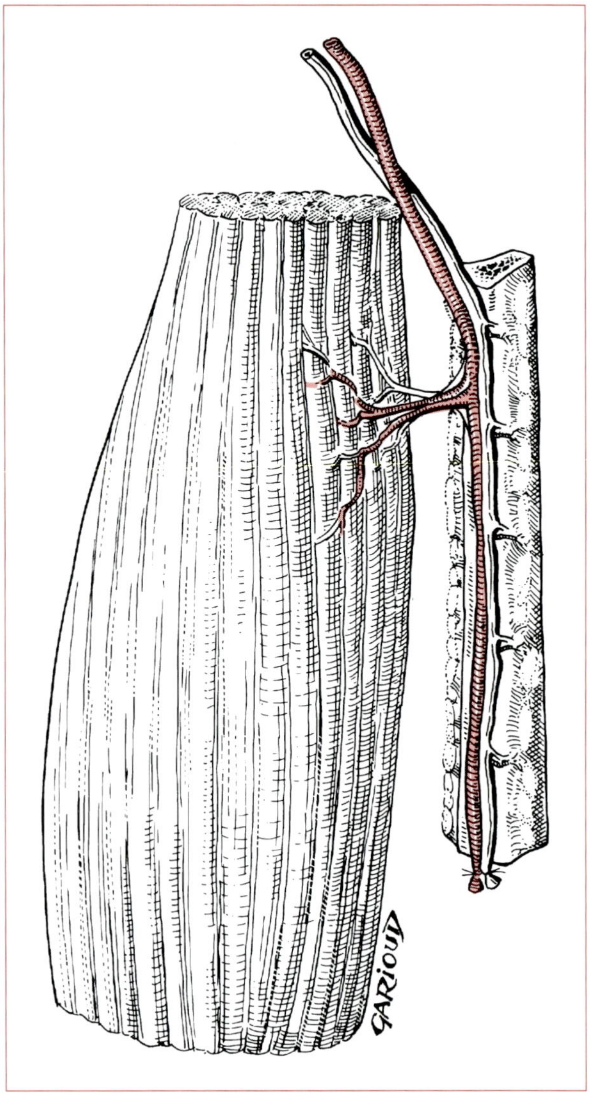

b

Fig. 21 *(a,b). The fibular and soleus flap.*

Fig. 22

(a) Long-standing infected bone defect of the left tibia
(b) Raising of the flap
(c) The large piece of soleus attached to the fibula
(d) Insetting of the flap
(e) Postoperative radiograph
(f,g) Result at 3 years
(f) Good coverage
(g) Healing.

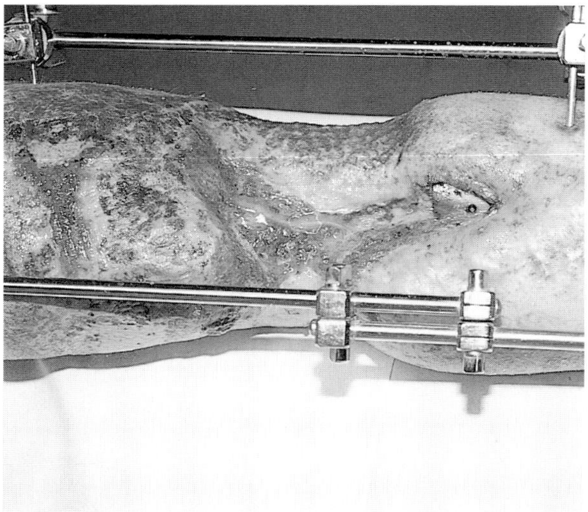

a

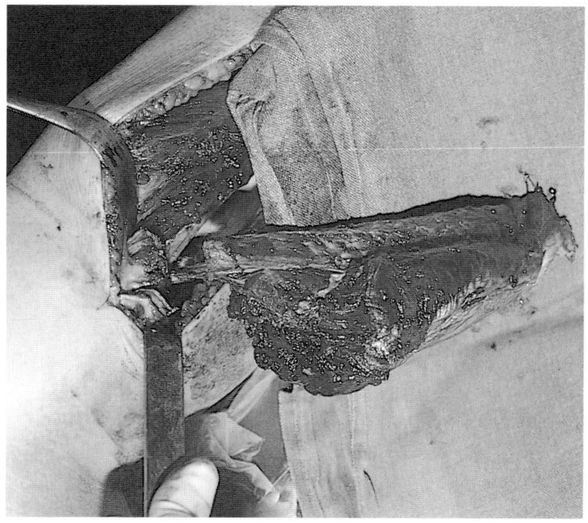

b

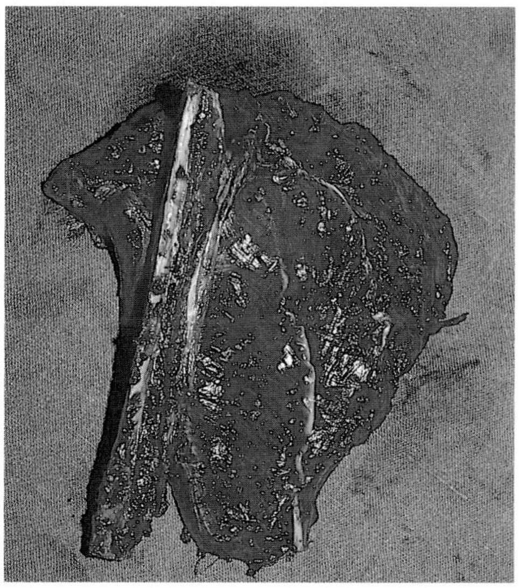

c

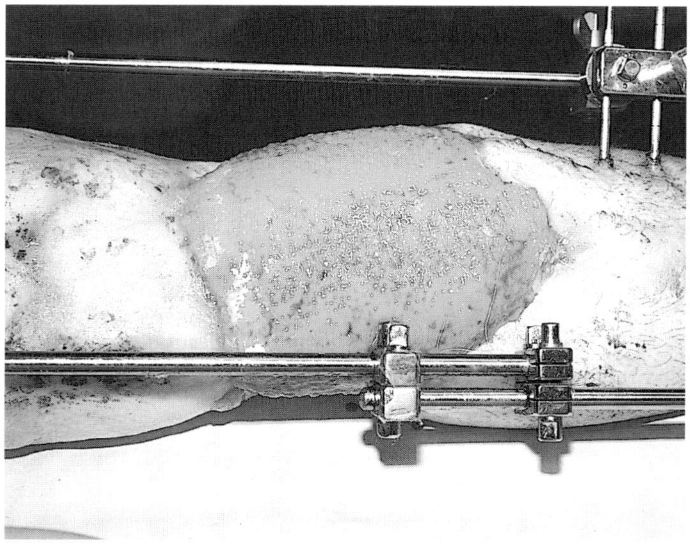

d

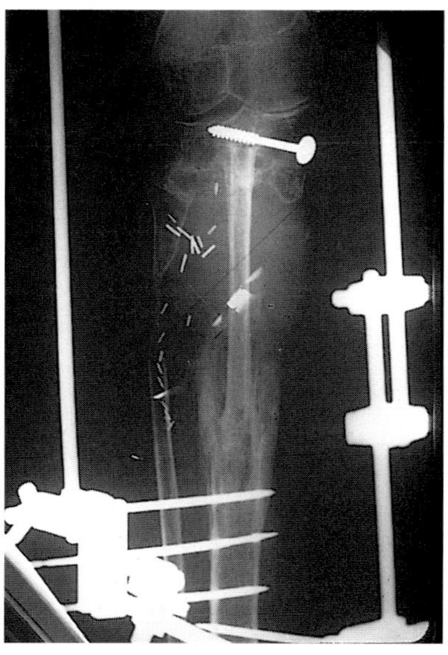

e

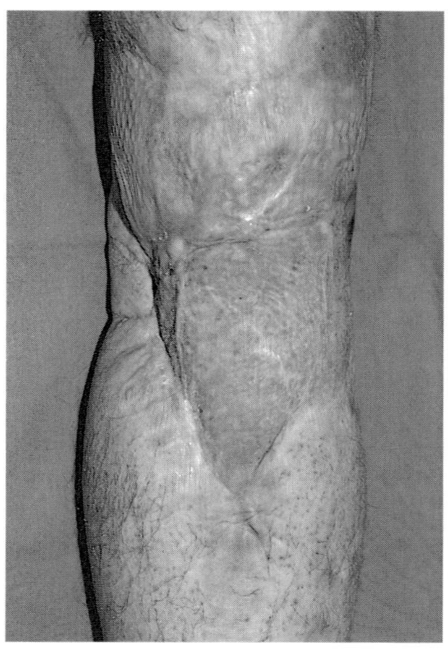

f

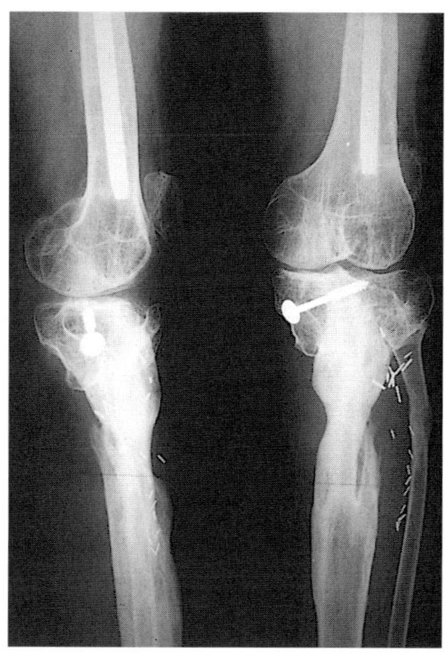

g

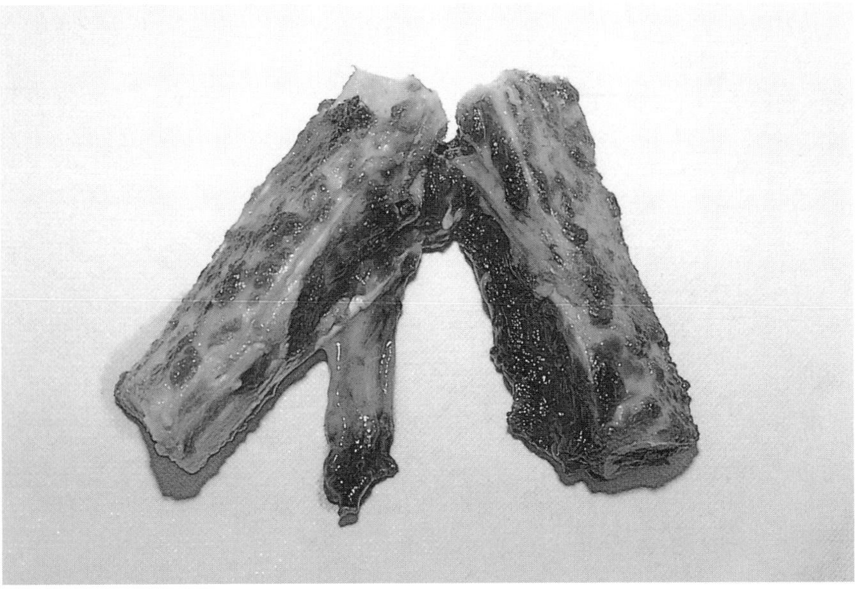

Fig. 23 *The fibula can be osteotomized if care is taken to protect the pedicle.*

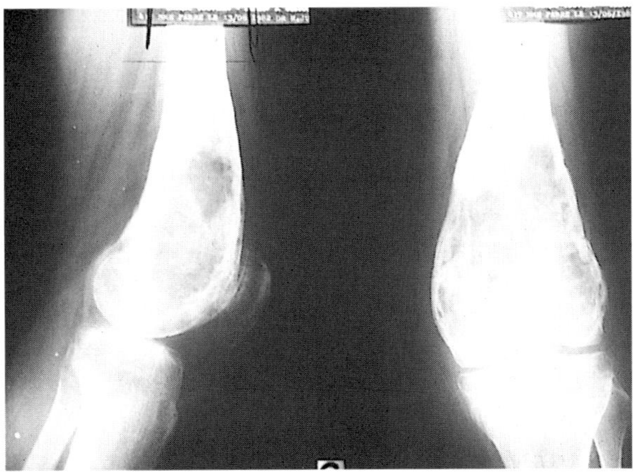

a

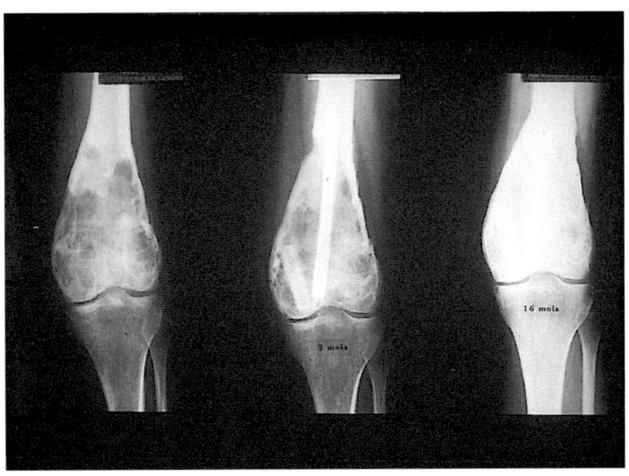

c

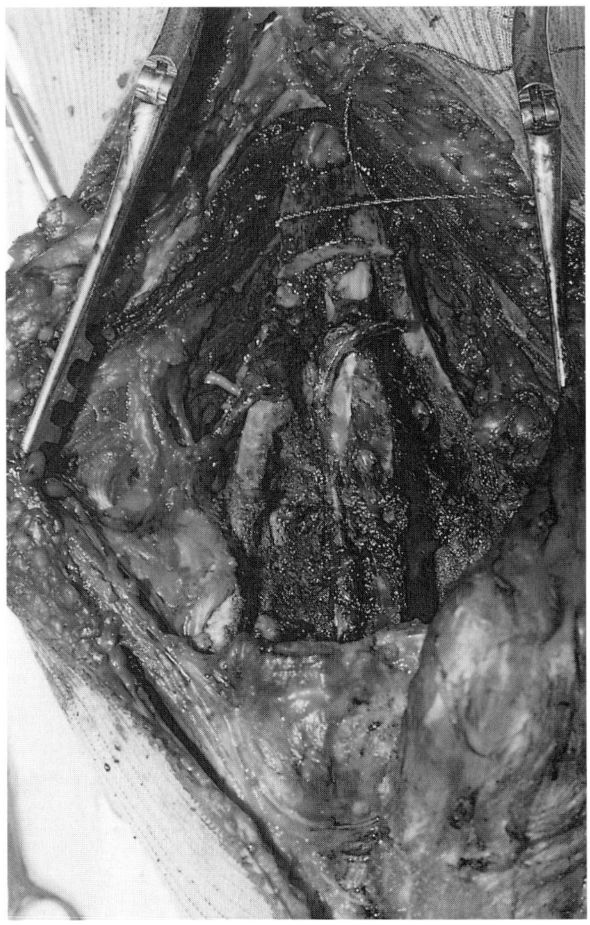

b

Fig. 24
(a) Giant cell tumor of the left femur
(b) Excision and filling with a 'double-barrel' fibula
(c) Progressive healing in 18 months.

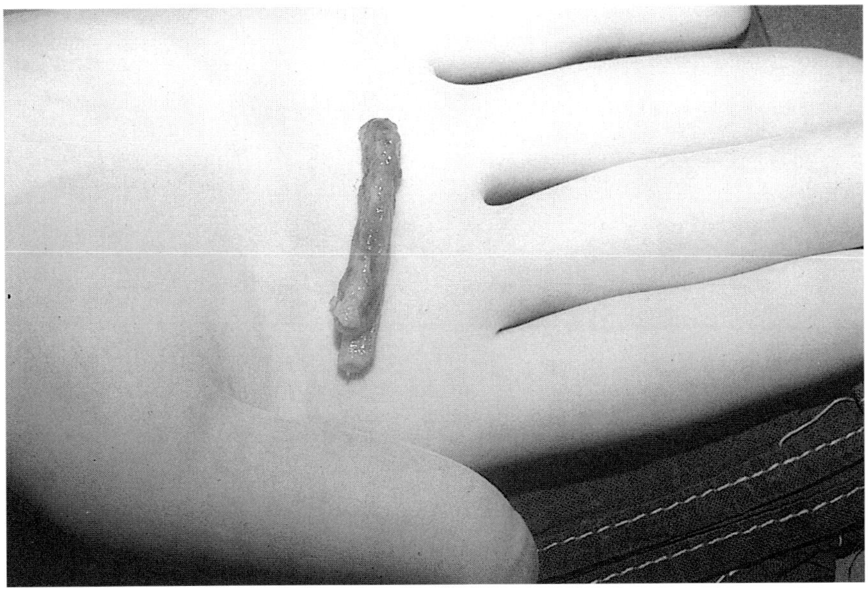

Fig. 25 *The fibula can be raised even in small children.*

Pedicle flap

The fibula can be used as a pedicle flap on the ipsilateral tibia. The dissection is identical, but, contrary to what one might expect, moving the fibula to the tibia is not easy. Crossing the interosseous membrane is tedious, and dangerous for the posterior tibial vessels and nerve and for the fibular pedicle itself. It also completely destabilizes the leg, as compared to an intact fibula.

There may be some rare indications for direct pedicle transfer of the fibula, but they should be weighed carefully against the difficulties of the procedure.

The fibula may be used as a reversed pedicle flap to reconstruct the lateral malleolus of the ankle. It is then the proximal artery and vein that are cut, and the dissection proceeds distally to the division of the peroneal artery. To lengthen the pedicle, it may be necessary to sacrifice one of the branches.

Fibular transfer in children (Fig. 25)

The main indication in children is for the treatment of congenital pseudarthrosis. It is then necessary to operate on these children very young.

Raising the fibula offers few differences from the technique described above. The only difference is the use of the periosteum sleeve. In young children, the periosteum is very thick and active. It is therefore a bonus to use a periosteal sleeve at the level of the bone extremities. On each side, the periosteum is cut 1.5 cm longer than the bone graft, and retracted in order to cut the bone. We then have on each extremity a periosteal flap that can be sutured over the recipient bone and will induce better healing.

The main difference with children is the problem of reconstruction of the donor fibula. Experience has shown that in a young child (under 9 years), absence of reconstruction of the fibula, or even pseudarthrosis, may induce a severe valgus deformity of the ankle on the donor side (see Chapter 16: Complications). It is then necessary to reconstruct the fibula after harvesting. Although several authors have used different types of synostosis (with screw or graft), we believe that the best method is reconstruction of the shaft.

An incision is made over the medial cortex of the tibia. A corticoperiosteal free graft will be taken to fill the defect. The periosteal flap is 2 cm longer than the defect, but the cortical graft is cut to the exact length. It is cut with a rotating saw.

A long Kirschner No. 18 wire is placed into the medulla of the remaining extremities of the fibula. The graft is applied in the defect. The periosteum is sutured, and the cortical graft sutured to the Kirschner wire with resorbable sutures. A non-weightbearing plaster is applied to the leg and thigh for 6 weeks, and then discarded.

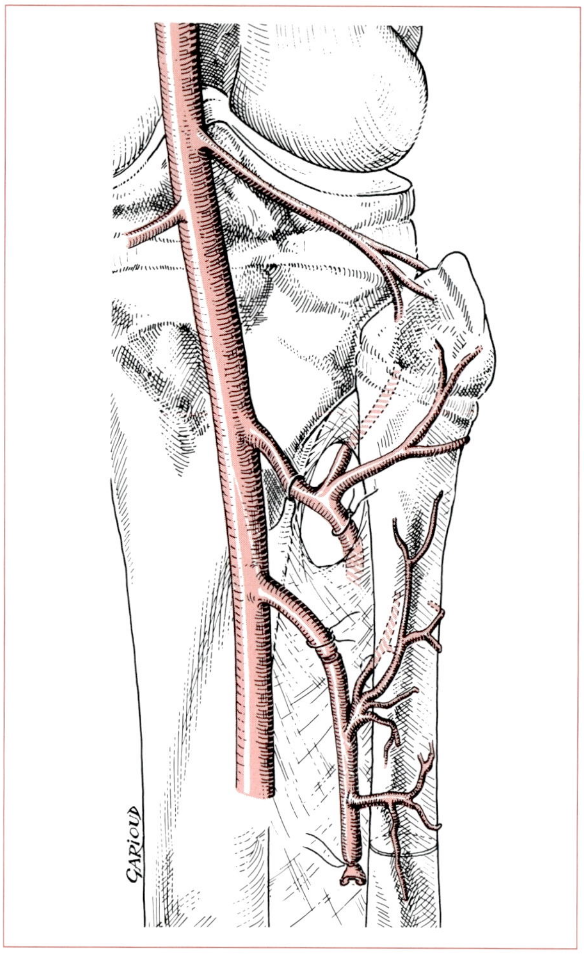

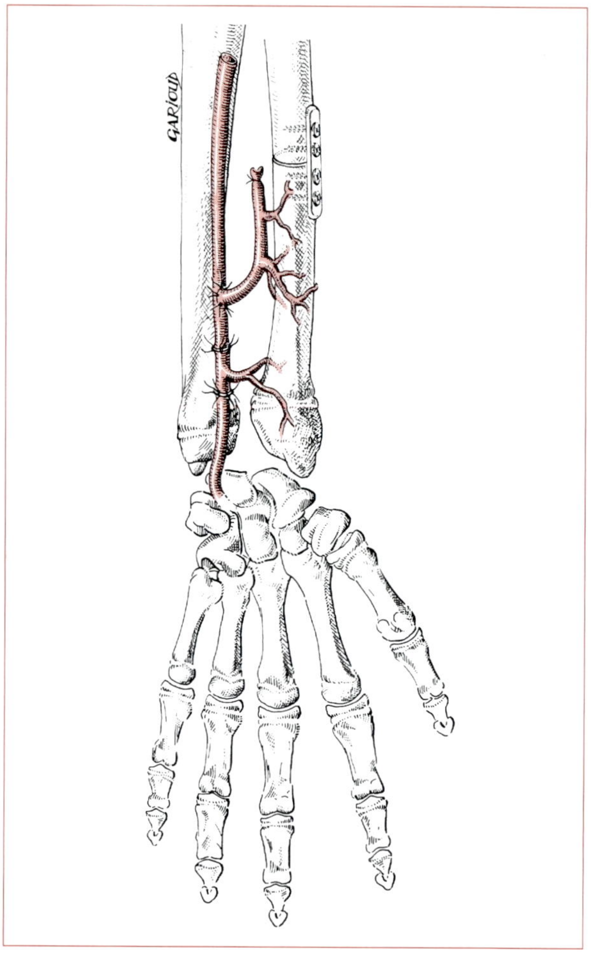

Fig. 26

(a) The epiphysis is vascularized by 3 nutrient systems. A piece of anterior tibial artery and the peroneal artery are dissected.

(b) The peroneal artery is sutured to the anterior tibial artery, which is used as a unique pedicle.

Transfer of the fibular epiphysis

As illustrated in Figs. 26a and 27, the vascularization of the epiphysis can be assured by branches of the anterior tibial artery. If in addition to the epiphysis we want to harvest a part of the diaphysis, it will be necessary to include the peroneal artery.

Dissection is long and tedious at the level of the fibular neck. The first and most important danger is to the lateral popliteal nerve, which must be protected. Then the dissection goes to the anterior tibial artery. Once the branches can be seen arising from this artery, they are too small to be anastomosed, and a piece 8–10 mm long of the artery is resected. The two extremities of the anterior tibial artery are anastomosed. If the peroneal artery has been taken, its proximal end is sutured to the portion of anterior tibial artery, so as to continue functioning with a single pedicle.

In reconstructing the donor area, care must be exercised not to provoke knee instability, and the lateral ligaments should be carefully repaired.

Anatomical basis

The peroneal artery is a branch of the peroneotibial trunk, arising 3–4 cm distal to the origin of the anterior tibial artery. It is almost constant; in a series of 100 cadaver dissections it was always present, and in a clinical series of over 300 transfers, the peroneal artery was absent in one case. It descends behind the tibialis posterior muscle, reaches the fibula, and runs parallel to the fibular diaphysis, lying between the tibialis posterior and the flexor hallucis longus muscles.

At the lower end of the fibula it divides into an anterior branch, communicating with the anterior tibial artery and a posterior branch, anastomosing with the posterior tibial artery.

The external diameter at the origin is 1.5–2.2 mm. It is accompanied by two venae comitantes, which are large vessels (2.5–4.0 mm).

Blood supply of the fibula

The blood supply comes from the periosteal vascularization and the nutrient artery (Figs. 27 and 28).

Periosteal vascularization

The supply comes from several direct branches of the peroneal artery and some musculoperiosteal branches.

These segmental branches are more numerous in the middle part of the bone, and number eight to nine over the length of the diaphysis.

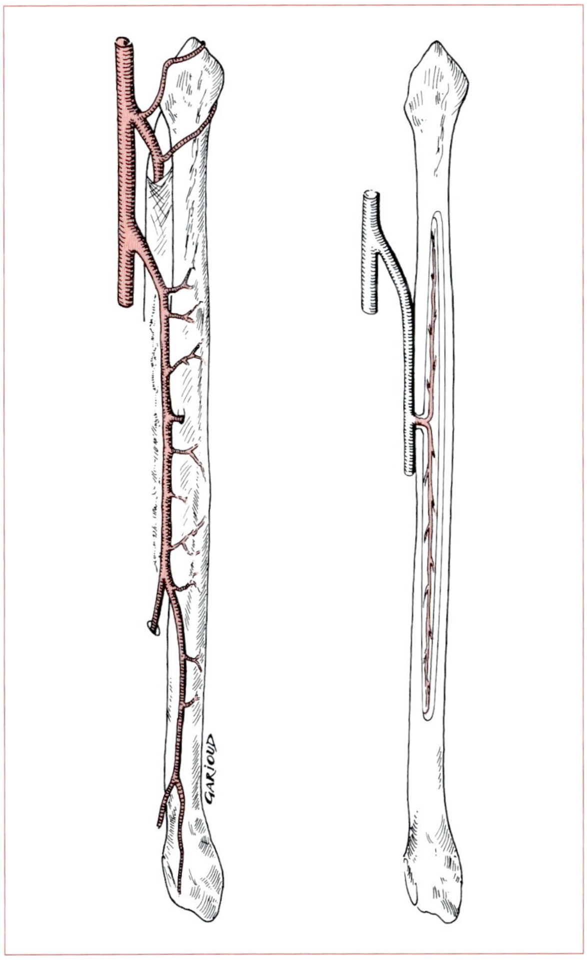

Fig. 27 *The fibula is vascularized partly by branches of the anterior tibial artery, but mainly by the peroneal artery. The nutrient artery enters the bone at mid-shaft, and develops into an ascending and a descending branch.*

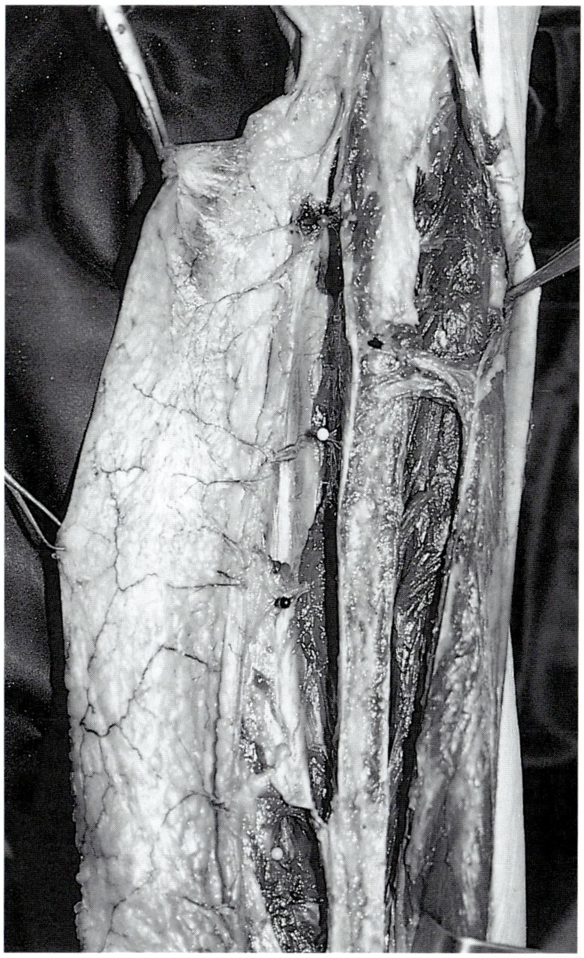

Fig. 28 *The injection shows the relations of the vessels, the bone, and the skin branches.*

There are enough direct periosteal branches to preserve the vascularization without keeping a muscle cuff around the bone.

On the anterior part of the fibula, some of these branches arise from the anterior tibial artery. In the lower part of the fibula some branches come from the anterior division of the peroneal artery.

The posterior tibial artery supplies a few branches to the medial surface.

The nutrient artery

The nutrient artery is the main source of vascularization of the bone. It always originates from the peroneal artery at between 6 and 14 cm from its origin. It can be a direct branch or a division of a musculoperiosteal artery.

The length of this nutrient artery is an average of 12 mm, with a diameter of 0.25–1.0 mm. It is usually unique, but in rare cases there may be two arteries (1%).

In 4% of subjects no nutrient foramen can be found.

The perforation occurs at mid-diaphysis, with a variation of 2.5 cm on either side. It is always on the posterior side of the fibula, close to the medial edge.

In the medullary canal, the artery divides into a short ascending branch and a long descending branch.

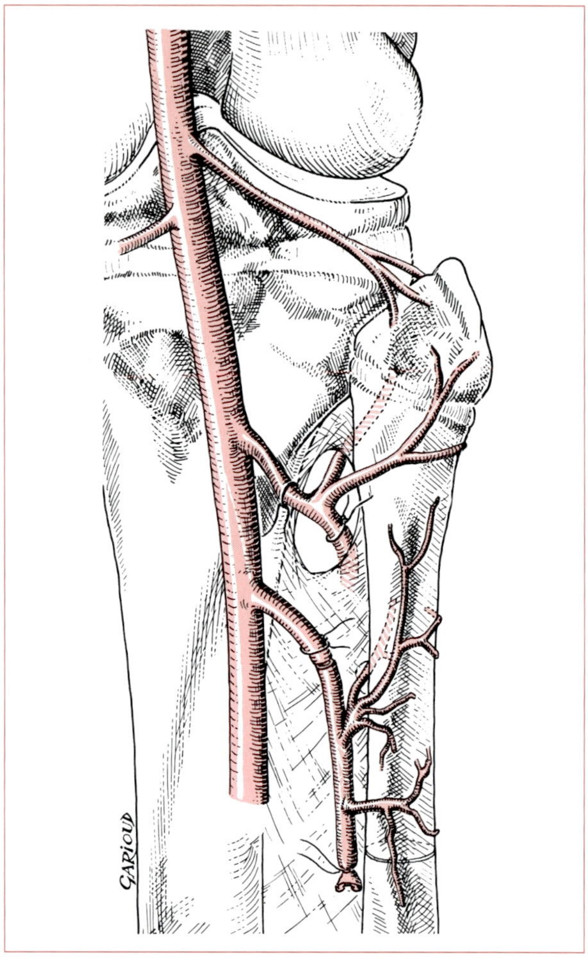

Fig. 29 *The vascularization of the upper fibular epiphysis is complex, with three vascular trees.*

The fibular proximal epiphysis

The proximal epiphysis is of much importance in attempts at growth plate transplantation. It has a complex vascularization (Fig. 29), which may explain the frequent failures to grow despite good apparent vascularity.

The proximal epiphysis is vascularized by two main systems.

The lateral inferior genicular artery

The lateral inferior genicular artery branches off the popliteal artery and courses towards the fibular head. It mostly supplies branches to the capsule that do not penetrate the bone, with some small anastomoses to the anterior recurrent tibial artery.

The anterior tibial artery

The anterior tibial artery (ATA) vascularizes the epiphysis with an anterior and a posterior network.

- *The posterior branch* (artery of the neck or posterior recurrent peroneal artery) branches usually from the origin of the ATA, but sometimes from the popliteal artery or the peroneotibial trunk.
- *The anterior branch* (anterior recurrent peroneal artery) is a constant and large vessel. It arises from the ATA after it has crossed the interosseous membrane. There are several anastomoses between the anterior and posterior systems, and with the lateral inferior genicular artery and the ascending branches of the peroneal artery.

Skin and soleus vascularization

The cutaneous branches

The peroneal artery vascularizes the lateral skin of the leg through five to eight direct fasciocutaneous branches.

The main branches are situated at the middle and inferior third of the fibula. They run inside or just posterior to the posterior intermuscular septum, and, when they reach the skin, anastomose between themselves.

There are also several (four to six) musculocutaneous branches, passing through the soleus muscle and reaching the skin close to the intermuscular septum.

The soleus branches

The lateral soleus is vascularized by one proximal main branch from the peroneal artery, another large branch at mid-leg, and several distal small branches. The entire muscle or a large piece of muscle can be vascularized by one single proximal pedicle.

Usually the main proximal artery branches from the peroneal artery immediately after the peroneotibial division, and before the peroneal artery reaches the fibula.

E. UPPER TIBIAL CORTICOPERIOSTEAL FLAP

This flap is small and purely cortical, and the chief indications for reconstruction of very small defects (Figs. 30–33).

Positioning

The patient is supine, with a tourniquet and an elevated buttock, allowing for internal rotation.

Incision

The incision is vertical, straight, and 15–20 cm long on the anterolateral part of the tibia. It starts 4 cm above the knee space and is centered on Gerdy's tubercle. The incision is made into the superficial fascia between tibialis anterior and extensor digitorum longus, and the proximal insertion of the two muscles are detached from the bone.

The recurrent anterior tibial artery and the two proximal nerve branches to the tibialis anterior are separated.

The anterior tibial vascular bundle is dissected over 7–10 cm up to the last musculoperiosteal branch to the tibialis anterior. The nerve is separated from the artery.

The corticoperiosteal flap is then designed on the cortex of the tibia. A flap up to 10 cm long can be harvested. The borders of the cortical flap are incised with an oscillating saw of small size, taking great care to avoid injury to the pedicle. The flap is then isolated on its vascular pedicle. If it is to be used as a free flap, the anterior tibial artery is ligated distal to the flap. After raising the flap, the proximal muscle insertions are used to cover the donor area and the area is closed over a drain.

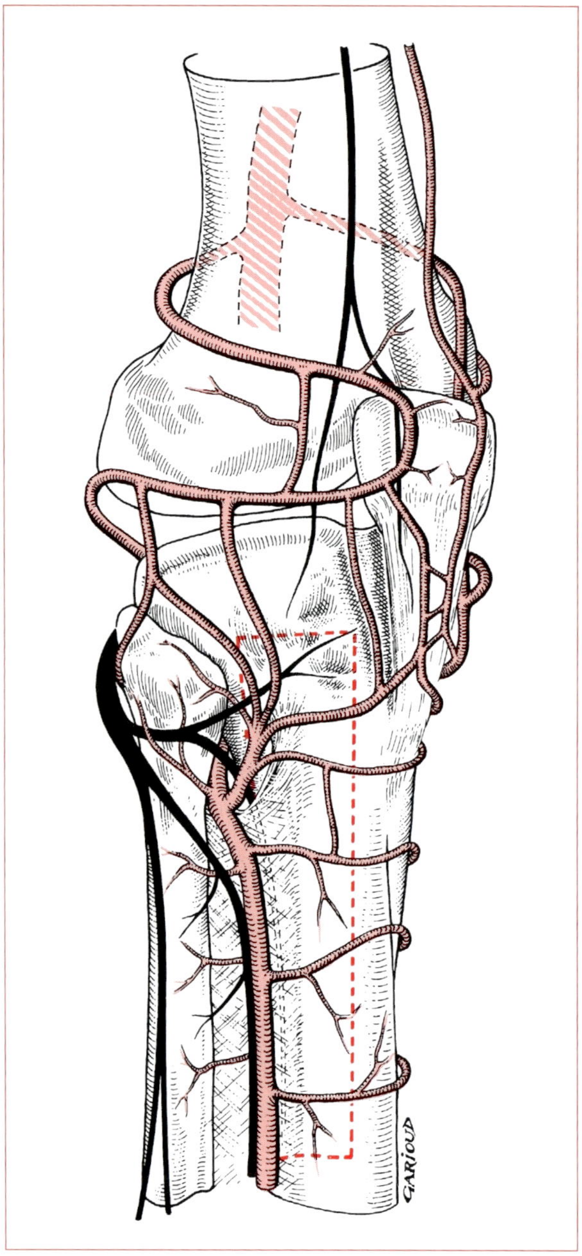

a

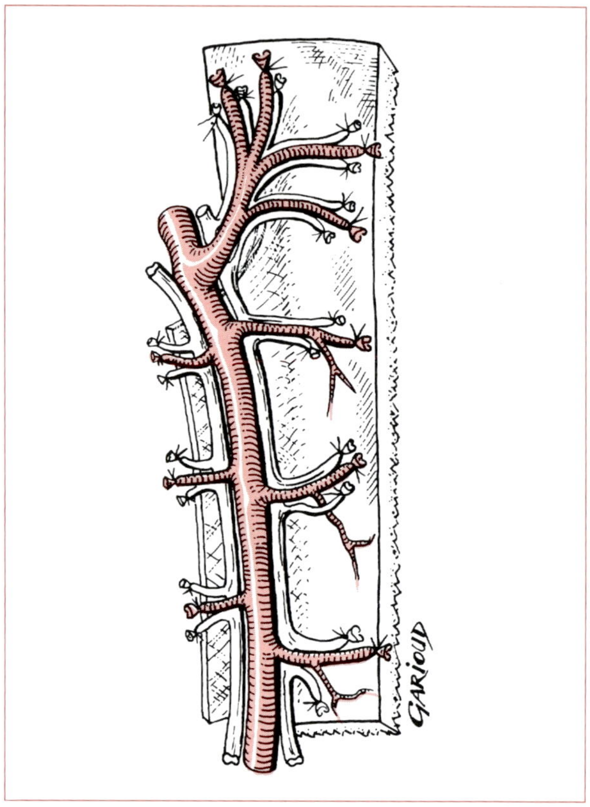

b

Fig. 30 *(a) The corticoperiosteal flap is vascularized by the branches of the anterior tibial artery. (b) A 10.0 × 3.5 cm flap can be designed and elevated.*

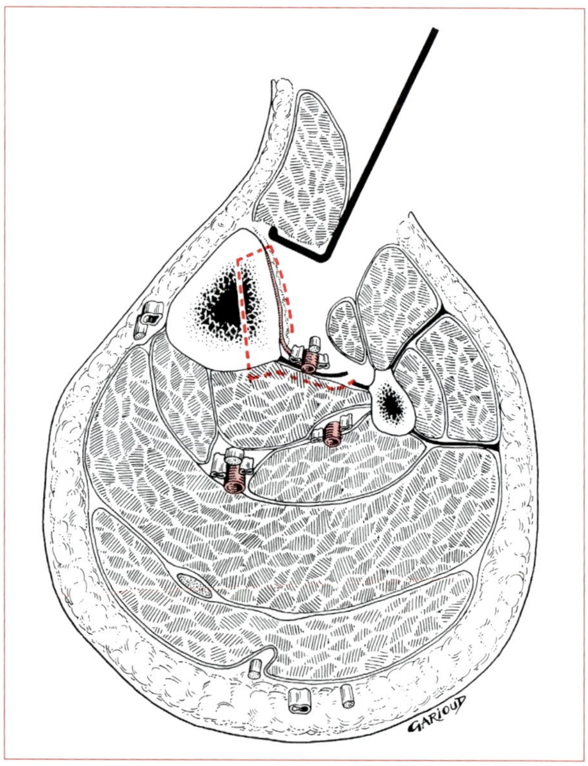

Fig. 31 *The approach is anterior, lifting the anterior tibial muscle. The lateral cortex will be raised.*

Fig. 32 *Clinical case.*
(a) Patient 26 years old. Open wrist fracture. Multioperated, infected. Two failed attempts to fuse the wrist.
(b) Raising a vascularized tibial bone graft
(c) The bone graft in place
(d) Healing at 7 months. No infection.

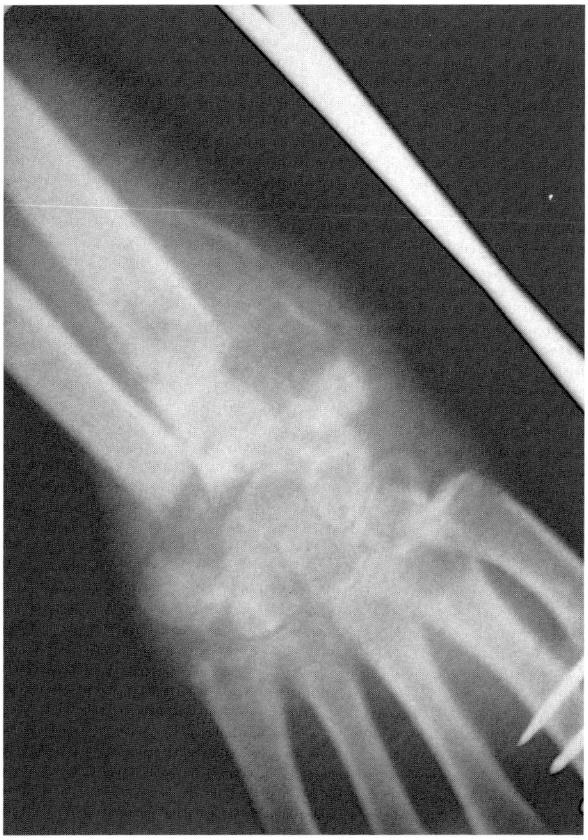

a

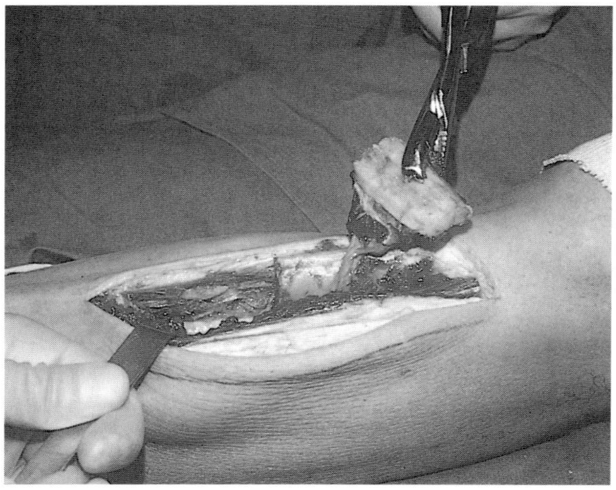

b

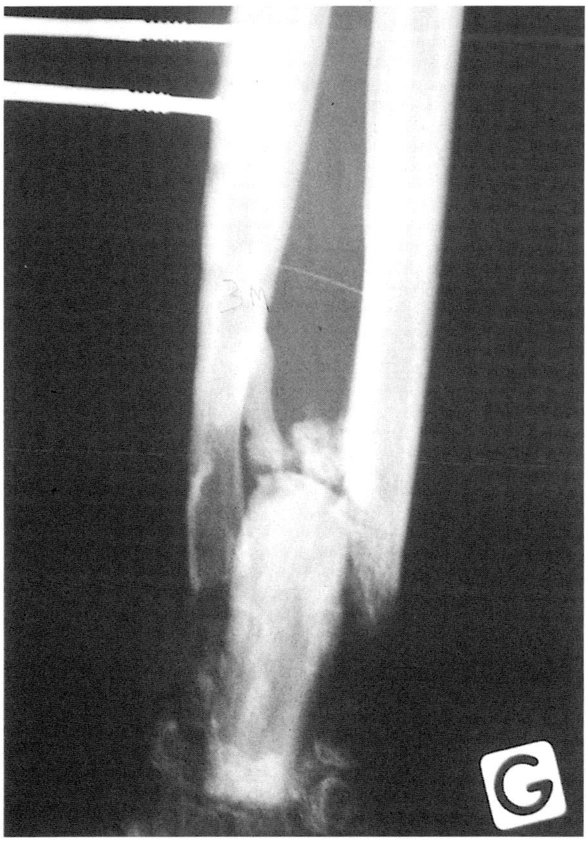

c

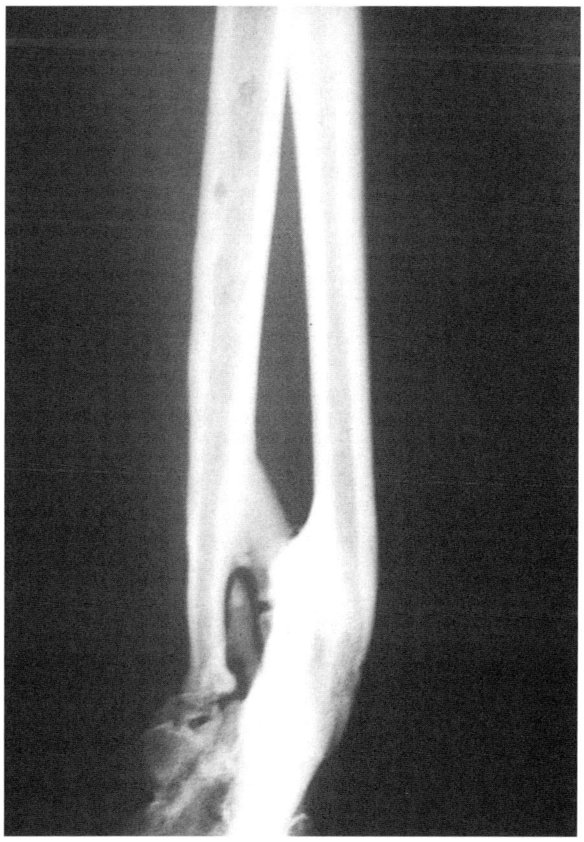

d

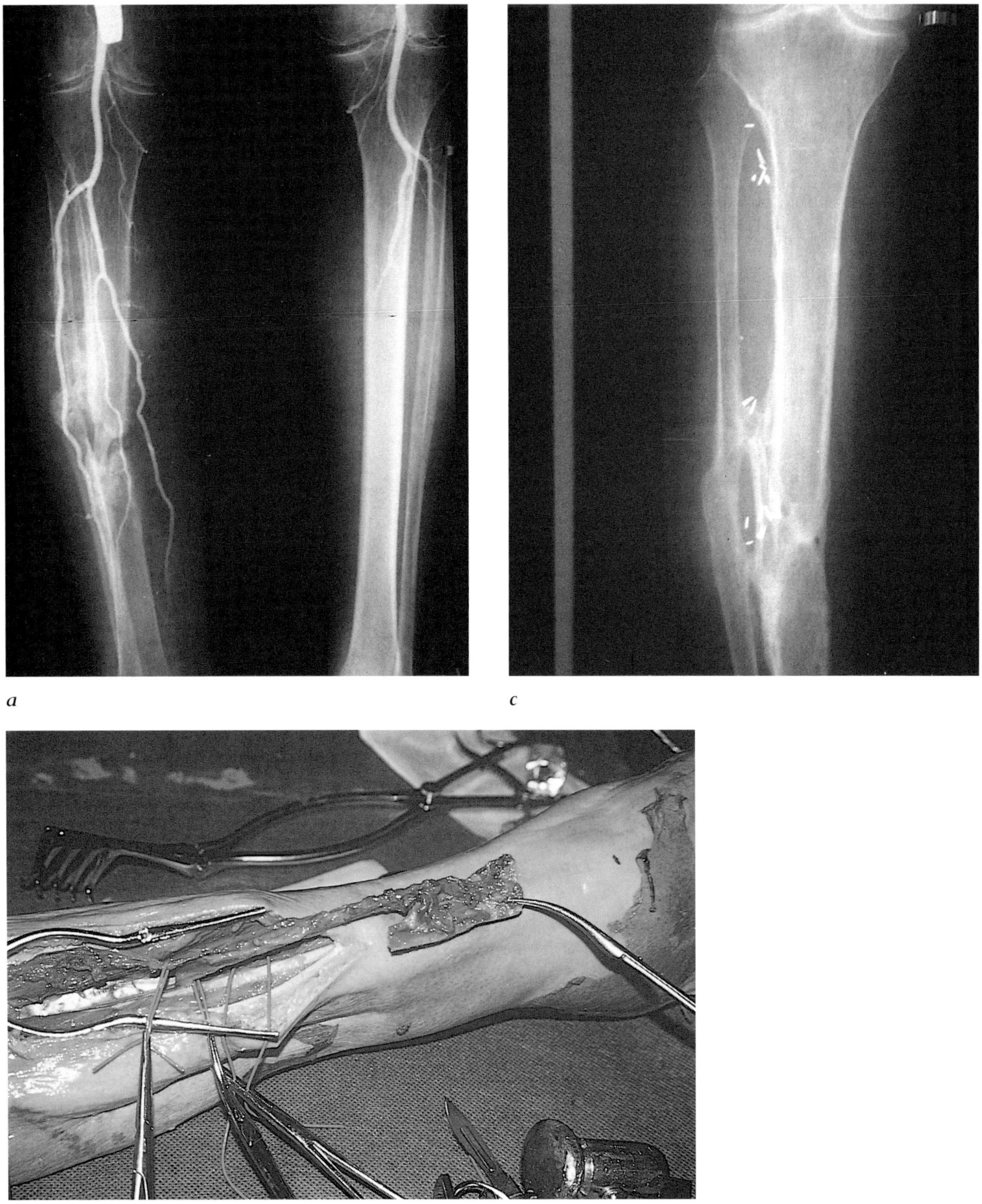

Fig. 33 *Clinical case.*

(a) Patient 39 years old. Infected tibial pseudarthrosis.

(b) A pedicle bone graft is raised on a reverse pedicle.

(c) Healing after 5 months.

F. SECOND METATARSAL OSTEOCUTANEOUS FLAP

Jamal Gousheh

Position and preparation

The patient is supine, with a slightly flexed knee and a tourniquet at the root of the limb.

Design

The bone graft is marked on the foot. If the length of the second metatarsal is not sufficient, it is possible to lengthen the graft by including the proximal toe phalanx, with an arthrodesis of the metatarsophalangeal joint.

The skin flap is designed over the graft according to the principles used for a dorsalis pedis flap. The vascular pedicle can be as long as necessary, depending on the recipient site.

Raising the flap

The incision starts with the medial border of the flap at the level of the lateral part of extensor hallucis brevis. Then the lateral skin incision is made and slightly elevated. During this dissection, the paratendon is protected and kept moist (Smith and Bellinger 1980). The extensor of the second toe is sacrificed. All the large longitudinal veins are protected until the end of the procedure, when it is possible to choose the vessel with the best venous outflow.

If the skin flap has to be reinnervated, it is possible to isolate the superficial branches of the peroneal nerve (usually two).

The first dorsal metatarsal artery is then dissected at the distal part of the first web space. If the basal toe phalanx is used, the collateral dorsal branch to the toe will be included.

The collateral ligaments of the metatarsophalangeal joint, the volar plate, and the deep transverse metatarsal ligaments are cut.

The lateral aspect of the second metatarsal is dissected extraperiosteally, leaving a thin layer of muscle fibers.

If the second toe has to be amputated, it is not necessary to preserve the flexor tendons and nerves.

The first dorsal metatarsal artery is dissected from distal to proximal, and on its medial side. It is often necessary to sacrifice a piece of interosseous muscle, especially if the vessel runs through it.

The extensor digitorum brevis tendon to the big toe is cut, and the deep proximal communicating branch is cut.

It is then possible to disarticulate the proximal metatarsal cuneiform joint. All the ligaments of this joint are cut, and the osteocutaneous flap is freed on its vascular pedicle. The artery is dissected to the exact length necessary, and it is next time to choose the best vein. The vascular pedicle is then cut.

Closure and postoperative care

The first and third metatarsal are approximated by a strong suture. The protected extensor tendons are disposed of over the donor area and grafted with a partial-thickness graft.

If the toe phalanx has been used, it is better to amputate the second toe. This is then filleted, and its skin is used over the donor area.

A toe over-dressing is applied, and the foot is protected by a splint for 12 days.

G. VASCULARIZED JOINT TRANSFERS

The exact role of vascularized joint transfers is not well established. Since 1967 (Buncke et al 1967) experimental and clinical reports have shown that although the transfer is possible, its function at long term rarely meets initial expectation, owing to stiffness and progressive joint degeneration in many cases.

Probably one of the most interesting indications lies in the reconstruction of children's joints: the growth plate transfer and the possibilities of remodeling give more hope of functional success.

Although most of the clinical reports deal with proximal interphalangeal (PIP) or metacarpophalangeal (MCP) joints from the foot, more recently the possibilities of pedicle distal interphalangeal (DIP) to PIP transfers (Foucher et al 1990) or heterodigital transfers have been presented.

Donor site anatomy

MCP and PIP joint transfers from the foot

Although free toe joint transfers have not been used frequently, their anatomy has been studied by several authors (Kuo et al 1984; Yoshizu et al 1984; Foucher et al 1990). Most of the time the PIP joint is used, as it is not so bulky, allows direct flexion, and can be transferred as a composite graft. The MCP joint is more bulky and has the disadvantage of having limited palmar flexion and excessive dorsiflexion. It can be used as a reversed graft, this transfer being slightly more complicated.

Metatarsophalangeal joint

Kuo (Kuo et al 1990) has studied its vascularization and has separated 3 groups:

- Group A (60%) The articular branch arises from the distal third of the first dorsal interosseous artery (FDIA).
- Group B (18%) The articular branch arises from the FDIA at the level where it plunges into the web. It is then a short artery.
- Group C (22%). When the FDIA is very deep and passes under the intermetatarsal ligament, the articular branches arise at this level.

In another study, Yoshizu et al (1984) found articular branches coming from both dorsal and plantar arteries.

Foucher (Foucher et al 1990) places the main emphasis on the role of the second dorsal interosseous artery.

The innervation of the second metatarsophalangeal (MTP) joint comes partly from the articular branches of the deep peroneal profundus nerve, and partly from the superficial peroneal nerve.

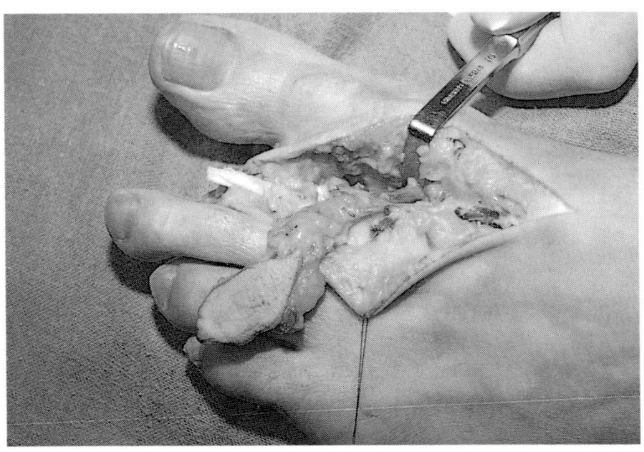

Fig. 34 Dorsal dissection and raising of the vascularized joint.

Interphalangeal joint

The vascular supply comes from the articular branches of the plantar digital artery. These branches arise proximal to the PIP joint, either directly from the digital artery or from the plantar transverse arch between the two arteries. This arch is located 8–10 mm proximal to the joint. The innervation of the PIP joint comes from branches of plantar digital nerves and the dorsal terminal branches of the peroneal nerves. The skin and tendons overlying the joint are also vascularized by the digital vessels. With one single pedicle it is possible to transfer a composite graft.

Procedures

Joint damage or destruction has been successfully treated by arthrodesis or arthroplasty, with or without prosthesis. Nevertheless, in a few selected cases these methods are not applicable or their expected results are not sufficient: these comprise children and young adults needing mobility and stability of the finger joint.

For these cases there may be some indications for vascularized joint transfers, either pedicled or with microvascular transfer.

The surgical anatomy of the foot donor areas is well known and recently clarified. It allows the transfer of either the MTP or PIP joints from the foot on long pedicles, which are dependable.

Since 1967 several authors have published their series of vascularized joint transfers. Their relatively small numbers show that the indications are still quite rare.

Surgical technique

Harvesting of the PIP joint from the toe has been well described by Tsai (Tsai et al 1982). Through a longitudinal dorsal incision on the foot, the dorsalis pedis artery and its branch, the first dorsal metatarsal artery (DMA), are dissected, as well as the dorsal veins (Fig. 34). The first DMA is followed to the web, and the medial collateral artery is dissected. A small island flap is designed on the dorsal medial aspect of the PIP joint.

The lateral collateral artery is preserved and the extensor mechanism is cut on each side of the joint. The DIP joint is disarticulated, and the proximal phalanx is osteotomized at the level of the mid-shaft.

The compound joint, skin, and tendon flap is isolated on its pedicle and ready for transfer.

In the hand, the toe PIP joint may be used for reconstruction of either the PIP or the MCP joints. Although for MCP reconstruction the toe PIP is small, it has the advantage over the toe MTP joint in that the latter has an excessive dorsal range of motion and needs to be rotated 180° to obtain a normal PIP range of motion.

It is possible to maintain the donor toe: this can either be done by accepting the shortening, or the defect can be bone grafted. Other authors prefer in some cases to amputate the entire second ray (Foucher et al 1990).

Some authors (Tsai and Hanna 1988; Tsai et al 1982, 1985; Foucher et al 1990) have used simultaneous transfer of two PIP joints from two toes, either on one or two pedicles. In that situation, it is possible to reconstruct one toe with the remnants of the second and third toes.

In some very selected cases it is possible to use a vascularized joint transfer from another finger of the same injured hand. It can be taken in multiple amputations from a nonreplantable digit or in an isolated destruction of the PIP joint exchanged with a mobile DIP joint. This technique of pedicled transfer of the DIP joint to the PIP defect has been described by Foucher. There are of course extremely few indications, as in many cases prosthetic replacement is much simpler.

Conclusion

Although the technique of vascularized joint transplantation is quite possible, as has been shown experimentally, the clinical results are often disappointing, and rarely superior to prosthetic replacement. The rare indications may lie essentially in joint reconstruction in children or young adults after traumatic injury to the finger joints.

Some publications have stressed the possibility of using the vascularized PIP joint in congenital defects either for substitution of an absent trapezometacarpal joint in Grade III aplasia of the thumb (Tajima) or for stabilization of radial club hand (Vilkki). These areas are promising but will need a long-term appraisal.

H. CHONDROEPIPHYSIS IN CHILDREN

Luc Téot

Tissue can be removed from any of three donor sites in a child without serious consequences for the growth or the overall function of the limbs: the upper fibular epiphysis, the iliac crest, and the lower part of the scapular crest.

The proximal fibular epiphysis

The proximal fibular epiphysis is a true epiphysis formed by a growth plate and a secondary ossification center, and presents a joint surface covered by aricular cartilage. Restrepo et al (1980) described three epiphyseal vascular sources, all of small diameter:

- the inferior genicular artery, providing the lateral branch coming from the popliteal artery and passing around the lateral tibial plate to reach the head of the fibula;
- the posterior tibial recurrent artery, originating from the anterior tibial artery at the branch of division with the peroneal artery, and penetrating the head of the fibula medially; and
- a direct artery, originating at the bifurcation of the popliteal artery, which supplies the medial portion of the fibular head, opposite to the tibial plateau.

Many variations can be observed. This epiphysis presents a very difficult scheme of vascularization for microsurgical transplantation, some sources coming from the anterior part of the epiphysis, others coming posteriorly. Each part of the epiphysis is supplied terminally by different vascular regions. The works of Nettelblad et al (1984) confirm the vascular separation into different territories. The mean growth of the fibula is about 35 cm between birth and the end of puberty; 70% of the growth occurs in the proximal end. The quantity of remaining growth in the proximal end of the fibula for each age can be evaluated from specialized charts.

The diameter of the proximal fibular epiphysis is 3–5 cm in the adult. The articular surface is orientated obliquely in the direction of the tibial plateau. It can be used for the replacement of long bones of the upper limb, such as the proximal humerus. Another application is to salvage growth potential in the partially damaged epiphyseal plate by side-by-side placement of the proximal fibula with the remaining physis remnant. In most cases, however, the exact physis alignment to the recipient site is not mandatory.

One of the main features of this bone is the length of diaphyseal bone that can be used. When transferring both the upper fibula and the fibular diaphysis, it is mandatory to revascularize both pedicles, i.e. the proximal epiphyseal vessels and the diaphyseal sources. This procedure considerably lengthens the surgery. Several authors chose to simplify the difficulties of keeping all the epiphyseal vessels and instead recommend use of the anterior tibial vessels only (Taylor et al 1988; Gupta 1995) (Fig. 35).

These difficulties are probably one of the causes of the unpredictable growth potential in some transplanted upper fibulae in clinical situations, reported in short series (1 cm/year) (Tsai et al 1986; Wray et al 1981; Sawaizumi et al 1991).

The iliac crest

The rounded cartilaginous ridge rising from the ilium can also be used as a donor site. Its thickness is limited, but the length of the removed fragment can vary. There is no organized articular surface. Growth

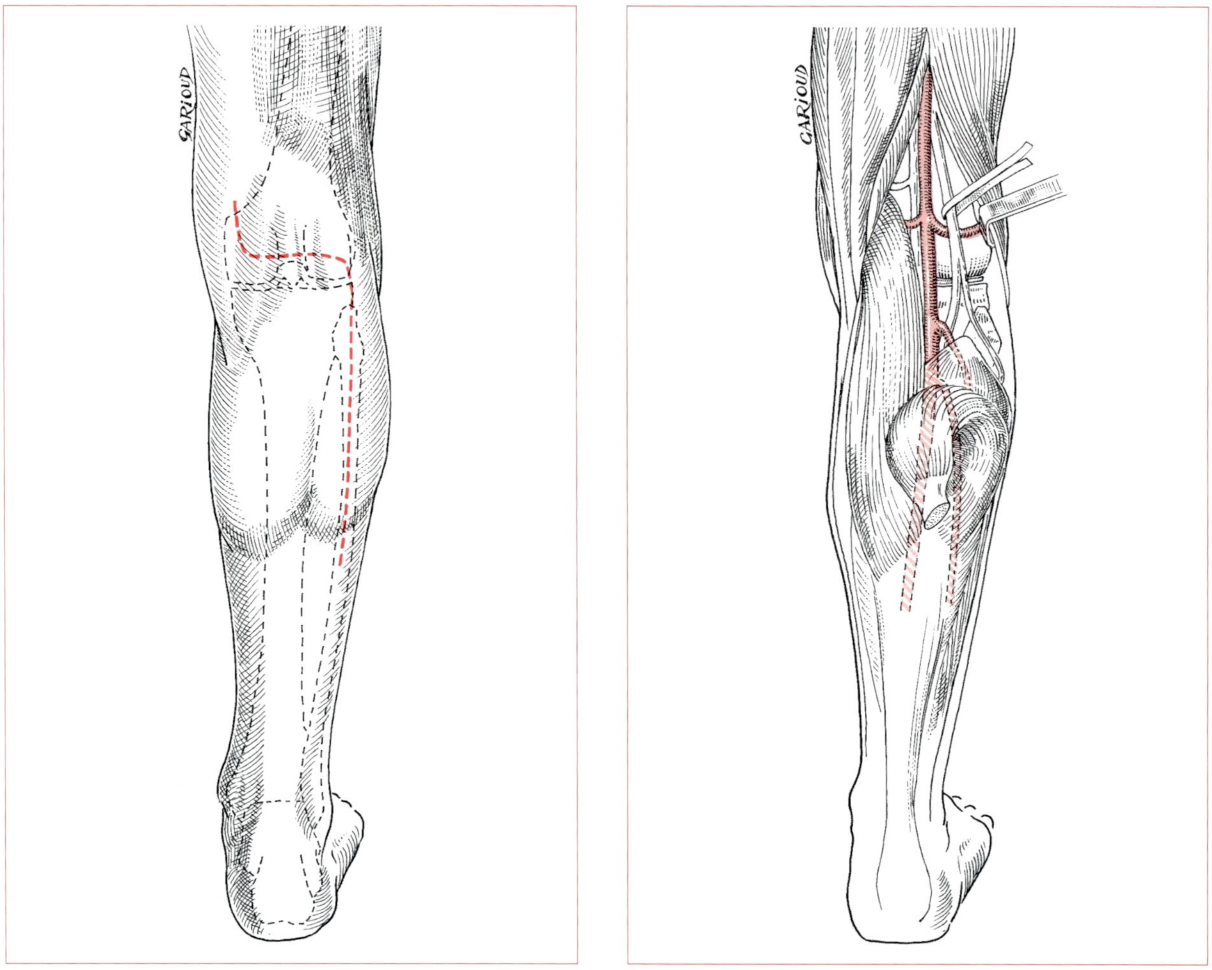

Fig. 35

(a) Outline of skin incision used for isolation of proximal fibula including physis.

(b) Isolation, mobilization and protection of sciatic nerve and branches.

occurs as in an epiphysis (Ponsetti 1970) during the first years of life, and then by the combined action of the abdominal and thigh muscles, as in an apophysis. Muscles are anchored on the iliac crest by a set of circular and penetrating fibers that have much in common with the Sharpey fibers. Recent studies of this apophysis (Téot et al 1992) have demonstrated that the deep circumflex iliac vessels pass along the posterior aspect of the iliac crest for 6 or 7 cm before continuing into the abdominal wall. This pattern is not present in the child, where the deep circumflex vessels cross the iliac crest perpendicularly, without passing on for any distance on the posterior aspect of the apophysis. They then give off vessels to each side, anastomosing with other sources coming from the superficial circumflex vessels. The muscular branch that runs within the abdominal wall originates from the femoral artery in the inguinal canal and ends on the metaphyseal slope of the anterior iliac spine, giving off an epiphyseal branch that runs along the top of the crest towards the deep circumflex iliac artery.

Branches arise from the lateral iliac artery, which originates from the second external branch of the internal iliac artery and runs along the iliac crest, giving off branches to the top of the crest and ending in the muscles of the lateral abdominal wall. This artery plays an important role in the vascularization of the iliac crest.

The epiphyseal circulation takes place from the dome of the crest, giving off 'teeth of a comb'-type ramifications that pass around the two aspects of the crest, medial and lateral. These ramifications give off perpendicular intraepiphyseal extensions.

Histologically, the growth plate presents a rather marked convex aspect. Its lateral limit is the perichondrial ring. The plate is 4 cm high at the end of growth. The maximal usable length of the diaphyseal portion is about 10 cm. Curvature of the pelvis restricts the use of the lateral and posterior portions. The ossification center is one of the latest to appear in the human, and its closure marks the end of the pubertal period in a child (Risser sign).

The ilium grows about 20 cm between birth and adulthood. Most of the growth occurs in the iliac crest.

The main problem with this growing apophysis is the future of the hyaline surface after its transplantation to an intra-articular position. In long-term experimental studies (2 years in the dog) we observed, by optical and electron microscopy, that a progressive arthritis was sometimes observed. It was concluded from these studies that the graft has to be located in an extra-articular position. The remodeling capacities of the transplanted epiphysis are excellent, and it adapts well to most situations, as in deepening the formation of a cup, in enlarging the acetabulum, or in replacing a deficient lower radius in a radial club hand.

In our clinical experience, this apophysis has a wide range of possibilities for replacing either a part of a tibial plateau or of a lower femoral growth plate, an epiphysis of a long bone of the upper arm, or the triradiate cartilage of the pelvic bone, or as an appositional growing structure for any site in the human body.

Clinical indications for the use of the iliac apophysis were described by the author and co-workers (in Brunelli: Téot et al 1988) after a large series of 18 cases, followed postoperatively over 6 years, and can be summarized as follows (Figs 36 and 37):

- for a radial club hand (post-traumatic or congenital);
- for a replacement of the lower humeral epiphysis;
- for the partial replacement of a large growth plate (lower femoral epiphysis); and
- as an island graft used as a material for enlarging the acetabulum in certain cases of paralytic hips that are difficult to cure by conventional means.

The lower portion of the scapula

The scapula is a classic flat bone, but it presents a lateral portion comparable to a corticodiaphyseal bone, whose distal end terminates in a large cartilaginous apophyseal area. It is 2.5 cm in diameter.

The anatomical and vascular characteristics of the diaphyseal portion have recently been described by the present author, who considers it to be a new donor site for vascularized bone (Téot et al 1981). The rich vascularity abundance of the region makes it a candidate for various composite transfers of skin, muscle, and bone, which constitute important new resources for reconstructive surgery of the limbs (Fig. 38).

The inferior angle of the scapula is covered by a wide chondroepiphysis in the young child.

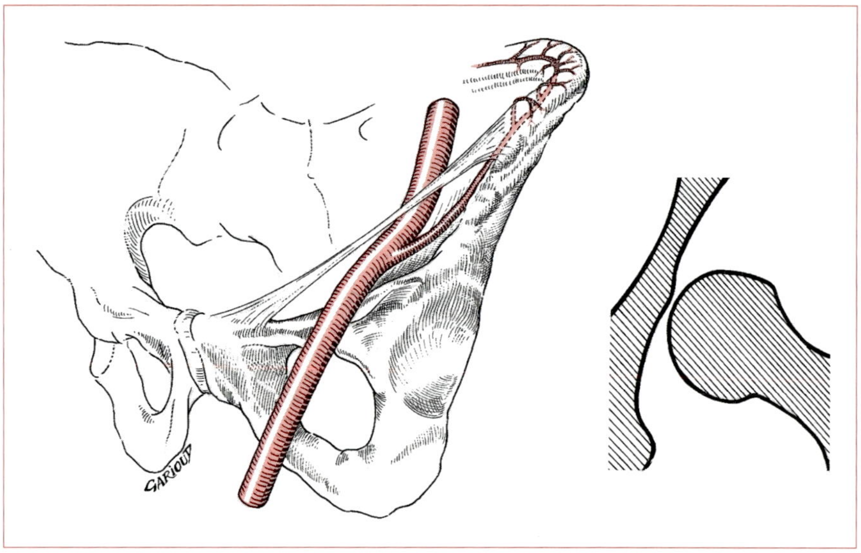

Fig. 36
Artist's depiction of dysplastic acetabulum with hip dislocation. Note deficiency of the cephelad bony coverage of the femoral head.

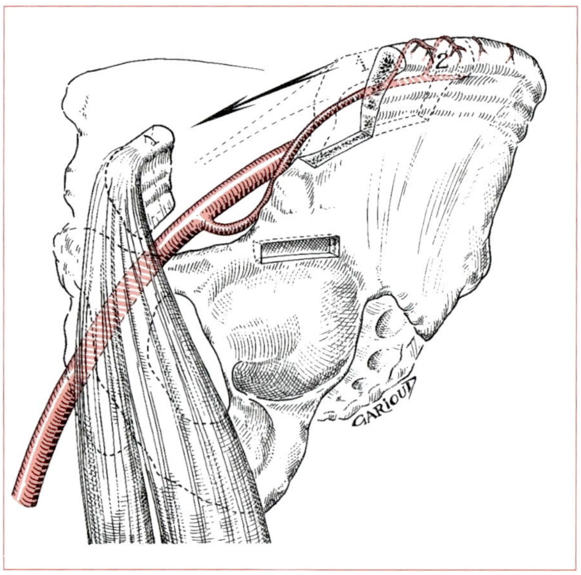

Fig. 37
(a) Use of the iliac apophysis as an island graft as a modified 'shelf procedure' to reconstruct the acetabulum.

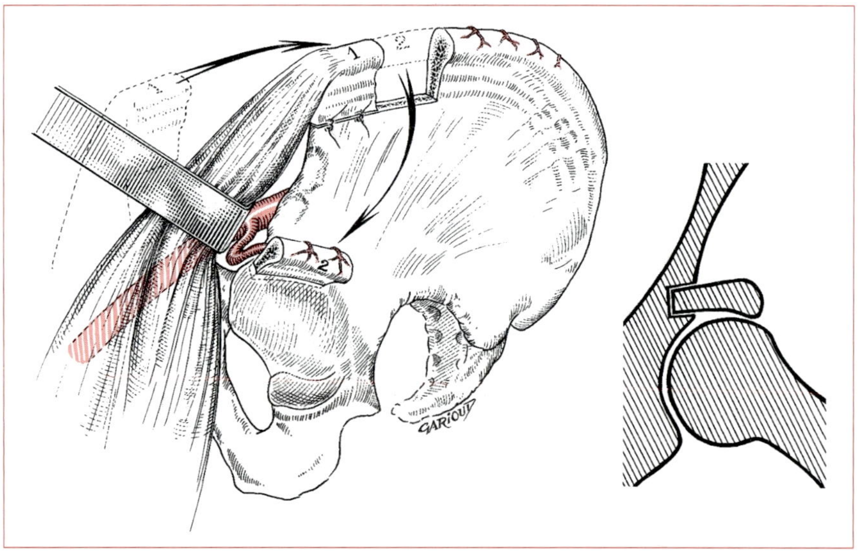

(b) Artist's depiction of postoperative modified 'shelf procedure'. Note improved bony coverage of femoral head.

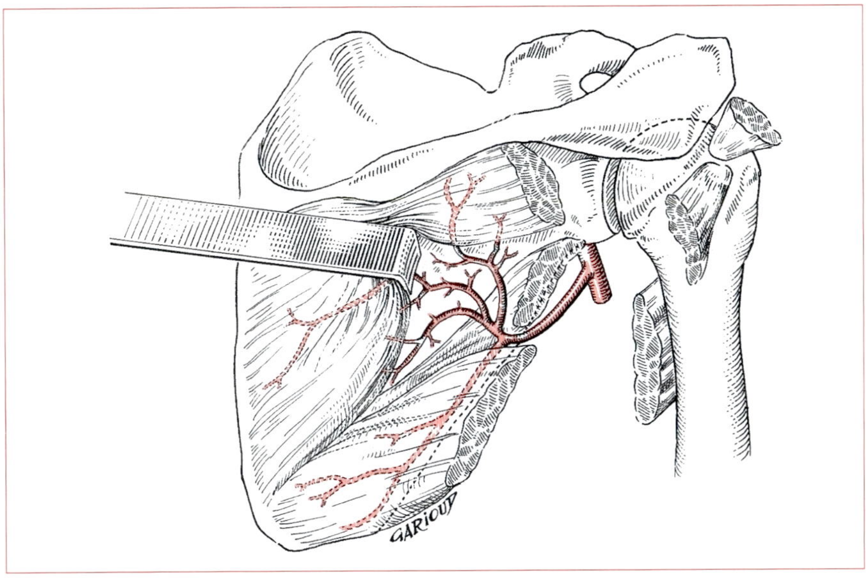

Fig. 38
Artist's depiction of vascular contributions from circumflex scapular vessels to scapular apophyseal region.

The epiphyseal vessels arise from a branch of a division of the circumflex scapular vessels, at the medullary foramen. These vessels pass along the scapular crest, and are distributed to the cartilaginous portion which supplies the lateral portion of the epiphysis, opposite to the diaphyseal segment, forming the scapular crest. The whole crest and its cartilaginous extension can be combined on the same vascular axis as is formed by the subscapular vessels.

The growth plate has long cellular columns comprising more than 30 superimposed cells, limited laterally by a thick perichondrial ring with abundant Sharpey fibers. The growth mechanism appears to depend essentially on muscular traction. The teres major, latissimus dorsi, subscapularis, and infraspinatus muscles are inserted on it. The hyaline cartilage is not covered by an articular surface. The considerable height of this zone is a good reflection of its extensive remodeling possibilities.

The growth and width of the scapula can be determined radiologically. Between birth and adulthood, the scapula grows about 8–10 cm. Almost all the growth occurs in the inferior part, since the superior portion of the scapula does not present an organized epiphyseal plate. Adaptation essentially involves changes in volume. In the adult the inferior angle of the scapula has a large oval bulge 9 cm long and 4 cm wide, where the powerful teres major muscle is inserted. The inferior apophysis of the scapula can be considered to be an important zone of chondrogenesis that can be adapted to many situations in spite of its initially limited thickness.

Experimental transplantations have confirmed these concepts (Téot et al 1986). The cartilaginous inferior angle of the scapula shows substantial adaptive power, and is able to double its cartilaginous volume over several months after replacing a much larger epiphysis such as the proximal end of the humerus.

I. VASCULARIZED PERIOSTEAL FLAP

Alain C Masquelet and Marie Claude Romaña

Bone reconstruction based on vascularized periosteum is not yet a routinely used procedure. Accounts of a few isolated clinical attempts have been published (Satoh et al 1983; Masquelet et al 1989; Sakai et al 1991; Crock and Morrison 1992), but without clarifying the indications. Moreover the development of vascularized periosteum transfer has been held back by the successful use of the fibula transfer (Östrup and Frederickson 1974; Taylor et al 1975) for the reconstruction of long bone defects.

For many years, we have been attempting to answer three questions that seem to us essential.

- Is the vascularized periosteum worthwhile in bone reconstruction, and should it be used?
- What are the potential donor sites for periosteal flap on the human body, and what is the source of the most reliable flap?
- What are the indications for vascularized periosteal flaps?

In order to answer the first and second questions we undertook in 1985 an experimental study and an anatomical investigation.

Our clinical experience, which began in the same year, has allowed us to identify some unquestionable indications and to discover objections to others. What we have to discuss thus falls into three sections:

1. the biological basis;
2. the periosteal flap donor sites, with their techniques of elevation; and
3. the clinical experience and the results.

The biological basis

Ollier (1867) was probably the first author to claim an osteogenic capacity for the periosteum, and the idea of using a periosteal transplant to produce new bone is not a new concept (Skoog 1967).

The crucial point is to establish whether the vascularized periosteum is better than nonvascularized periosteum in bone production. Although free nonvascularized periosteal grafts are able to promote bone formation (Uddstromer 1978), it is now incontestable that the osteogenic capacity of a revascularized periosteal graft is considerably more significant. The vascular supply is a determinant factor.

Even the earliest work gave evidence of this. Ritsila et al (1972), using free nonvascularized periosteal graft in rabbits, noted that bone formation is better after implantation in well-vascularized muscle than after implantation in fascia. The same conclusion was asserted by King (1976), who stated that 'the behaviour of pedicled periosteal flaps is predictable, provided they retain an adequate blood supply'.

The role of vascularization was definitively affirmed by the experimental studies based on transfers revascularized by microsurgical techniques. Finley et al (1978), using dogs, demonstrated the osteogenic capacity of a revascularized periosteal graft; but Acland (1978) and Puckett et al (1979) emphasized the role of weight or stress in bone formation. Several works during the last decade have been useful in clarifying the conditions for using a periosteal transfer. Van den Wildenberg et al (1984), working on adult African pygmy goats, concluded that the osteogenic capacity of vascularized periosteum varies with donor site, and that tibial periosteum gives more bone formation than rib periosteum. Takato et al (1986) showed in rabbits that a vascularized periosteal graft resulted in a significant amount of new bone formation, even when not subjected to stress or weight. These authors also stated that the osteogenic capacity of the periosteum is dependent on blood supply, and that a vascularized musculoperiosteal flap is better than a simple periosteal flap.

On the other hand, Jaroma and Ritsila (1988) used in combination a free nonvascularized periosteal graft wrapped around a cancellous bone graft. The whole transplant was buried into muscle. The authors demonstrated that the periosteal graft partially inhibits the resorption of cancellous bone, and results in new bone formation. However, the use of fascia instead of periosteum does not inhibit the resorption of cancellous bone. Isolated cancellous bone grafts transplanted in muscle are resorbed. Clinical observations indicate that, even after prolonged contact, cancellous bone grafts show marked resorption, especially if the recipient site is poorly vascularized.

Hypothesis

Therefore the results of all this earlier experimental work logically suggest that the association of a vascularized periosteal flap with a cancellous bone graft would be the best procedure to produce cortical new bone. We tested this hypothesis on rats (Romaña and Masquelet 1990). Twenty 6-week-old Wistar rats were used. Both hindlegs and the left foreleg were exposed and prepared, and three procedures were performed on each rat during a single initial operation (Fig. 39).

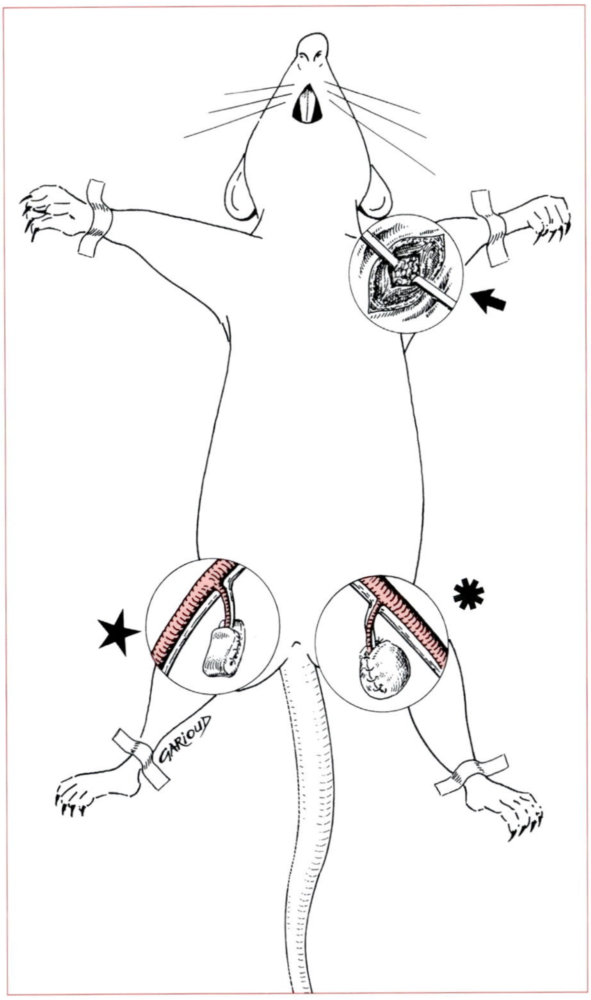

Fig. 39 Experimental work. Three procedures are performed on each rat (MC Romaña et al 1990). Procedure 1 (asterisk): a vascularized musculoperiosteal flap is wrapped around small pieces of cancellous bone graft harvested from the ipsilateral knee metaphysis. Procedure 2 (star): the vascularized musculoperiosteal flap is sutured on itself. Procedure 3 (arrow): small pieces of cancellous bone, harvested from the right knee metaphysis, are buried into triceps muscle.

Procedure

On both hindlegs a vascularized musculoperiosteal flap was raised from the lower third of the femur, pedicled on the descending genicular artery. This artery supplies the articular muscle of the knee and the periosteum of the lower third of the femur (see technique of elevation). A slip of musculoperiosteal tissue was harvested from the anteromedial part of the lower femur, remaining pedicled on the descending genicular artery.

- On the right hindleg the flap was sutured on itself, with the cambium layer inside.
- On the left hindleg the musculoperiosteal flap was wrapped around a small amount of cancellous bone harvested from the upper extremity of the tibia.
- On the left foreleg the same quantity of cancellous bone was buried into muscle.

Observations

Thus we were able to observe the behaviour of three implants:

- the cancellous bone graft isolated in striated muscle;
- the vascularized musculoperiosteal flap alone; and
- the cancellous bone graft enclosed in vascularized musculoperiosteal flap.

The results were statistically significant, and were chiefly assessed by radiologic and histologic observation (Figs 40, 41).

- The association of the vascularized musculoperiosteal flap with cancellous bone resulted in a significant amount of compact bone formation. This newly formed bone was typically cortical.
- Bone formation from the vascularized musculoperiosteal flap alone was inconsistent and of little value.
- The cancellous bone graft isolated in muscles resulted in fibrous tissue or necrotic bone.

Conclusions

This experimental work, when considered in conjunction with other previous work, suggests to us several interesting and worthwhile conclusions from a clinical point of view.

1. The role of the blood supply in bone formation from a periosteal flap is well established.
2. However, a periosteal flap alone is not sufficient to induce a quantity of bone sufficient to treat

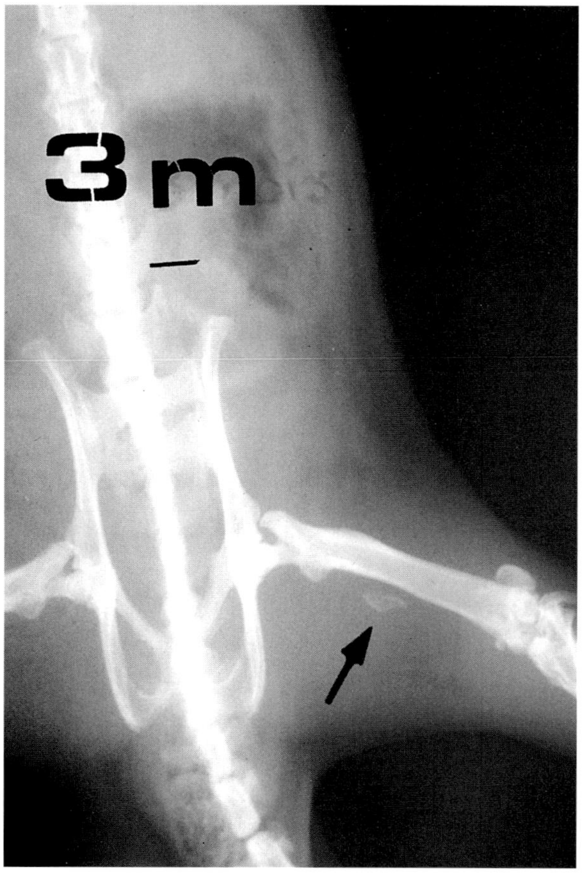

Fig. 40 *Radiographic control at 12 weeks (Procedure 1). Compact bone formation can be seen. Resorption is less than half of the initial volume of cancellous bone graft.*

atrophic nonunion or to reconstruct long bone defects. It is highly recommended that one should use a conventional bone graft in association with a periosteal flap, especially when there is a bone defect. The musculoperiosteal flap can be tubulized and filled up with cancellous bone graft to reconstruct a long bone defect.

3. In an early work, Axhausen (1956) observed that free periosteum of an adult dog could proliferate and induce bone formation in muscle only when small pieces of cortical bone were left attached to the periosteum. Therefore we think that the musculoperiosteal flap should be raised with small pieces of bone, favoring new bone formation from periosteum, and we conclude that a bone reconstructive procedure using periosteum should

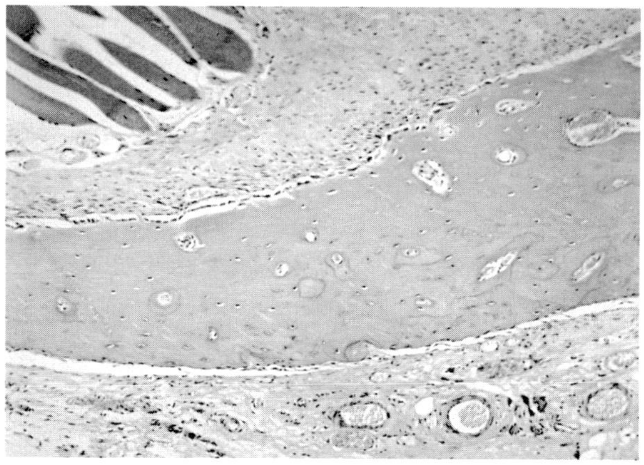

a

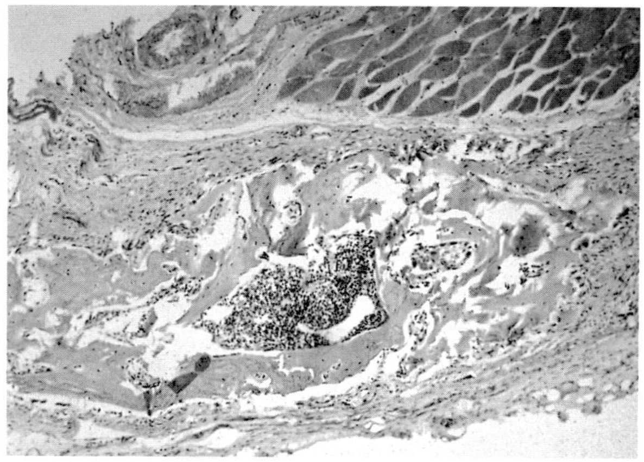

b

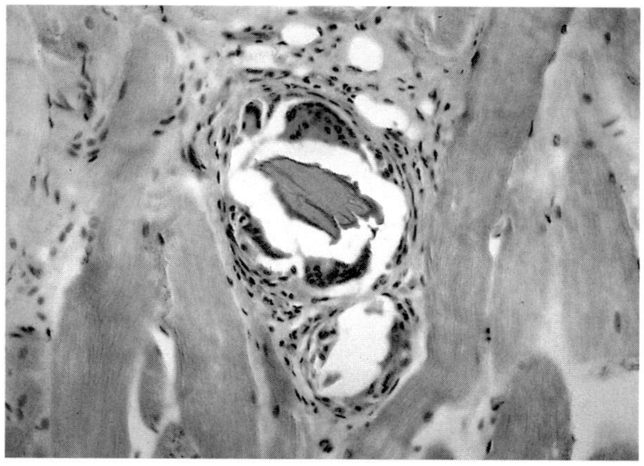

c

Fig. 41 *Histologic findings.*
(a) Procedure 1: new compact bone formation, with the typical structure of a haversian system with live cells.
(b) Procedure 2: new bone formation was of little importance. Osteogenesis and resorption are very active.
(c) Procedure 3: histologic observation of a small piece of necrotic bone at a resorption stage; the bone is surrounded by giant cells.

involve a vascularized musculocorticoperiosteal flap that should be sufficiently supple and versatile to be tubulized or wrapped around a conventional cancellous bone graft.

Vascularized periosteal flap donor sites

In order to create a clinical application with a potential capacity for reconstructing bone with periosteum, an anatomic study was undertaken and brought to a successful conclusion by Penteado et al (1990).

The periosteum in the adult is a fine membrane whose surgical elevation may be rather difficult. So for practical and biological reasons it is easier and better to raise an osteoperiosteal flap by detaching fine cortical flakes with the periosteum. Further, the inclusion of a muscle or a part of a muscle, resulting in a musculo-osteoperiosteal flap, improves the capacity of the flap for revascularization.

The study was done on twenty-five fresh specimens, injected with colored latex. The injection was made into the subclavian and the external iliac arteries, and the dissection involved all four limbs.

The potential donor sites for periosteal or musculoperiosteal flaps were checked out on the upper and the lower limbs, and only those flaps were retained that were supplied by an artery of sufficient caliber to allow dissection of the pedicle or microsurgical anastomosis.

Upper limb

Three donor sites were studied:

- the distal third of the humerus;
- the shaft of the ulna; and
- the shaft of the radius.

Humerus

The flap is located on the distal third of the humerus, and can be raised on the anterior, the posterior, and the lateral aspect of the bone.

It is supplied by the deep brachial artery, which constitutes the pedicle of the flap (Fig. 42).

The deep brachial artery divides into its anterior and posterior branches at the junction between the middle and the distal thirds of the humerus. The anterior branch accompanies the radial nerve in the bicipital groove. The posterior branch, which is the one which concerns us, descends between the triceps and the brachioradialis, and participates in the periarticular network of the elbow. During its course it gives off small branches to the triceps, to the periosteum of the humerus, and to the overlying skin, forming the basis of the lateral arm flap.

The elevation of a periosteal flap requires the complete extraperiosteal detachment of the brachioradialis and partial release of the brachialis and triceps muscles.

The posterior branch of the deep brachial artery, which is contained in a septum inserted on the humerus, is left in continuity with the periosteum, and the dissection of the pedicle must be made by proceeding up to the origin of the deep brachial artery after ligation of the anterior terminal branch.

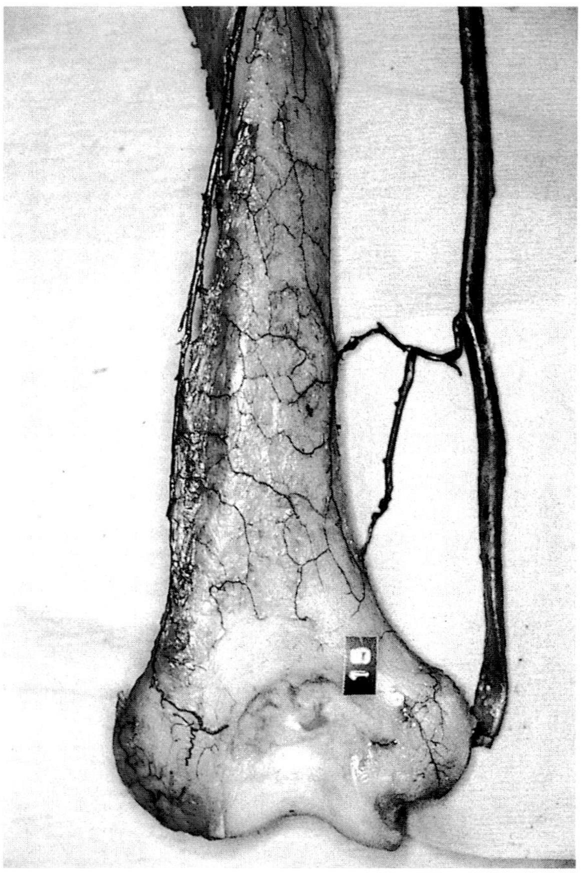

Fig. 42 *Anatomic study of the blood supply to the periosteum of the lower third of the humerus (C V Penteado et al 1990).*

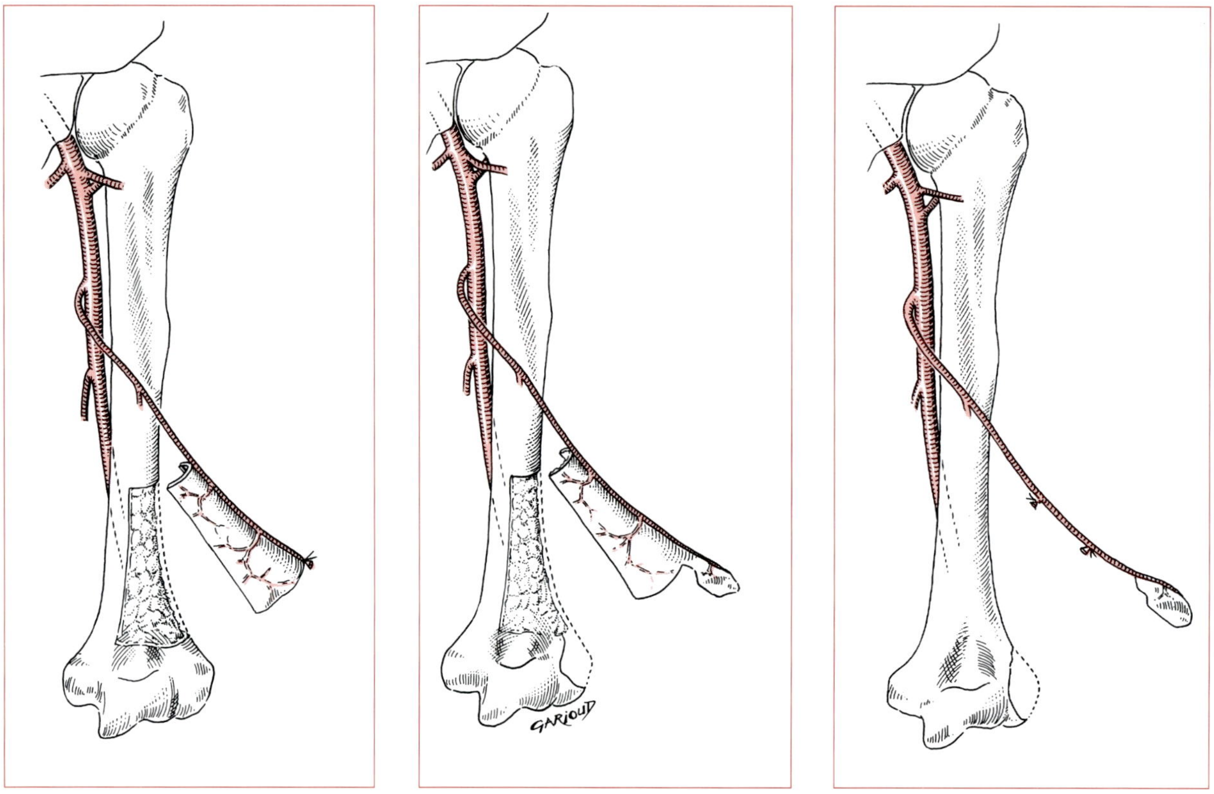

a *b* *c*

Fig. 43 *Different types of flaps raised on the deep brachial artery:*
(a) periosteal or musculoperiosteal flap;
(b) osteoperiosteal flap; and
(c) vascularized transfer of the lateral epicondyle.

The periosteum of the anterior, posterior, and lateral aspects of the humerus is raised. The flap may include a fine muscular layer (a musculoperiosteal flap), a distal corticocancellous block from the lateral epicondyle, or a cortical layer from the humeral shaft (osteoperiosteal or musculo-osteoperiosteal flap). The length of the pedicle should allow one to reach the upper end of the humerus (Fig. 43).

Radius and ulna

The blood supply to the periosteum of the radial shaft is remarkably constant. The proximal fourth of the radius, including the tuberosity, is supplied by a branch issuing from the common interosseous artery or by the recurrent interosseous artery.

The distal three-fourths are supplied by the anterior interosseous artery, which gives off four to six periosteal branches to each of the anterior and posterior aspects of the bone.

The blood supply to the periosteum of the ulna is derived, for the most part, from the anterior interosseous artery, which gives off three or four branches to the anterior and posterior aspects of the ulna. The posterior interosseous artery has very little part in supplying the ulnar periosteum. Our conclusion concerning the forearm is that the vascularization of the periosteum of the two bones depends almost entirely on the anterior interosseous artery.

Surgical approach to this artery is difficult, and involves the sacrifice of numerous muscular branches. Nonetheless, it is theoretically possible to raise a periosteal flap on one or other forearm bone that remains pedicled on its nutrient small arteries without interrupting the continuity of the anterior

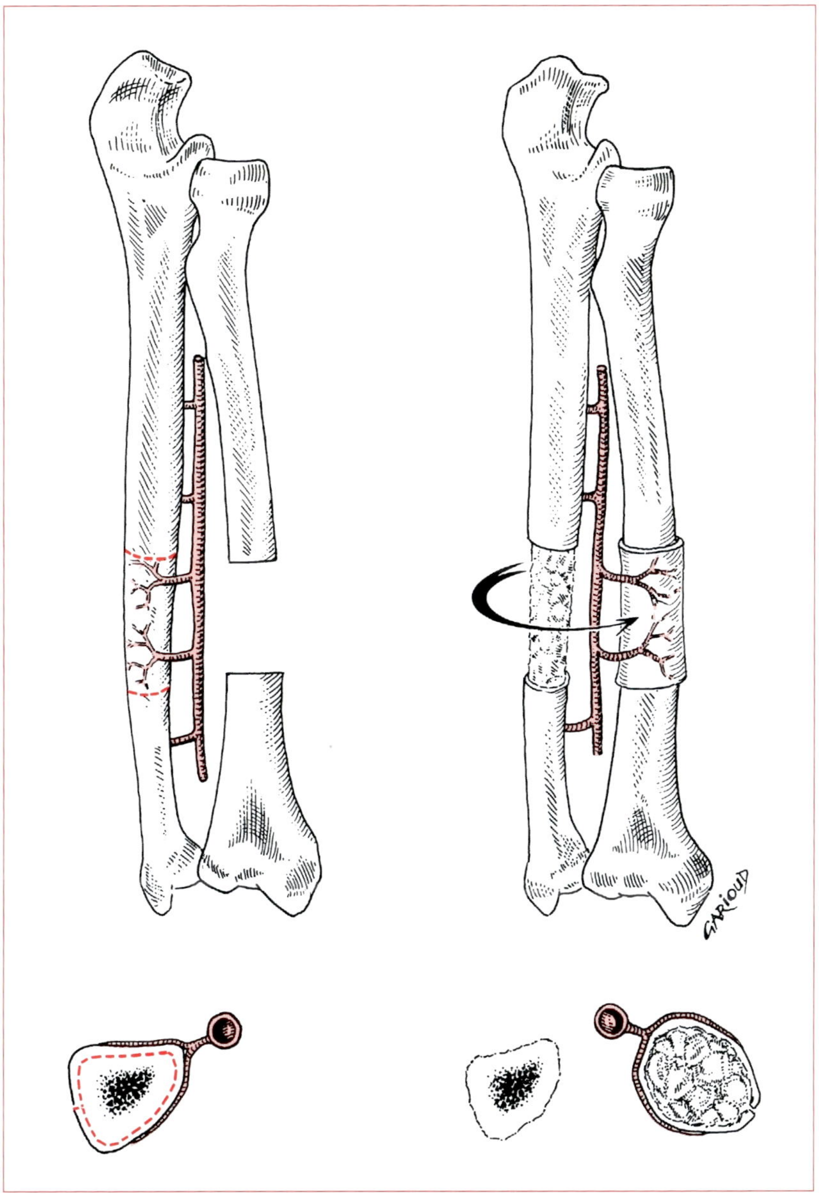

a ***b***

Fig. 44 *(a) The periosteum of the ulna is supplied by the anterior interosseous artery.*
(b) The diagram shows the possibility of raising a periosteal flap from the ulna to treat a defect of the radius by simple translation of the flap without interruption of continuity of the anterior interosseous artery.

interosseous artery. The flap may then be translocated on to the other segment by simple rotation (Fig. 44).

Lower limb

The lower limb is the principal donor site for periosteal flaps. Three sites were determined:

- the iliac fossa;
- the distal third of the femur; and
- the shaft of the tibia.

Iliac fossa (Fig. 45)

The iliac fossa is a clinically used donor site (Satoh et al 1983; Masquelet et al 1989). The main arterial trunk is the deep circumflex iliac artery, which arises from the external iliac artery and supplies the iliacus muscle and the periosteum of the inner surface of the ilium.

A very large musculocorticoperiosteal flap can be raised from the ilium and pedicled on the deep circumflex iliac artery. It is necessary to include a

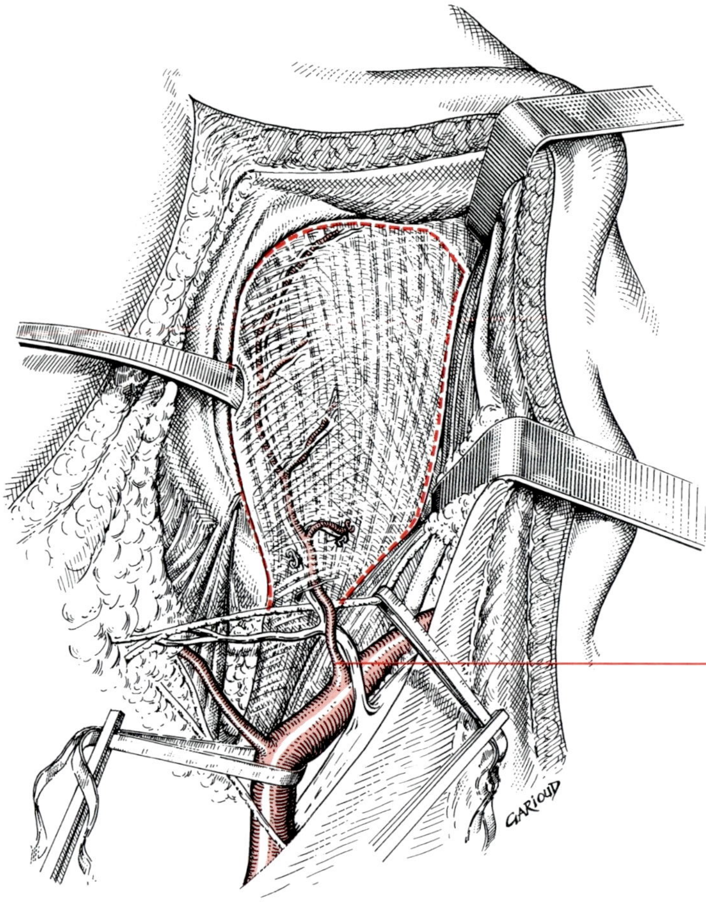

a

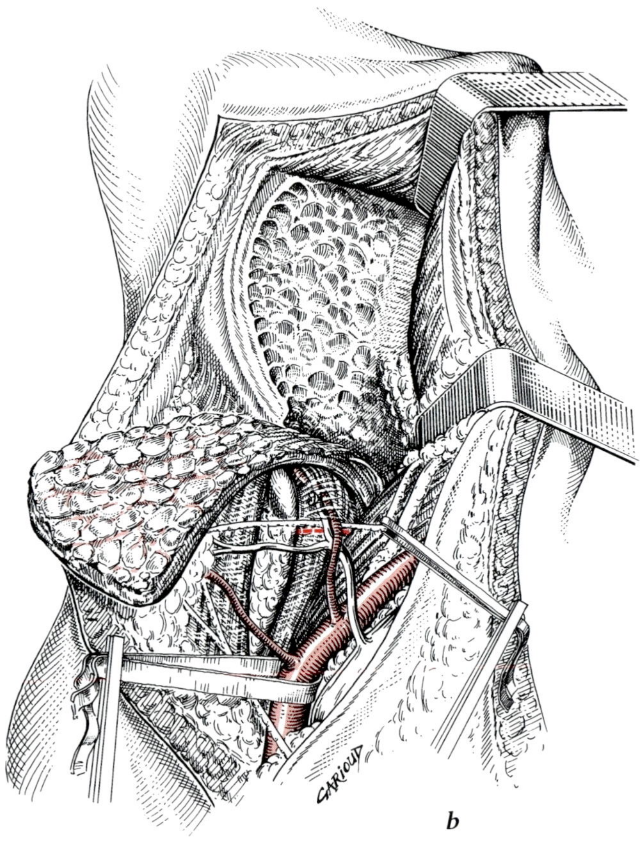

b

Fig. 45 *Osteomusculoperiosteal flap from the inner aspect of the ilium (a). The flap is supplied by the deep circumflex iliac artery, and can be used either as a pedicled or as a free flap. The arc of rotation of the island pedicled flap allows it to cover the proximal third of the femur (b).*

part of the iliacus muscle to provide vascular supply to the periosteum. This flap can be used as a pedicled flap to undertake bone reconstruction of the upper third of the femur or as a free flap. The flap is sufficiently supple to be tubulized and filled up with cancellous bone.

Femur

The periosteum of the femoral shaft is richly vascularized by numerous arteries. The lateral femoral circumflex artery, through its descending branch, supplies the anterior, lateral and medial aspects of the upper half of the femur. However, approach to the upper part of the femur and the lateral femoral circumflex artery is difficult, and this site cannot be routinely used to raise a flap.

It is in fact the distal third of the femur that is regarded as the site of choice (Masquelet et al 1989; Sakai et al 1991). The predominant flap is raised on the anterior and medial aspect of the lower third of the femur. The site of elevation includes the distal portion of the shaft, the metaphyseal region, and the extra-articular portion of the epiphysis.

The flap is nourished by the articular branch of the descending genicular artery (DGA). The DGA rises from the femoral artery just proximal to the adductor hiatus. The common trunk is rather short (average: 2 cm), and divides into three branches:

- a muscular branch to the vastus medialis muscle;
- a cutaneous branch that joins the saphenous nerve and passes beneath the sartorius muscle; and
- an articular branch that courses along the adductor magnus tendon until its femoral insertion on the medial condyle. At this level the articular branch anastomoses with the proximomedial collateral artery and runs upwards to reach the metaphysis of the femur. It divides into numerous small branches that supply the periosteum and the articular muscles around the knee.

The pedicle is isolated at the origin of the DGA (Fig. 46). The muscular and the cutaneous branches (saphenous artery) need to be ligated and severed.

Different kinds of flaps can be raised:

- a periosteal flap, which is very thin and not of interest;
- a thin osteoperiosteal flap including small flakes of cortical bone or an osteoperiosteal flap with a compact piece of cortical cone detached from the medial aspect of the femur; and
- a musculo-osteoperiosteal flap, created by including a portion of the muscles around the knee.

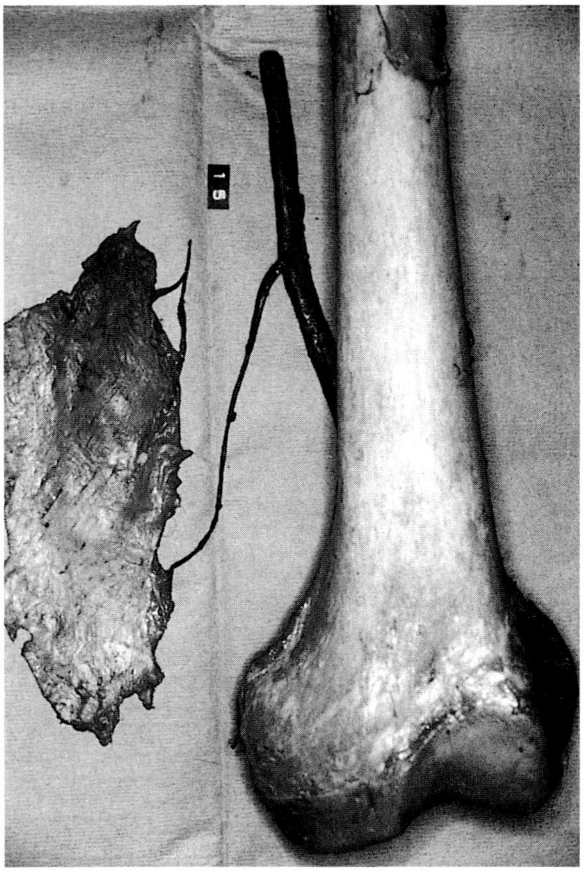

Fig. 46 *Anatomic preparation, showing the musculo-periosteal flap from the distal third of the femur. The flap is pedicled on the descending genicular artery (C V Penteado et al 1990).*

In our clinical experience the most frequently used has been a thin corticoperiosteal flap.

The operative procedure (Fig. 47) is as follows:
(*a*) The patient is supine and the lower limb is externally rotated. A tourniquet is applied at the root of the thigh. The skin incision is outlined on the relief of the adductor magnus tendon. (*b*) The deep fascia is incised, exposing the posterior border of the vastus medialis and the tendon of adductor magnus. (*c*) The vastus medialis is released from the distal aponeurosis

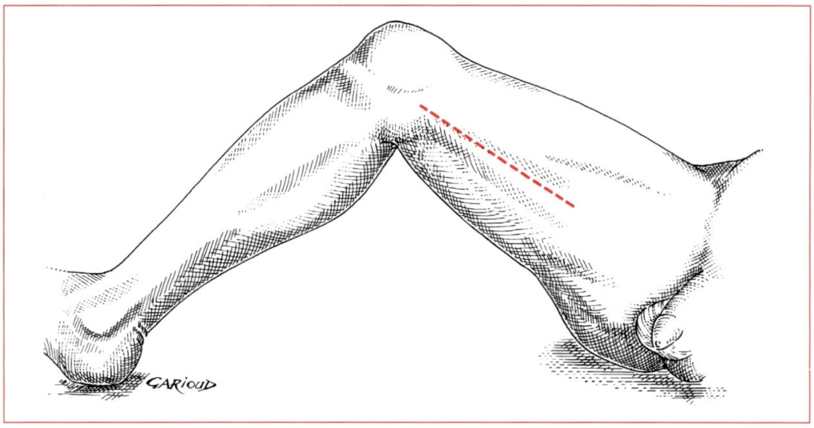

a

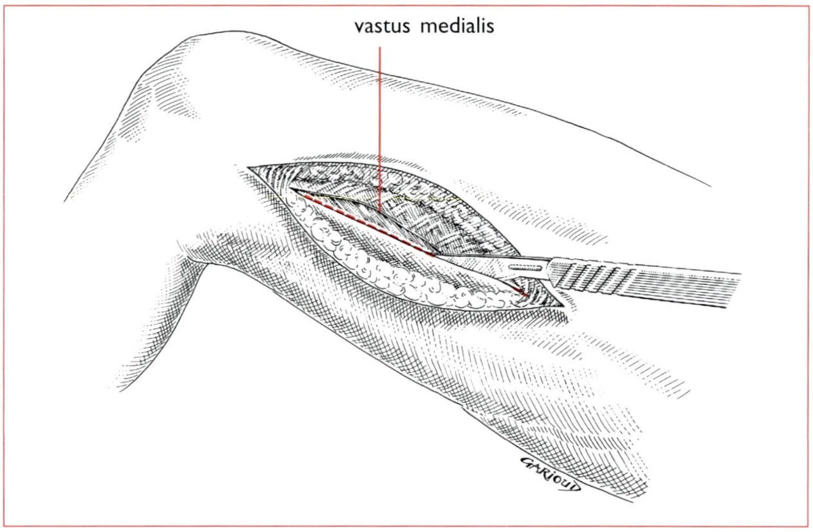

b

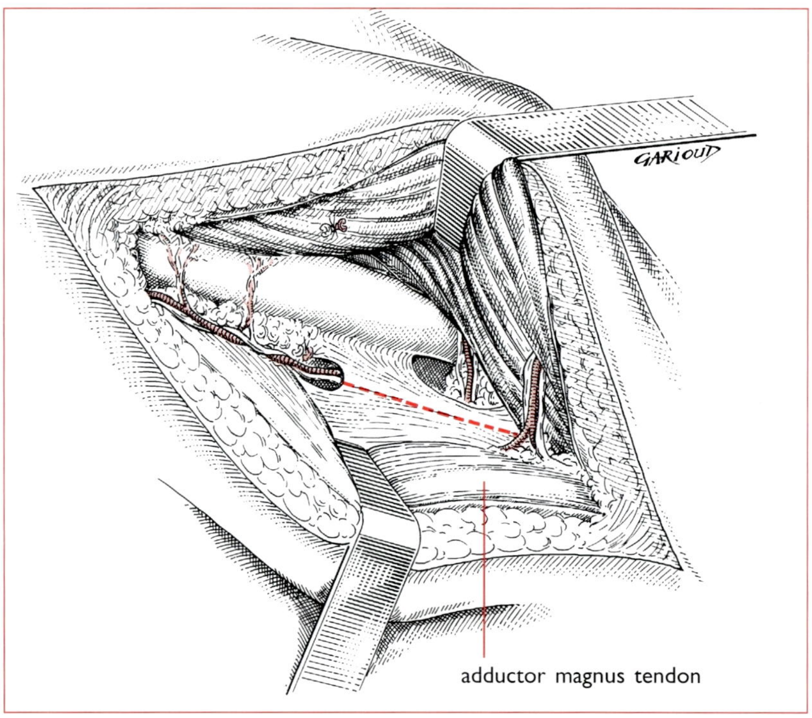

c

Fig. 47(a–e) *Surgical elevation of a corticoperiosteal flap from the distal third of the femur (see text, page 97).*

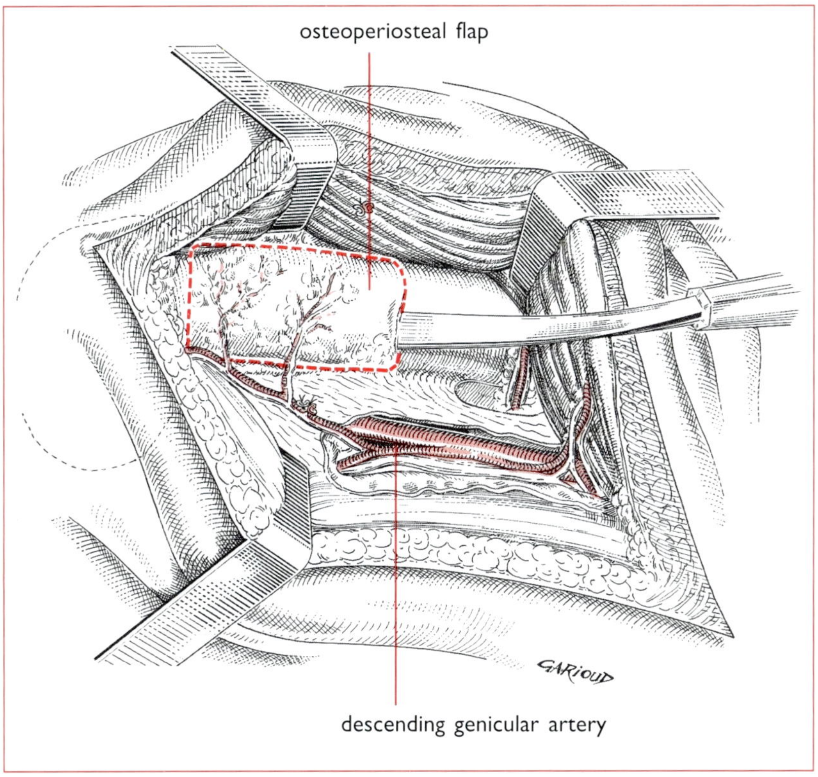
osteoperiosteal flap
descending genicular artery
GARIOUD

d

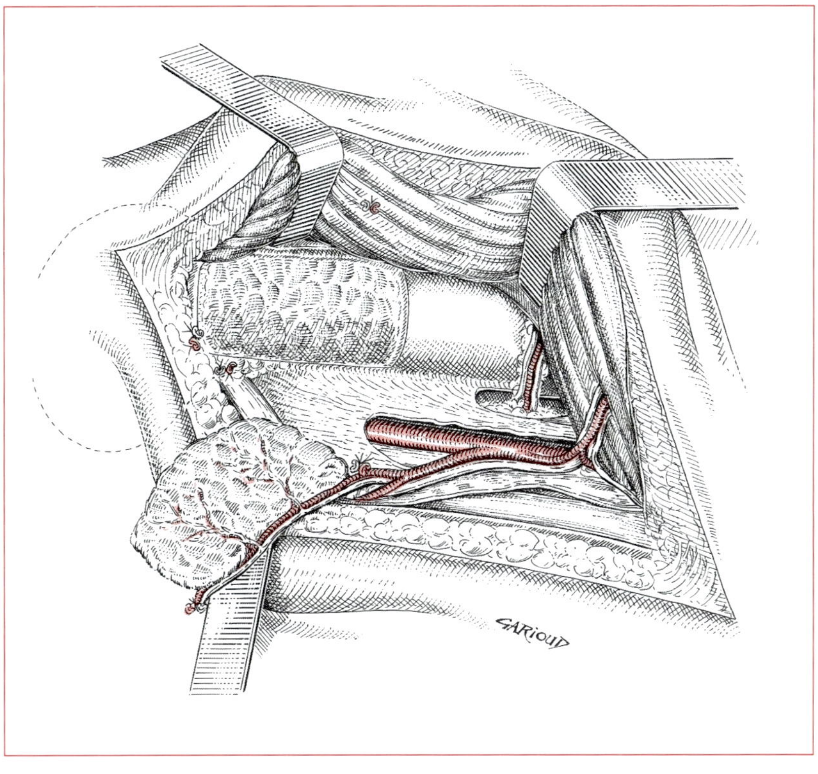
GARIOUD

e

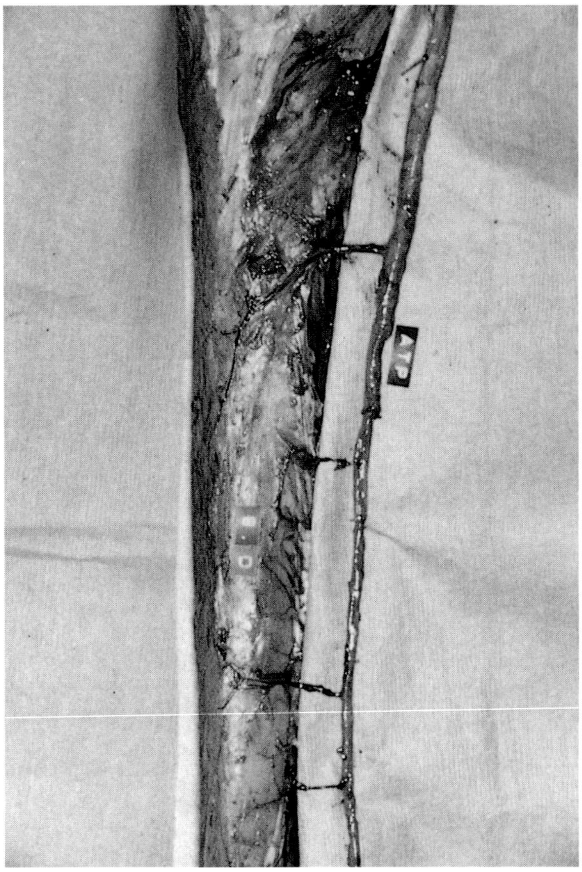

Fig. 48 *Blood supply to the periosteum of the tibia (C V Penteado et al 1990).*

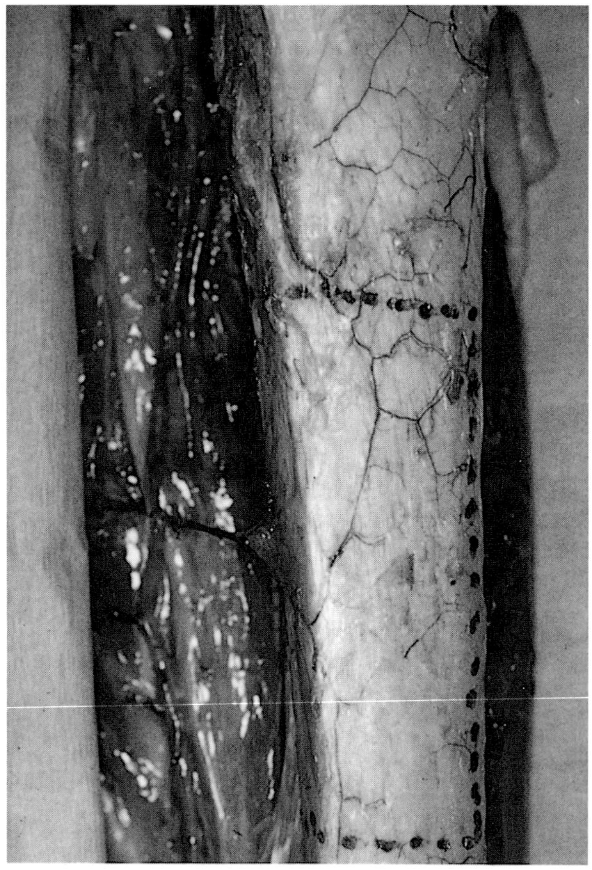

Fig. 49 *Theoretic possibility of raising a limited periosteal flap from the tibia (C V Penteado et al 1990).*

of the adductor magnus muscle. The articular branch is often included in a fibrous tunnel, which should be incised to expose the origin of the descending genicular artery. (*d*) The metaphyseal region of the femur is exposed. The vascular pattern of the area is identified. The anastomosis of the articular branch with the proximomedial collateral artery is ligated and severed. When it is not included, the muscles about the knee should be sharply released to expose the underlying periosteum. Small arterioles should be diathermied. The periosteal flap is outlined on the femur and the periosteum is incised with a knife. Small pieces of cortical bone remaining attached to the flap are raised with a sharp curved chisel. (*e*) The flap is raised. Its size is about 10 × 5 cm. It can be modeled according to the indications of the recipient site. The saphenous artery and the muscular branch to the vastus medialis should be ligated anteriorly to raise the pedicle. The arc of rotation of the pedicle allows the flap to cover the middle third of the medial aspect of the femur.

We used this flap as a free flap; the caliber of the vessels (1.5–2 mm) is sufficient for microsurgical anastomosis. Blood supply is reliable, and the flap is supple enough to be tubulized. Reconstruction of long bone defects about 10 cm in length can be performed with this flap in association with cancellous bone graft.

Tibia

The periosteum of the tibia is nourished by multiple arterioles issuing from the anterior and the posterior tibial arteries, but mainly by the anterior tibial artery (Baselga 1986; Penteado et al 1990; Crock and Morrison 1992; Fig. 48).

Long periosteal flaps can be raised from the lateral aspect of the tibia and isolated on the anterior tibial artery. However, the sacrifice of the anterior tibial artery is prejudicial to the vascularization of the muscles of the anterior compartment of the leg, and the tibia cannot be considered as a potential donor site for a free periosteal flap.

On the other hand, the numerous arterioles allow the raising of limited rotational periosteal flaps while preserving the integrity of the main vascular axis (Fig. 49).

The periosteum of the lateral aspect of the lower fourth of the tibia may be raised either on the lateral malleolar artery or by retrograde flow on the ramus perforans of the peroneal artery, in order to cover the medial aspect of the lower tibia.

These two arteries are of small caliber, and unsuitable for transfers with microsurgical anastomoses.

Clinical experience and results

Since 1985 we have operated on 19 patients. Our first impression is that indications are limited, and it is necessary to be very selective. In our opinion it is not worthwhile to treat an ordinary post-traumatic long bone nonunion by a vascularized cortico-periosteal graft.

Our series and their results have shown both the limits to and well-founded indications for this procedure.

The patients have been distributed amongst four pathologies:

- long bone reconstruction;
- post-traumatic recalcitrant nonunion;
- congenital pseudarthrosis; and
- cranioplasties.

Long bone reconstruction

This short series concerns three children (one of 12 and two of 13 years) who presented with long bone defect of the ulna. The defects were of between 8 and 10 cm.

In the three cases we used a free thin cortico-periosteal vascularized flap from the femur as described above.

The flap was filled up with autologous cancellous bone graft and revascularized at the recipient site.

In two cases bone healing was achieved in less than 3 months (Fig. 50). In the other case bone formation was impaired, probably by occlusion of the vessels of the flap owing to postoperative compression of the limb.

Bone reconstruction of the upper limb is a good indication for vascularized periosteal flap in children and when the recipient bed is poorly vascularized.

This procedure is an alternative to vascularized fibula transfer, which cannot be carried out without risk in regard to ankle function.

Post-traumatic recalcitrant nonunions

Five patients have been operated on, and the long bones concerned were femur, humerus, and tibia. Four patients had had several previous conventional bone grafts without success, and their nonunions were considered as recalcitrant.

Femur

Two nonunions of the middle third of the femur were treated by a proximally based pedicled flap from the distal third associated with cancellous bone graft (Fig. 51).

One case of nonhealed arthrodesis of the hip was treated by a pedicled musculoperiosteal flap from the inner aspect of the iliac bone.

These three cases healed in 4 months or less.

Humerus

One patient presented with a post-traumatic nonunion of the proximal third of the humerus. No previous conventional bone graft had been attempted. Bone healing was achieved in less than 3 months with a proximally based pedicled periosteal flap from the lower humerus associated with a cancellous graft.

Tibia

One case of pseudarthrosis and necrosis of the tibial tuberosity resulting from a Maquet's procedure was treated by a distally based pedicled flap from the lower femur as described by Hertel and Masquelet (1989). Healing was achieved 3 months later.

We believe that recalcitrant bone nonunion is a good indication for use of a musculoperiosteal flap

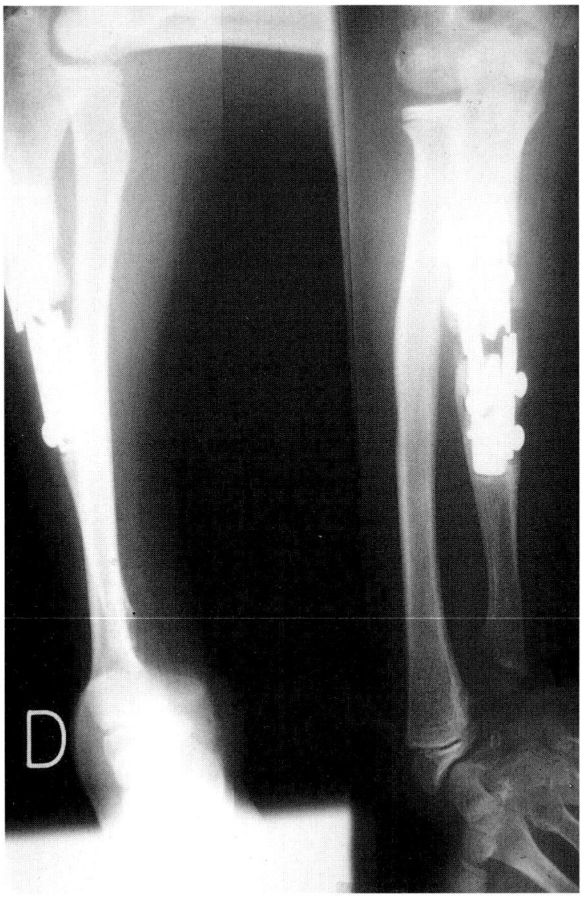

a

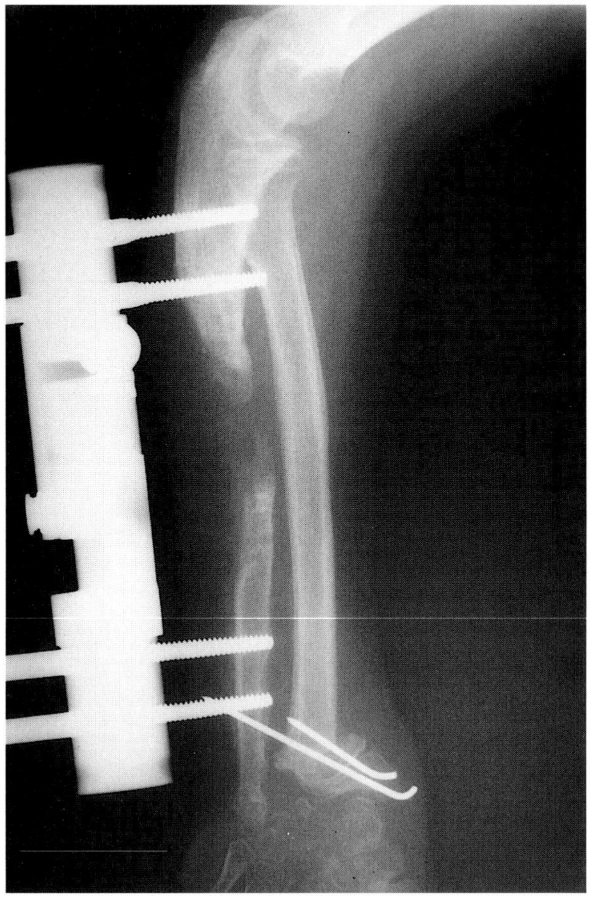

b

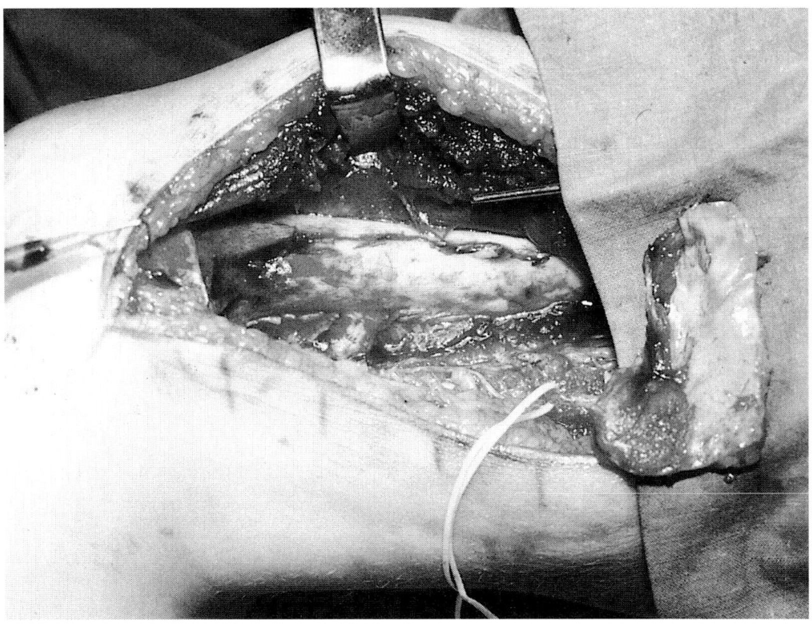

c

Fig. 50 *Reconstruction of the ulna following a failure of lengthening of the bone.*
(a) Radiologic aspect
(b) The bone extremities are excised. The distal end of the radius is osteotomized and the ulna is stabilized by an external device.
(c) The bone defect is repaired by a tubulized corticoperiosteal flap raised from the lower third of the femur. The tube is filled up with cancellous bone graft. Microvascular anastomoses are performed on the recipient site.
(d) Radiological aspect 3 months later
(e) and (f) Clinical result.

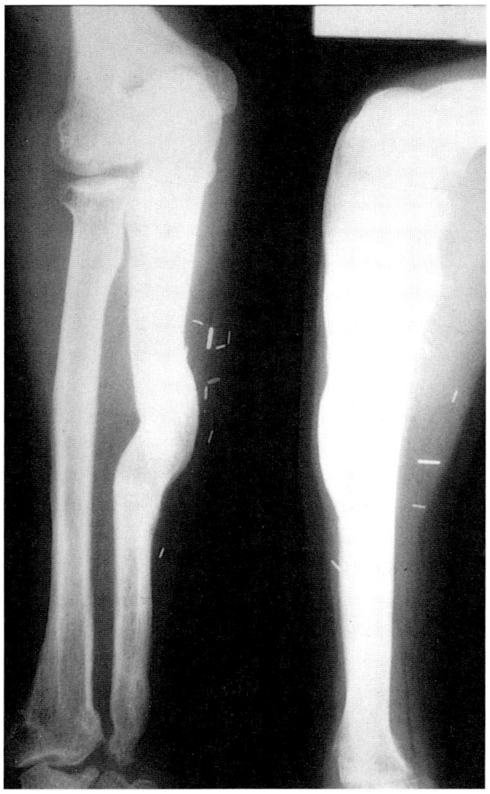

d

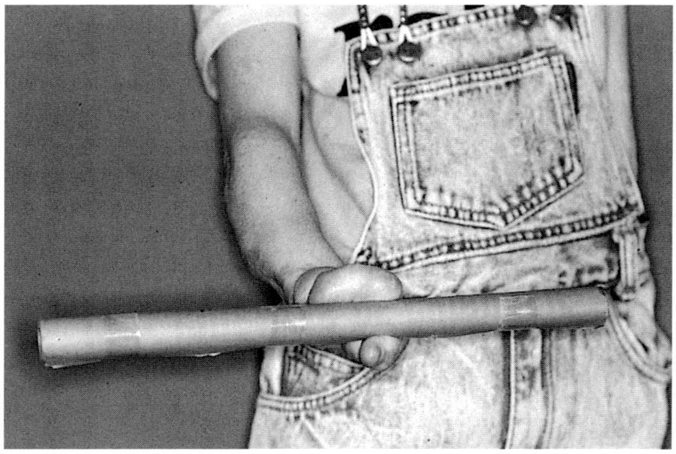

e

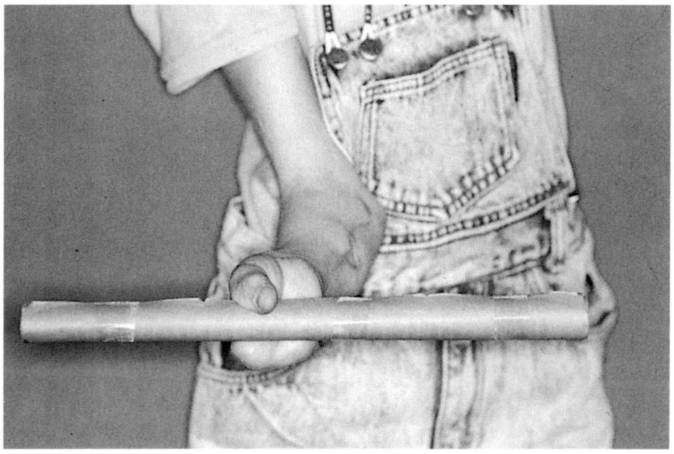

f

Fig. 50 *continued*
(d) Radiologic aspect 3 months later
(e) and (f) Clinical result.

wrapped around cancellous graft. This procedure should be reserved for cases that have previously been treated unsuccessfully by conventional procedures.

Congenital pseudarthrosis of the long bones

The treatment of congenital pseudarthrosis is always a challenge. Recently advances have been recorded with the use of fibula transfer or the Ilizarov method.

We have attempted to treat this regional disease by excising the dystrophic area and repairing the defect with a tube of vascularized periosteum filled up with cancellous bone.

Fibula

Three cases of pseudarthrosis of the lower fibula were treated.

The flap was raised from the ipsilateral tibia, pedicled on the anterior tibial artery, without interrupting the continuity of the vascular axis. One case was a complete failure. In the other two other cases, reconstruction and bone healing were achieved in less than 3 months, but a recurrent pseudarthrosis occurred at the distal part of the reconstruction 18 months later.

Tibia

One case of pseudarthrosis of the tibia was treated with a distally based pedicle flap. The flap was raised on the proximal tibia, in an area that was judged to be free of disease. The flap was distally pedicled on the anterior tibial artery after ligature of the proximal portion of the artery. This case was a complete failure, and was reoperated on with the Ilizarov method.

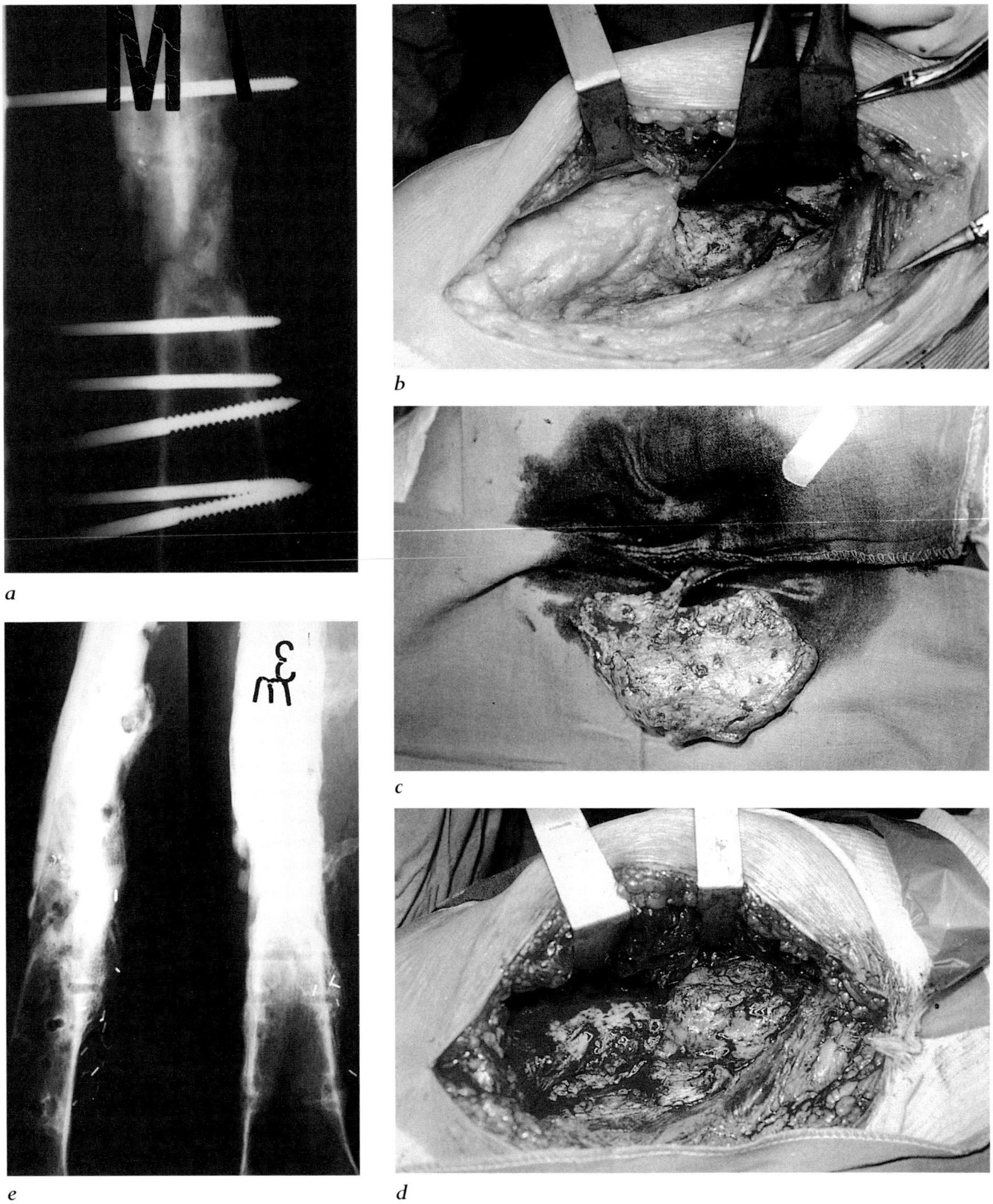

Fig. 51 *Atrophic nonunion of the mid-shaft of the femur, which has previously been treated by several conventional bone grafts.*
(a) X-ray tomography
(b) Preoperative aspect (medial approach)
(c) Musculoperiosteal flap raised from the lower third of the femur and pedicled on the descending genicular artery.
(d) The flap is wrapped around the site of the nonunion. The bony space has been filled up with cancellous bone graft.
(e) Radiologic aspect 3 months later. The bone is well healed.

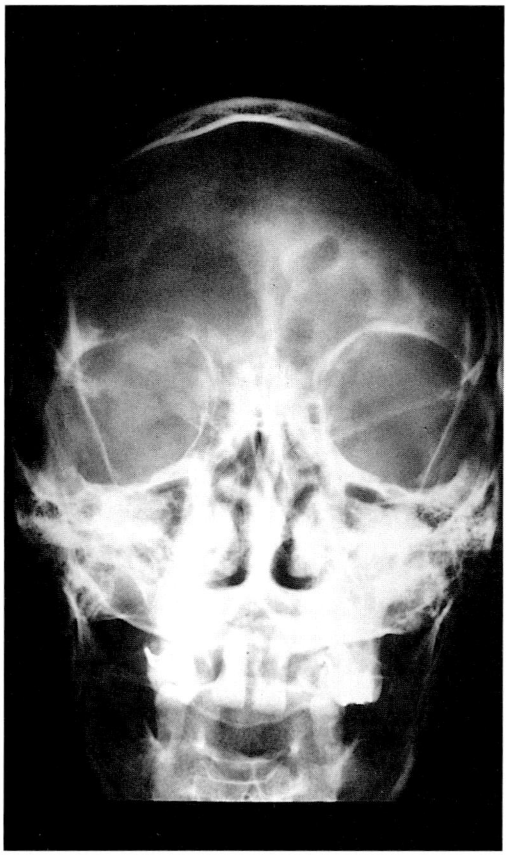

a

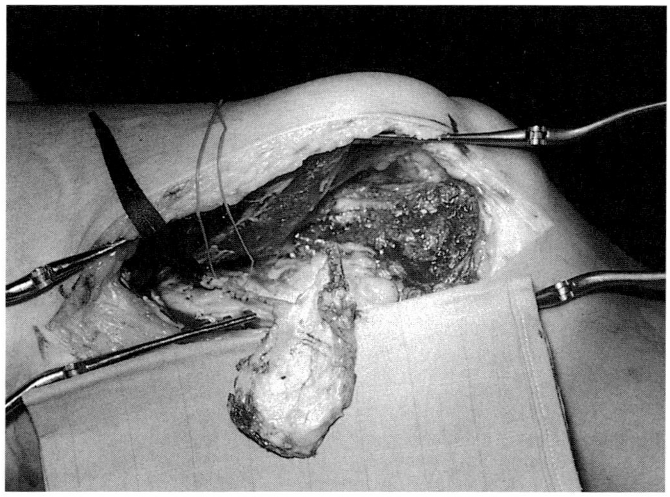

b

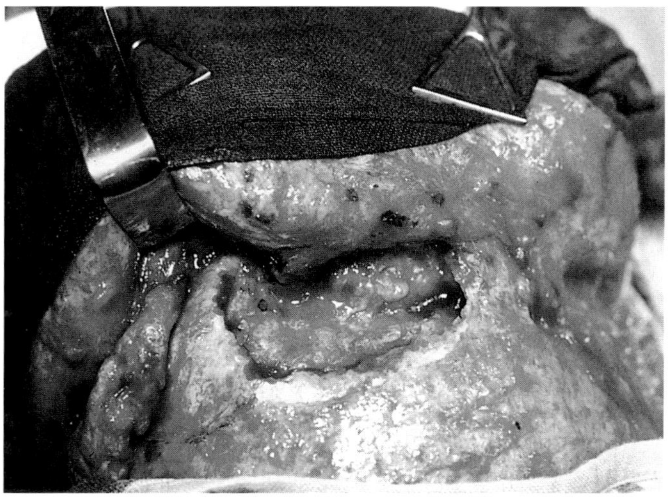

c

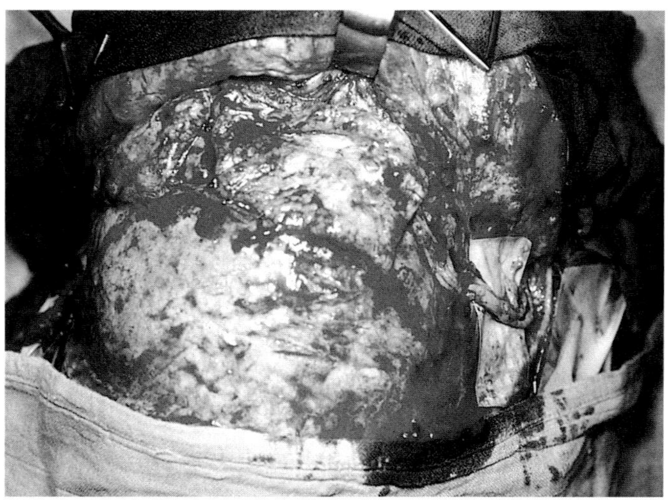

d

Fig. *52 Defect of the frontal bone.*
(a) The patient has been operated on several times. Failures of the surgical attempts were due to recurrent infection.
(b) Elevation of a thin corticoperiosteal flap on the descending genicular artery.
(c) Peroperative aspect of the skull defect.
(d) The flap on the recipient site. Microvascular anastomoses are performed with the temporal vessels (a vein graft was needed).

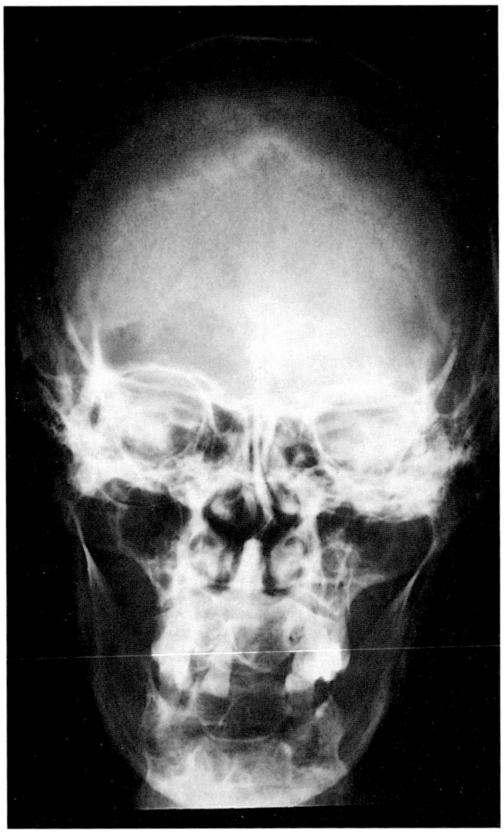

e

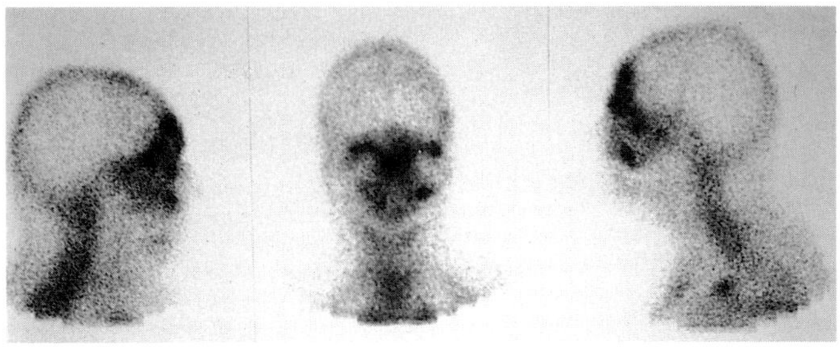

f

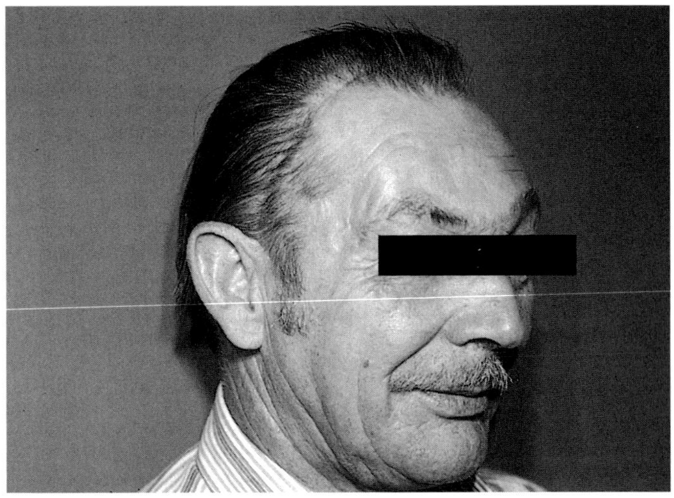

g

***Fig.** 52 continued*
(e) Postoperative radiographic control 3 months later.
(f) Good viability of the transfer assessed by bone scanning 3 months later.
(g) Clinical aspect. No recurrent infection 3 years later.

Radius
One case of pseudarthrosis of the radius was treated by the same procedure. The flap was raised on the lower femur and revascularized at the recipient site. Reconstruction and bone healing were achieved in 3 months, but follow-up is only of 10 months' duration.

Results were disappointing. Several points should be emphasized in this specific frame of pathology. In the reconstruction of the fibula the failure was due to a recurrence of the pseudarthrosis at the lower extremity of the reconstruction.

This final outcome should be compared to the results obtained with vascularized fibula transfers. While the same final issue was noted in several cases, the pseudarthrosis of the tibia was a complete failure, and we believe that a periosteal flap should not be raised on the ipsilateral tibia, because congenital pseudarthrosis is a local disease that probably involves the periosteum.

Cranioplasties
The management of large skull defects is difficult, and often complicated by the proximity of the sinus cavities of the frontal bone, which can be responsible for recurrent infections.

Classic materials (polymerized resins, metallic prostheses, nonvascularized bone) have to be removed in cases of chronic infections.

In six cases of post-traumatic defects of the frontal or temporal bone that had been previously treated by classic procedures without success we used a free revascularized thin corticoperiosteal flap from the lower femur (Lapierre et al 1990; Masquelet et al 1989; Fig. 52).

In all cases, bone healing was obtained in less than 3 months, and the long-term viability of the osteoperiosteal flap was assessed by bone scanning. The final cosmetic and functional result was good in all cases, and no recurrent infection was noted (follow-up: 1.5–5.0 years).

Cranioplasties that have been unsuccessfully treated by other procedures are probably one of the best indications for the use of a free osteoperiosteal flap from the femur.

The flap is very supple and can be matched to the defect. The vessels are anastomosed to the temporal vessels.

11. Surgical techniques: recipient sites and mandibular reconstruction

A. TIBIA

Most often vascularized bone transfer to the tibia is carried out for the purpose of reconstructing a diaphyseal defect. Occasionally onlay vascularized bone transfer is done for special cases of persistent nonunion without a substantial bone defect. At times distal tibia to talus or calcaneus reconstruction may be necessary for reconstructions of distal tibial defects associated with ankle joint destruction. These three recipient site situations differ in approach and will be discussed separately.

Tibial diaphyseal defect

Often the patient requiring tibial diaphyseal reconstruction has an associated anterior or anteromedial wound or soft tissue defect as a result of prior surgery or trauma. However, if this is not the case, the tibial defect should be exposed by an anteromedial incision. This will allow ample access to the proximal and distal tibial remnants. For this exposure, assuming the contralateral fibula or iliac crest is the donor site, the patient is most easily positioned in the semilateral decubitus position with a soft roll under the opposite buttock. If the ipsilateral fibula or iliac crest is chosen as the donor site, a standard supine position is best. Either the anterior tibial or posterior tibial vessels may be selected as the recipient vessels. The anterior tibial vessels are conveniently located for end-to-end anastomosis when the surgeon is dealing with a relatively pristine soft tissue bed or fresh defect. However, in patients with a chronic and fibrotic defect, as is typical in patients with osteomyelitis, the anterior tibial vessels are either extensively damaged or heavily embedded in scar tissue, which may preclude their use as recipient vessels. Because of this, frequently the posterior tibial artery and the accompanying veins are the recipient vessels of choice. Even in heavily scarred wounds, the posterior tibial vessels are separated from the tibia by a layer of muscle tissue, which in most patients protects the vessels from regional fibrosis. The posterior tibial vessels are most easily exposed by mobilizing the soleus muscle in a posterior direction from the medial aspect. If the posterior tibial artery is selected as the recipient vessel end-to-side anastomosis is advised. This is particularly true in patients known to have disruption or injury to the anterior tibial artery. The venous anastomoses may be end-to-end to either the accompanying posterior tibial venae comitantes or to the saphenous vein. Regardless of the selection of recipient vessels, the most ideal placement of bone graft should be in line with the long axis of the bone (Fig. 1; Chapter 13 Fig. 2). In most patients the fibula is selected in preference to the iliac crest because of its linear diaphyseal configuration, which lends itself well to intramedullary bone placement. Specific techniques of bone fixation will be discussed in the next section. Whenever possible the osteosynthesis site between the proximal and distal tibial ends and the transferred bone segment should be augmented by a cocoon of iliac cancellous bone autograft (DeBoer et al 1990).

Postoperatively, rigid immobilization by using either a cast or an external fixator and strict

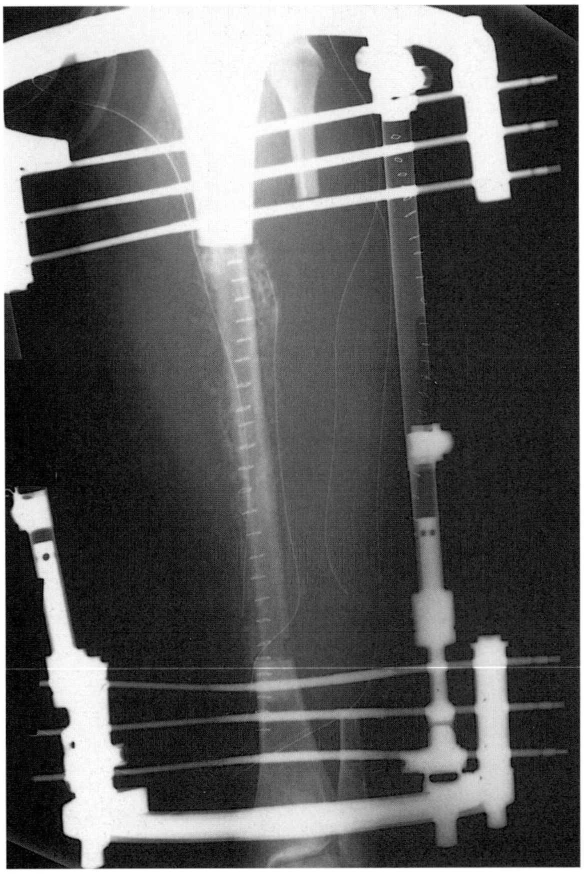

Fig. 1 *Note the placement of the fibular bone graft in line with the tibial axis for reconstruction of a tibial diaphyseal defect. For maximal bone surface contact intramedullary placement within the tibia is preferred.*

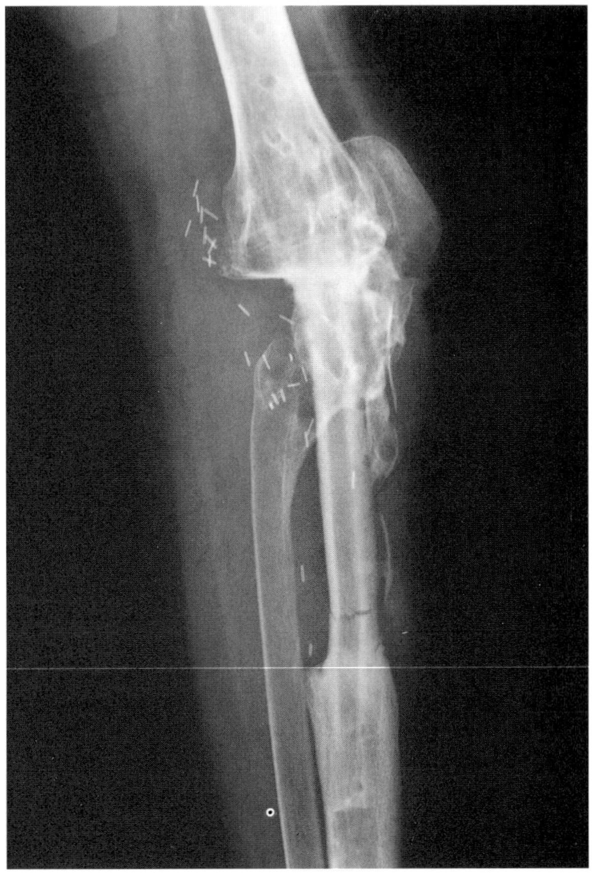

Fig. 2 *AP radiograph of the tibia, illustrating union at both ends of the transferred fibula but at a stage prior to sufficient fibular hypertrophy for unprotected weightbearing.*

nonweightbearing is recommended, until union with radiographic confirmation is present at both bone ends. On average, this requires about 3 months (Fig. 2). When union at both ends of the transferred bone segment is confirmed, the patient may progress to partial weightbearing using either a patellar tendon bearing cast or orthosis. This should be continued until adequate hypertrophy and remodeling of the bone occurs, which may require a period of an additional 3 to 9 months (Fig. 3). If union is not achieved by 6 months following surgery, further iliac bone autografting of the nonunion site with stable internal fixation using a compression plate is advised.

Onlay use of vascularized bone graft

The use of a vascularized bone graft as an onlay graft to the tibia is indicated for extraordinary nonunions of the tibia. Most commonly this situation exists in patients without a bone defect, but with a tibial nonunion that is unlikely to heal with a nonvascularized bone autograft. This may be seen in patients with fracture-related postradiation osteonecrosis (Rock and Wood 1991), or nonunion of a large diaphyseal allograft (Clinkscales et al 1991), or in select cases of tibial nonunion that has failed to heal with prior autografting and/or electrical stimulation. For onlay application the ipsilateral fibula is utilized as a graft immobilized on the peroneal arteriovenous pedicle

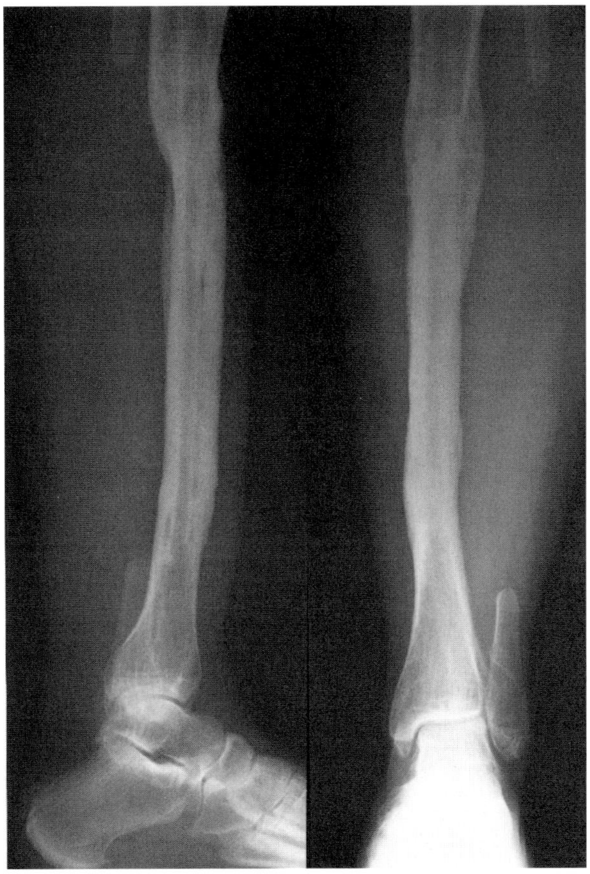

Fig. 3 *AP radiograph of the tibia, illustrating sufficient hypertrophy of the transferred fibula to permit unprotected weightbearing (8.5 months postoperative).*

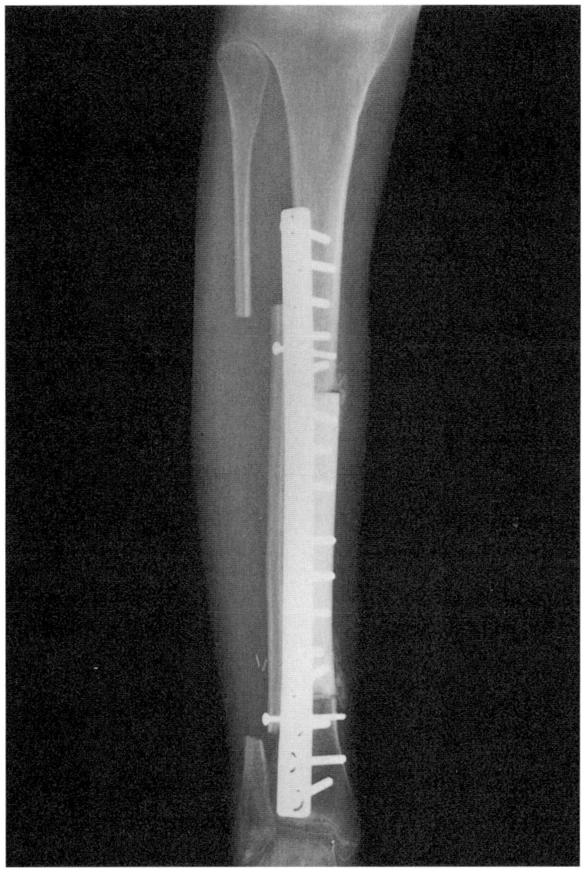

Fig. 4 *Nonunion of a tibial diaphyseal allograft treated only by an ipsilateral pedicled fibular graft – immediate postoperative radiograph. Note that the fibula segment spans the host bone from proximal to distal.*

(Fig. 4). For this procedure, the patient should be placed in a semilateral position with a soft roll under the ipsilateral buttock. A lateral incision over the fibula extending from the fibular neck to a point about 5 cm proximal to the lateral malleolus is made. This incision is used both to isolate the required length of fibula and to gain access to the lateral aspect of the tibial nonunion site. The length of fibula to be isolated is somewhat arbitrary, but typically should include at least 5 cm both distal and proximal to the tibial nonunion site. This length of fibula is isolated precisely as is required for free fibula isolation, but, in most cases, does not require ligation of the distal peroneal artery and vein. After complete isolation of the desired length of fibula, the lateral aspect of the tibia is easily exposed by anterior retraction of the peroneal muscles and muscles of the anterior compartment of the leg. The lateral surface of the tibia for a length that corresponds to that of the isolated fibula segment is subperiosteally exposed. The periosteum over the anterior lateral surface of the fibula segment is similarly elevated. The fibula is then rotated and shifted in a medial direction so as to oppose the exposed bony surfaces of the tibia and fibula respectively. Fixation is accomplished by a bone screw passing from the fibula through both cortices of the tibia at both the proximal and distal ends. The fibula screw holes should be over-drilled in order to

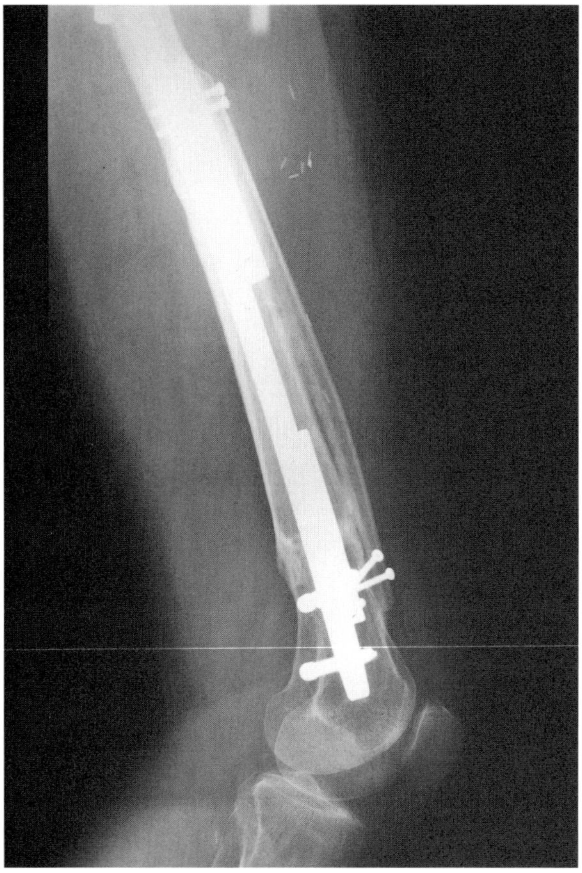

Fig. 5 *Radiograph demonstrating unequivocal evidence of union between fibula and femur when used as an onlay graft. Note the confluence of new bone formation between fibula end and adjacent bone.*

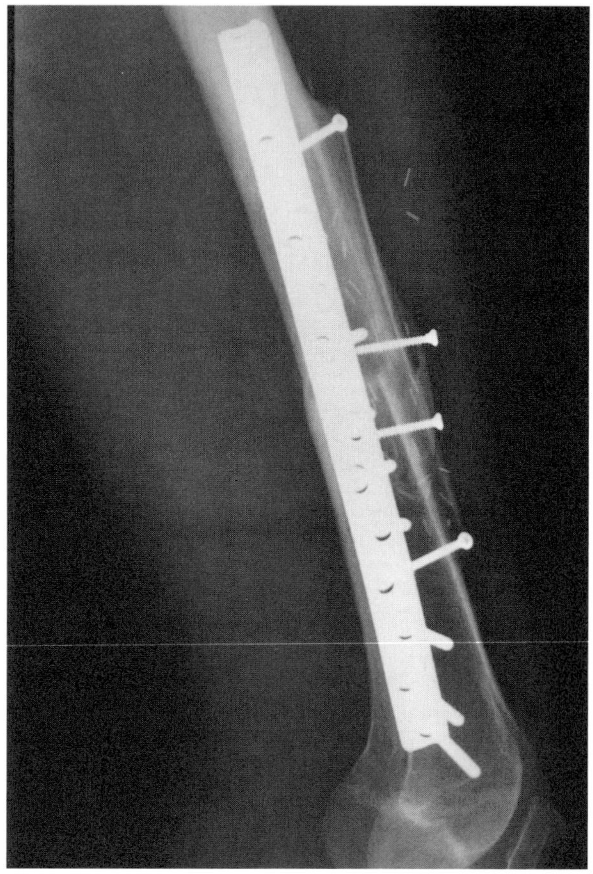

Fig. 6 *Radiograph demonstrating the union of fibula to femur; note the appearance of uninterrupted bone between the fibula segment and the femur.*

provide a lag screw effect and avoid the risk of bone surface distraction.

Postoperatively, nonweightbearing cast immobilization should be continued for at least 3 months. Progression to partial weightbearing in a patellar tendon bearing cast or orthosis may be initiated thereafter, provided there are radiographic signs of progression to union. This may be difficult to judge in such constructs. A definite sign is the radiographic evidence of bone confluence between the fibula end and the adjacent tibia, much like flowing wax or viscous fluid (Fig. 5). Full weightbearing in a cast or orthosis may be permitted after 6 weeks' partial weightbearing provided there are no clinical or radiographic signs of fracture instability. One may see progressive obliteration of space between the opposing fibular and tibial surfaces (Fig. 6). Some protection should be continued during full weightbearing until the original tibial nonunion site demonstrates radiographic evidence of union.

Distal tibial–ankle fusion reconstructions

If the distal tibia articular surface is destroyed in association with a defect of the distal tibia, reconstruction of the bony deficiency and either tibiotalar or tibiocalcaneal fusion is required. In most such instances, there is an associated skin defect. Thus a compound flap including soft tissue is either

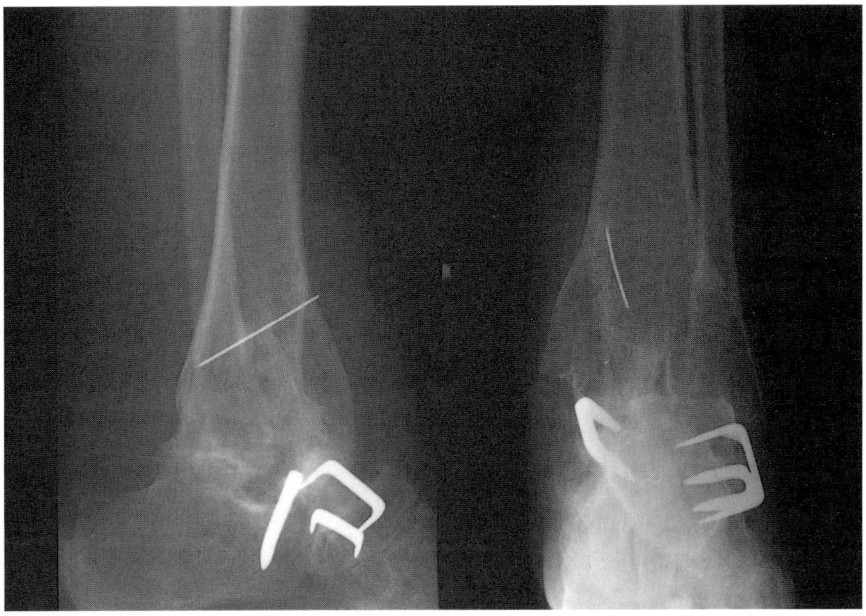

Fig. 7 *Lateral radiograph demonstrating tibiotalar fusion following reconstruction by transfer of vascularized iliac crest segment.*

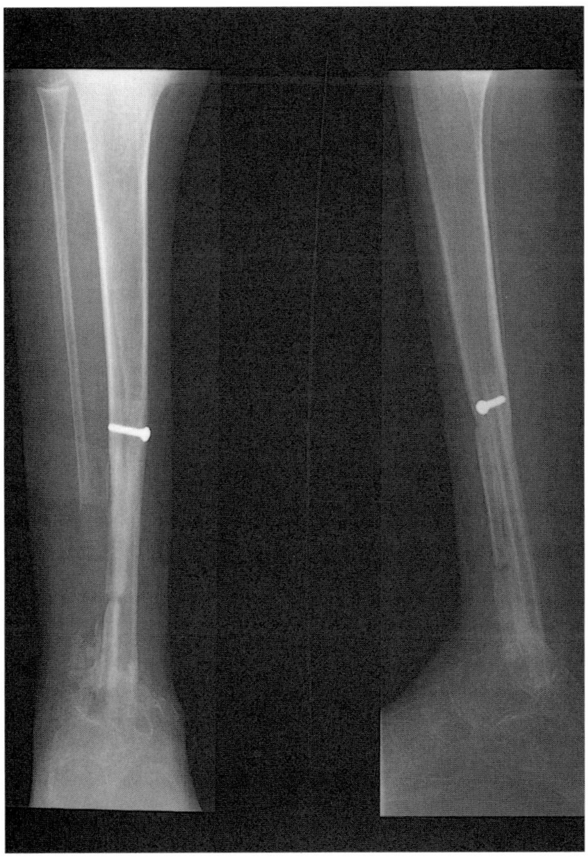

Fig. 8 *AP and lateral radiographs demonstrating tibiotalar fusion following reconstruction by transfer of vascularized fibula segment.*

necessary or preferred. Depending upon the length and size of both bone and soft tissue loss, either an osteocutaneous iliac crest (Fig. 7) (based on the deep circumflex iliac artery) or fibula (Fig. 8) may be useful.

The patient should be positioned either supine or semilateral, with the involved limb down. If an open wound is not already present, exposure of the ankle and distal tibia is gained by direct anterior incision. If an open wound already exists, the exposure should utilize it. The proximal tibial end should be exposed subperiosteally. Distally, the dome of the talus (or calcaneus if the talus is absent) should be exposed and debrided of articular cartilage to the cancellous bone lying deep to the subchondral bone surface. The posterior tibial artery and accompanying veins are preferentially used. In most patients the anterior tibial vessels are either damaged, absent, or heavily embedded in scar tissue. The posterior tibial artery and veins are exposed in either the proximal aspect of the wound by a posteromedial incision directly over their course or by extending the defect wound in a proximal and posteromedial direction. Because many patients with distal tibial destruction have only a posterior tibial artery blood supply to the foot, end-to-side arterial anastomosis should be planned. Venous anastomosis may be either end-to-end or end-to-side. Bone placement should be intramedullary within the tibia, whether using fibula or iliac crest as the donor bone. Distal coaptation to talus or calcaneus should aim for maximal bone-to-bone contact. When using iliac crest this is achieved by shaping the iliac bone segment to the size and shape of the talar dome. For a fibula, a hole in the talar done down to but not through the subtalar joint is made to permit the doweling of the fibula into the talus. Fixation should be carried out by whatever means will provide stability for the particular situation. Usually an external fixator is indicated. Proximally, intramedullary placement with a transcortical screw fixation across tibia and transferred bone segment is usually appropriate. Distal fixation for fibula transfer can be achieved by a screw across the talus which engages the distal end of the transferred fibula. If iliac crest is used, placement of cerclage wires through the talus and iliac crest is appropriate. If tibial–calcaneal fusion is carried out, distal fixation may be accomplished by one or multiple Steinmann pins passed through the heel pad and into the iliac bone segment. Aftercare is essentially the same as that described earlier in the chapter following reconstruction of a tibial diaphyseal defect.

B. FEMUR

Recipient site techniques for the femur may be broadly divided into those involving femoral shaft reconstruction and those involving distal femur replacement with knee arthrodesis. The latter technique is most often required in patients with resection of malignant lesions of the distal femur or in patients undergoing limb salvage by knee fusion for an infected knee joint endoprosthesis. The extent of the complexities and difficulties encountered in the course of femoral reconstruction is somewhat dependent upon the degree of the patient's obesity. For either technique of femur reconstruction the patient should be positioned supine. The ipsilateral fibula should be selected as the donor bone unless it is absent or damaged, in which case the opposite fibula can be utilized. The iliac crest is recommended only in those patients who have a femoral defect largely confined to the distal metaphysis or in those patients lacking a fibula donor site option.

Femoral shaft reconstruction

For patients undergoing femoral shaft reconstruction, usually a two-incision technique is recommended. A lateral incision should be used for exposure of the femoral defect. Through this incision preparation of the femoral defect, fibular placement, and internal fixation are most easily accomplished. The proximal and distal ends of the femur should be exposed sufficiently to define the cortical circumference and intramedullary canal. At least a portion of the surface of the proximal and distal femoral ends should be exposed subperiosteally for a sufficient length to allow placement of internal fixation hardware. Scar tissue interposed between the two bone ends within the femoral defect should be sharply excised, so that the transferred bone segment may be easily placed within the defect.

Following preparation of the recipient bed a medial incision overlying the course of the sartorius muscle is made (Wood 1990b). This incision may be localized along an axis that runs between the anterior superior iliac spine and the adductor tubercle of the femur, and is carried through subcutaneous tissue to the fascia overlying the sartorius muscle. Posteriorly the greater saphenous vein is identified within the subcutaneous tissue as a possible recipient vein site. Whether it is used or not is dependent upon the size and quality of the veins accompanying the femoral artery. Therefore, once identified, the greater saphenous vein should be tagged with an elastic loop, but not transected distally until a decision is made to use it. The sartorius fascia is then incised and the muscle reflected posteriorly, exposing Hunter's canal and its contents – femoral artery, veins and the saphenous nerve. The femoral artery and one or two accompanying veins are then isolated over a 3- to 4-cm length. This process may require ligation and sectioning of some arterial branches and venous tributaries from the femoral vessels. Once the vessels are isolated, the soft tissue interposed between them and the femoral defect is incised over a length sufficient to pass two or three fingers between the medial and lateral wounds. If the accompanying femoral veins are not ideal for anastomosis, the greater saphenous vein previously isolated along the length of the medial incision should be ligated distally and sectioned. The fibula, once isolated, is exposed subperiosteally at

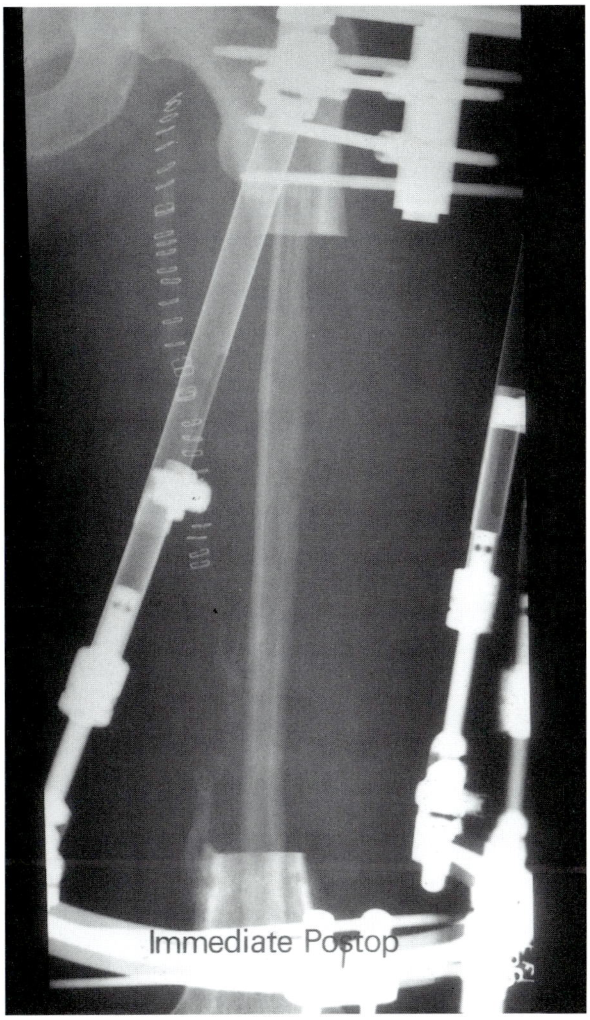

Fig. 9 *AP radiograph illustrating fibula segment placed within femoral intramedullary canal for diaphyseal reconstruction.*

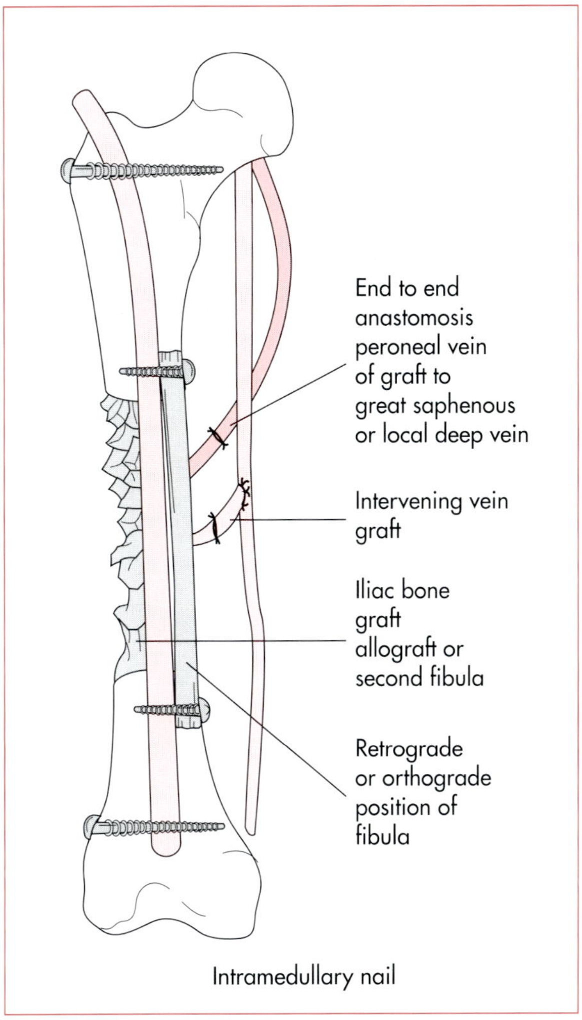

Fig. 10 *Schematic drawing illustrating fibula placement as an onlay graft adjacent to an intramedullary nail used for stabilization (from MB Wood: Atlas of Reconstructive Microsurgery (Wood 1990a)).*

both ends, and then placed into the distal and proximal femoral intramedullary canal through the lateral incision (Fig. 9; Chapter 13 Fig. 8). Some reaming of the femoral intramedullary canal using a power burr may be necessary.

If intramedullary nail fixation of the femur is elected then the fibular segment should be placed between the proximal and distal femoral remnants by an inlay technique, using a power burr to create a trough along the anteromedial aspect of the femur (Chapter 13 Fig. 6). Fixation of the fibula either within the medullary canal or as an inlay graft should be accomplished by use of a single transcortical screw at each end (Fig. 10). This step may be eliminated if a compression plate is used (to be discussed). After fixation the pedicle is manually passed in a medial direction through the soft tissue channel previously developed. End-to-side anastomosis between the peroneal arterial pedicle of the fibula and the femoral artery is carried out. Either end-to-side or end-to-end anastomosis of one or more veins from the fibula either to veins accompanying the femoral artery or to the greater saphenous vein is recommended. Whenever possible, additional cancellous iliac

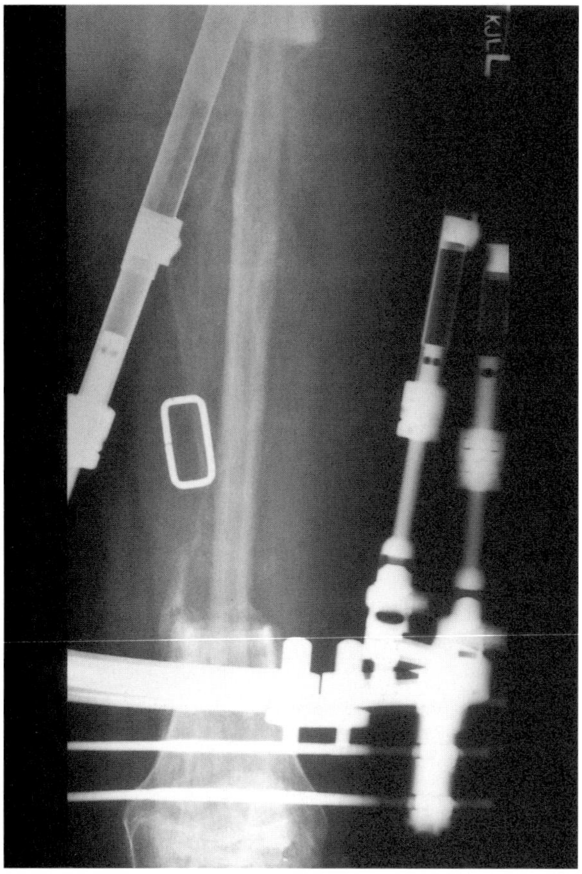

Fig. 11 *AP radiograph illustrating union between the fibula and the distal femur 3 months postoperatively, but with insufficient hypertrophy to permit full unrestricted weightbearing.*

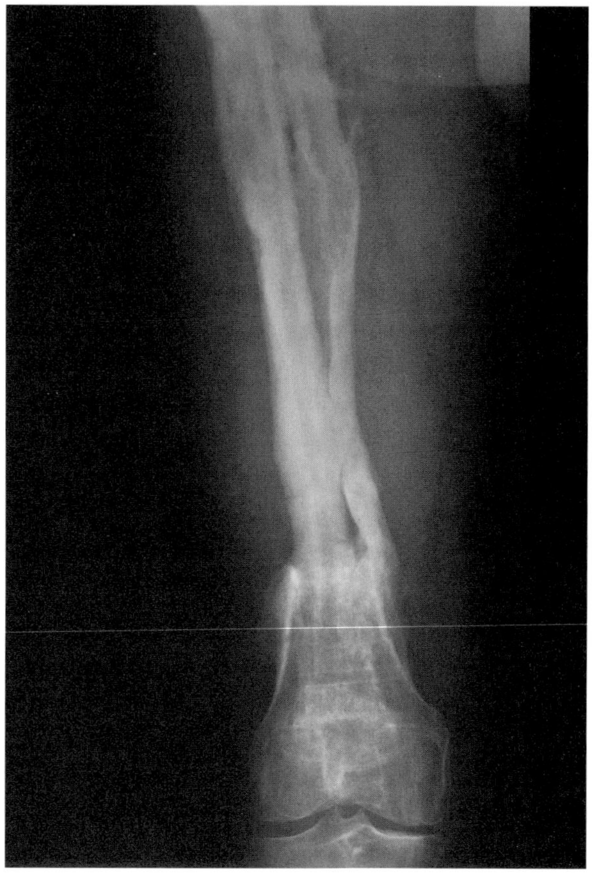

Fig. 12 *AP radiograph of the patient depicted in Fig. 11, demonstrating the development of hypertrophy of the transferred fibula segment by 11 months postoperatively adequate to permit full weightbearing.*

autograft should be placed about both proximal and distal osteosynthesis sites and along the shaft of the transferred fibula if sufficient material is available. Suction drains should be placed in the depths of both the medial and lateral wounds, and a layered subcutaneous tissue and skin closure should be accomplished using a technique of surgeon's preference. If stable internal fixation is not achieved, or if a biplanar external fixator is not used, the use of a hip spica cast and strict nonweightbearing for 3 months is advisable. Nonweightbearing should be continued

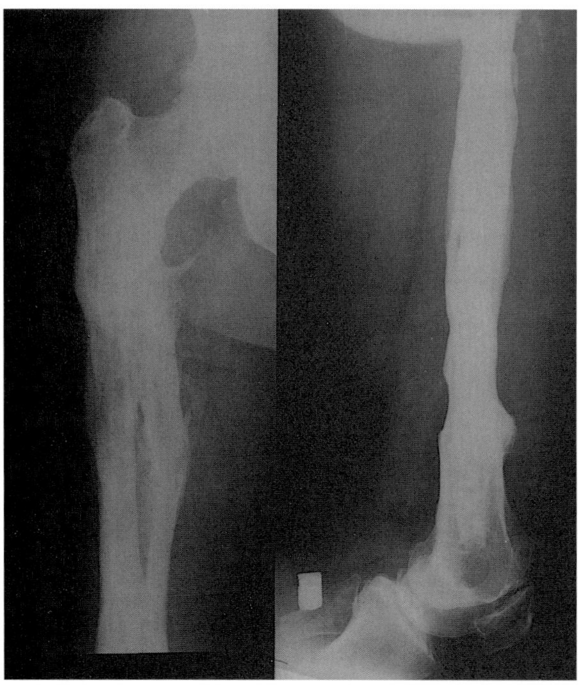

Fig. 13 *AP radiograph of the patient depicted in Figs 11 and 12, illustrating the healing of the femoral construct 7 years postoperatively.*

until there is radiographic evidence of union at both ends of the transferred fibula (Fig. 11). This may require as long as 6 months. Once union occurs, partial weightbearing, progressing to full weightbearing depending on the rate of fibular hypertrophy, may be initiated (Figs 12, 13). At times a hip spica cast with foot and ankle free is used to facilitate full weightbearing if the rate of bone hypertrophy is slow. On average, return to full activity, including complete weightbearing without support, requires 17 months (Han et al 1992). If bone union is not achieved in the 6 months following surgery, further bone grafting using iliac autograft at the nonunion site, possibly with application of a compression plate, is advised (Figs 14, 15).

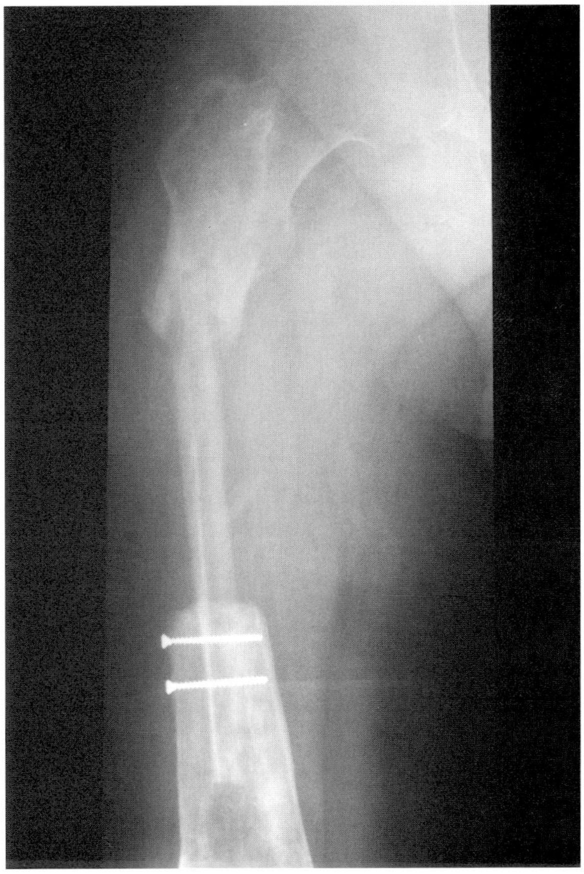

Fig. 14 *AP radiograph of a femur reconstructed by vascularized fibula transfer, seen 6 months postoperatively. Note the obvious nonunion proximally.*

Distal femur reconstruction with knee arthrodesis

A femoral defect in conjunction with loss or destruction of the knee articular surface is most easily managed by the use of the ipsilateral fibula rotated proximally on its intact vascular pedicle. The turned up fibula may be used as a single or double construct (Fig. 16), depending upon the defect length. If a double fibula construct is employed care is necessary to avoid injury to the nutrient artery when osteotomizing the bone. One segment should contain the nutrient artery (endosteal blood supply) and the second should be based on a thick periosteal and soft tissue pedicle. If the femoral defect extends more proximally than the metaphyseal flare and includes loss of more than 10 cm of distal femur, it may be difficult to make up more length with a pedicled fibula turn-up. In such a case free microvascular transfer is recommended. An anterior or anteromedial incision is used to expose the distal femur and the proximal tibial remnant. Usually this incision will already be present as a result of prior tumor excision or infected knee endoprosthesis removal. The fibula is exposed through a lateral incision and isolated in a manner identical to that previously described for free

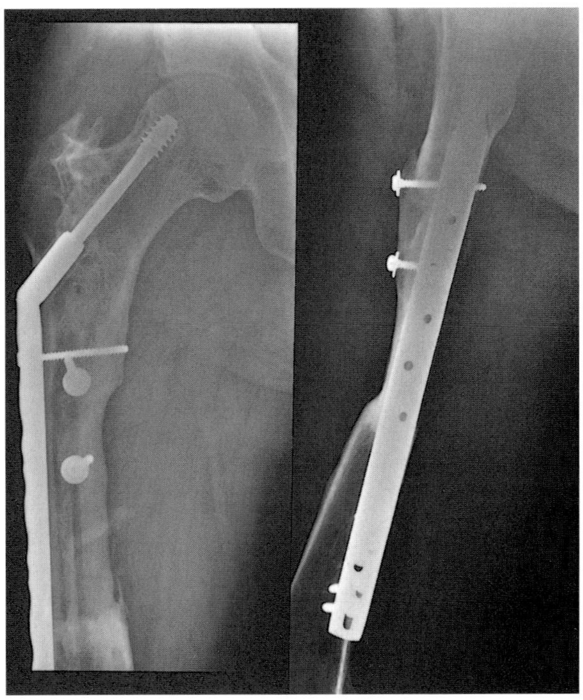

Fig. 15 *AP radiograph of the femur depicted in Fig. 14 3 years following readjustment at 6 months after fibula transfer by internal fixation and onlay cortico-cancellous iliac autograft.*

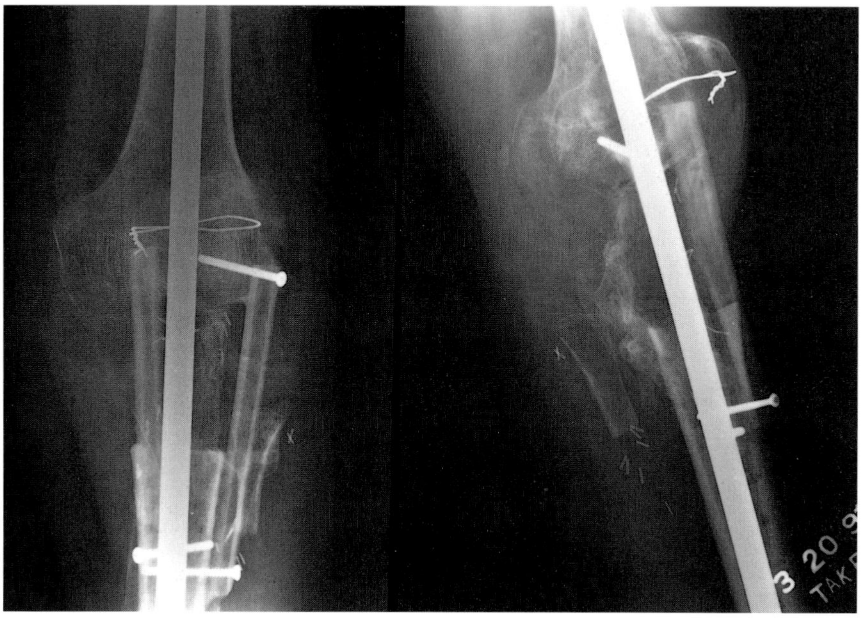

Fig. 16 *AP radiograph of a distal femur reconstruction for infected total bone arthroplasty using an ipsilateral 'double-barrel' fibula turn-up to provide a femoral tibial arthrodesis.*

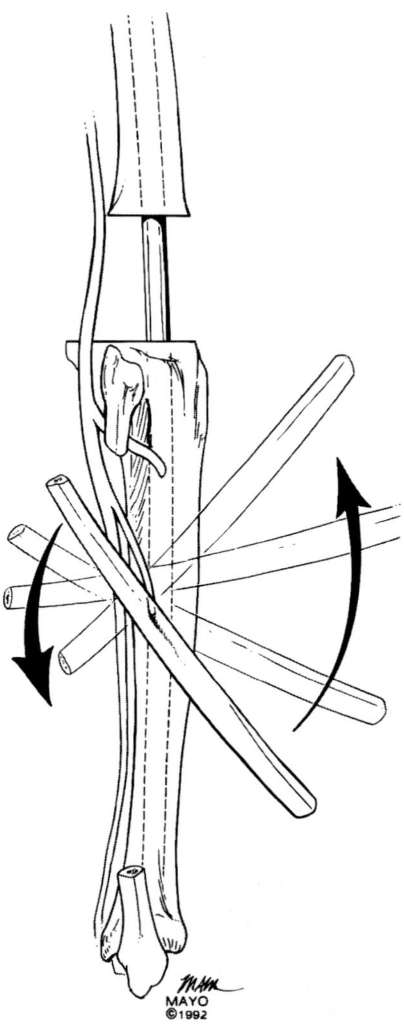

Fig. 17 *Schematic drawing illustrating the axis of rotation for ipsilateral vascularized fibula 'turn-up' (from Rasmussen et al).*

transfer. The axis of rotation for a fibula turn-up with intact vascular pedicle is a point approximately 8–10 cm distal to the fibula head. Thus a surprisingly long segment of fibula requires isolation (Fig. 17).

In most cases, in order to provide the maximum versatility for this procedure, the distal fibular osteotomy is planned at a point just proximal to the distal tibiofibular syndesmosis. Axial rotation of the fibula is complicated by the presence of the peroneal nerve and intervening muscles of the anterior and peroneal compartments. This can be addressed in most patients by passing the fibula deep to the elevated peroneal and anterior compartment muscles. Distal extension of the anterior incision and elevation of the tibialis anterior muscle off the surface of the tibia may be necessary to provide sufficient room for rotation of the fibular segment. Following rotation the peroneal vascular pedicle to the fibula must be carefully scrutinized for kinking, traction, or compression. If these occur, release of tethering fascial bands about the vessels or interosseous membranes should be carried out. Coaptation of the fibula to the tibia below and the femur above is most easily accomplished from the anterior incision. In most patients an intramedullary rod across the femoral–tibial defect or an external fixator is used for stabilization. In such cases an anterolateral trough should be fashioned in tibia below and femur above to permit an inlay positioning of the fibula across the bone defect. If a double-barrel construct is used the second segment based on the periosteal flap is similarly managed, with placement along the antero-medial aspect of the defect. Fixation of fibula to femur or tibia is accomplished by a single transcortical screw or a short compression plate with screws at each end. The defect should be supplemented by a large amount of cancellous autograft. If insufficient autograft is available to obliterate the bony void, allograft bone may be used in addition.

Wound closure over suction drains may then be carried out in a manner of surgeon's preference. If there is difficulty closing the anterior wound, as may be the case with chronically infected defects, some means of soft tissue transfer is necessary. This may be accomplished by including a peroneal-artery-based fasciocutaneous flap or a segment of soleus muscle with the transferred fibula, or by transposition of one or both heads of the gastrocnemius muscle with skin grafting. Postoperative management for patients with this form of reconstruction is identical to that described for a femoral shaft defect.

C. FEMORAL HEAD

Vascularized fibula transfer to the femoral head may be indicated for avascular necrosis of the femoral head prior to marked collapse or secondary articular degenerative changes. This procedure requires use of an intraoperative image intensifier. The patient is positioned in the lateral decubitus position with the affected limb in the elevated position. The entire lower limb including the iliac crest is prepared. A standard anterolateral approach to the hip is used. The dissection is deepened through fascia lata and tensor fasciae femoris muscle to expose the underlying greater trochanter. The lateral femoral circumflex artery and the accompanying veins are then identified deep to the rectus femoris and adjacent muscles. The attachment of the rectus femoris muscle from the ilium is detached and retracted distally to facilitate exposure. The vessel selected for anastomosis is the ascending branch of the lateral femoral circumflex artery and its accompanying vein. Once identified, it is isolated and secured with a microvascular occlusive clamp and sharply sectioned. Following this, using an image intensifier, a guide pin is passed from the lateral cortex of the femur just distal to the greater trochanter into the femoral head. Care should be taken to avoid penetration of the articular surface of the femoral head. The guide pin should reach the superior aspect of the head and contact the bone infarct. If there is a focal area of subchondral femoral head collapse, the tip of the guide pin should be placed in the epicenter of the collapse site. The importance of correct guide pin site placement cannot be overemphasized. Following satisfactory guide pin placement a cannulated drill bit is passed over the pin and advanced to a point just deep to the affected subchondral bone. Articular surface penetration should be meticulously avoided. The drill hole is then used to permit either manual or burr-assisted curettage of the femoral head to include the entire area of the affected bone. Adequacy of femoral head curettage can be determined by injecting radiographic contrast material into the femoral head drill hole, and then observing the size and location of the contrast material pool on the image intensifier (Yoo et al 1992). Once adequate femoral head curettage is achieved, cancellous bone is obtained from the adjacent iliac crest. The graft is firmly impacted into the femoral head to obliterate the curetted cavity to a level of about 5 mm deep to the subchondral bone. The adequacy of the bone graft placement can be confirmed by a second injection of radio-opaque contrast material into the femoral head drill hole and visualization of the contrast agent pool.

An 8- to 10-cm length of fibula with its attached vascular pedicle is then isolated and harvested as previously described. The distal end of the fibula is introduced into the femoral head via the lateral drill hole. It is necessary to ensure that the prepared drill hole is sufficiently large to permit passage of the fibula without compression or damage to the vascular pedicle attached along the length of the fibular segment. The fibula is then impacted using several gentle blows from a mallet, attempting to make firm contact with the previously placed layer of cancellous bone graft lying just deep to the subchondral bone

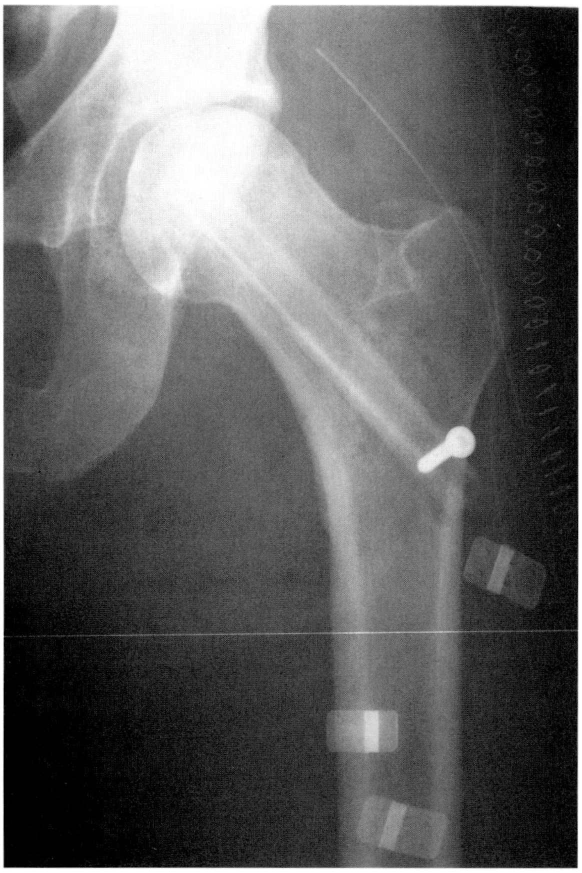

Fig. 18 AP radiograph of a proximal femur following fibula transfer for avascular necrosis of the femoral head (immediately after surgery).

within the femoral head. Fixation of the fibula in this position is accomplished by passing a single Kirschner wire or screw from anterior to posterior in the base of the femoral neck, which engages the fibula (Fig. 18). It is, of course, important to protect the vascular pedicle of the fibula during the process of screw placement Finally, revascularization of the fibula is accomplished by end-to-end anastomosis of the previously isolated ascending branch of the lateral femoral circumflex vessels to the pedicle artery and at least one vein supplying the fibula. Wound closure is carried out by approximation of the fascia lata using interrupted absorbable 2-0 sutures over suction drains. The subcutaneous tissue and skin are closed by the technique of surgeon's preference.

Repair of the detached origin of rectus femoris is not advised, and may compress the vascular pedicle. Postoperatively strict nonweightbearing is required for 3 months. Thereafter, ambulation should be restricted to partial weightbearing for 3 additional months. Full weightbearing may begin at 6 months following surgery, but complete resumption of all activities should be avoided until 1 year postoperatively.

D. PELVIS/SPINE

The use of vascularized fibula for pelvis or spine reconstruction is only rarely indicated. Specific guidelines regarding recipient site management are therefore not warranted. In all cases the principles of selection of healthy recipient vessels, mechanically optimal bone segment placement for weightbearing, and stable internal fixation should be adhered to. For the use of spine stabilization the fibula should be used as an inlay graft into the remaining vertebral bodies. For pelvic reconstruction of defects of the ilium, either iliac crest or fibula may be used, depending upon the size and shape of defect. In patients who have undergone internal hemipelvectomy with

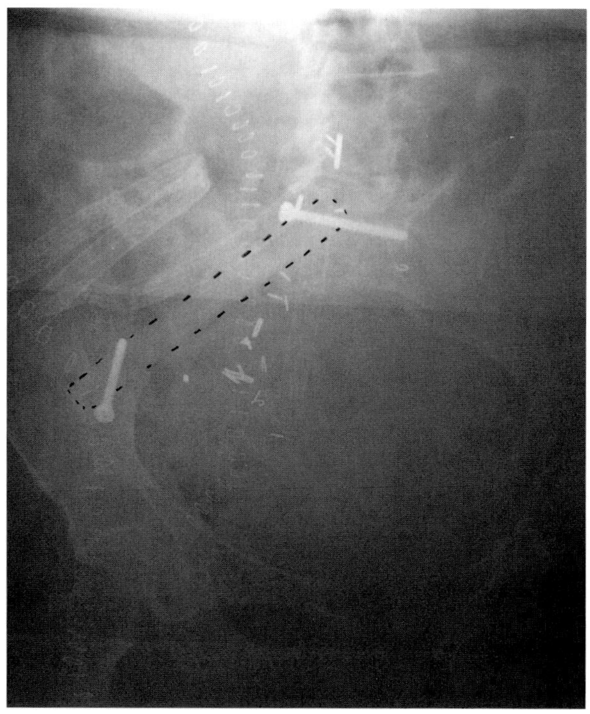

Fig. 19 AP radiograph of a pelvis following internal hemipelvectomy and reconstruction using 'double-barrel' fibula transfer (immediately after surgery).

complete resection of the ilium, double-barrel fibula has been used effectively (Fig. 19). In such cases the fibula is fixed anteriorly to the supra-acetabular bone margin and posteriorly to either the remaining sacrum or the S1/L5 vertebral body. Postoperative care in all such patients should be individualized.

E. FOREARM

For reconstruction of either radius or ulna the fibula is well suited by virtue of its size and shape. Occasionally the iliac crest may be useful for repair of bone defects involving the distal radius and carpus. Virtually all patients requiring vascularized bone reconstruction of the forearm have long diaphyseal defects. The recipient site considerations for both radius and ulna are similar.

The patient is positioned supine with the upper limb positioned on a lateral side table. For the radius a classic Henry incision along the radial border of the forearm is recommended. This permits access to both the distal two-thirds of the radius and the radial vascular bundle of the forearm. For ulnar defects an incision that begins proximally over the subcutaneous border of the ulna and extends distally in a palmar direction provides adequate exposure to both the ulna and the ulnar vascular bundle of the forearm. Through either incision the bony defect of radius or ulna is exposed with subperiosteal elevation of both the proximal and distal bone ends. For both radius and ulna the respective forearm vascular bundle is similarly isolated. The forearm bone ends should be freshly resected to produce either a straight transverse osteotomy or a step-cut osteotomy. The author prefers the former, believing it is associated with less bone-end necrosis from thermal injury resulting from a power saw. After determining the size of the forearm bone defect a fibula of equal dimensions based on its vascular pedicle is isolated and harvested. Both ends of the fibula are shaped to complement the respective proximal and distal osteotomies of the forearm bone. Once maximum bone contact is obtained internal fixation using a compression plate at both ends is

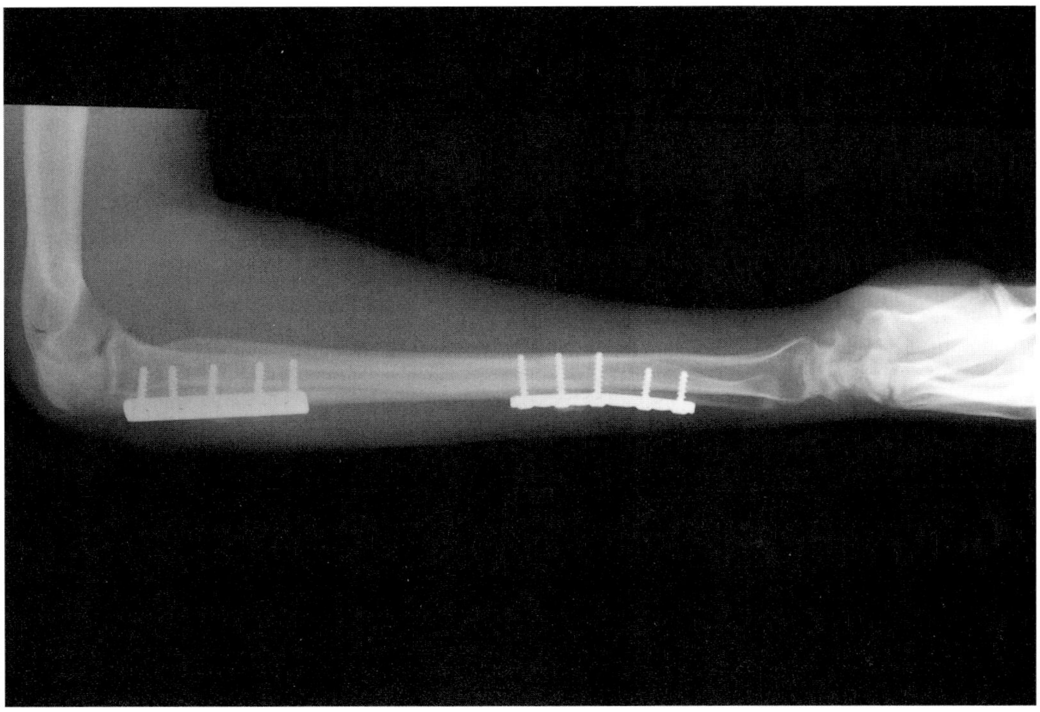

Fig. 20 *Radiograph of a forearm illustrating ulnar reconstruction by vascularized fibula transfer and compression plate fixation at each end.*

carried out (Fig. 20). The proximal–distal orientation of the transferred fibular segment may be either orthograde or retrograde, depending upon which position allows easiest vascular pedicle orientation for anastomosis. Revascularization is accomplished by end-to-end repair of the peroneal artery from the fibula to the radial artery for reconstruction of the radius or to the ulnar artery for ulnar reconstruction and by corresponding venorrhaphy. If only a single artery in the forearm is patent, the arterial anastomosis may be carried out in an end-to-side manner. Additional bone graft about the fibular osteosynthesis sites is not always required, because of space considerations and the risk of promoting radioulnar synostosis. Suction drains should be placed in the depths of the wound, and direct skin closure should be accomplished in a manner of surgeon's preference.

Postoperatively, assuming stable internal fixation, an above-elbow cast should be employed for 6 weeks. This should be followed by 6 weeks' use of either a below-elbow cast or a removable orthosis. If union is present after 3 months, immobilization may be discontinued. If, however, radiographic union cannot be confirmed at 3 months, continued cast or splint immobilization is indicated. It should be emphasized that the end point of support for forearm reconstruction is union. Hypertrophy is both unnecessary and rarely seen, because the fibula in its normal state coincides closely with the diameter of the forearm bones.

F. HUMERUS

The major applications for humerus reconstruction are for reconstruction of lengthy shaft defects and replacement of the proximal humerus with associated shoulder fusion (scapulohumeral arthrodesis). Except in unusual cases the fibula is the preferred donor bone for transfer, because of its size and configuration. For reconstructions of humeral shaft defects the patient is positioned supine and the contralateral fibula is preferentially used. However, for those defects involving the proximal humerus or when scapulohumeral arthrodesis is planned, surgical access to the spine of the scapula may be necessary. Thus the patient should be placed in a semilateral position with the affected side up and the ipsilateral fibula selected for transfer. In such cases the use of a draped mobile stand (Mayo stand) is useful to support the upper limb during the course of surgery. For all humerus reconstructions arterial revascularization of the transferred fibula is preferentially carried out to the brachial artery in an end-to-side manner. Venous anastomosis may be done either end-to-side to the accompanying brachial vein or end-to-end to a smaller brachial vena comitans or to the cephalic vein. The recipient vascular pedicle in the upper limb is most easily accessed closer to the elbow than to the shoulder, because of limb-positioning considerations. Thus the fibula should be oriented in a retrograde manner, with its vascular pedicle in a distal position relative to the upper limb.

Humeral shaft reconstruction

Preferentially the defect of the humerus is exposed through a lateral approach. If there is an existing wound or previous incision it may alternatively be used for access to the humerus. In all patients it is safest to identify, isolate, and protect the radial nerve during the course of the procedure. For mid-humeral defects identification and protection of the musculocutaneous nerve is also advised. In a similar manner to that described for the tibia or femur, the proximal and distal ends of the humeral defect are exposed about their circumference. For most patients intramedullary placement of the fibula with proximal and distal bone fixation using either transcortical screws or short compression plates at either end is preferred (Figs 21, 22). When this is the case the intramedullary canal of both the proximal and distal humeral segment may require reaming over a distance of 2–3 cm in order to accommodate the diameter of the fibula within the humeral medullary canal. The proximal and distal ends of the transferred fibula should be subperiosteally exposed for a corresponding distance. Sufficient subperiosteal exposure of the proximal and distal ends of the humerus should be made to permit transcortical screw placement or compression plate application. In very obese patients or in those with extreme osteoporosis, fibula fixation by transcortical screws or compression plates may be difficult to achieve or to support adequately with a cast during the postoperative period. In such patients a locked intramedullary rod may be preferable as a means of internal fixation. When intramedullary rod fixation is used the fibula should be applied as an inlay graft in the manner described for the same situation in the femur.

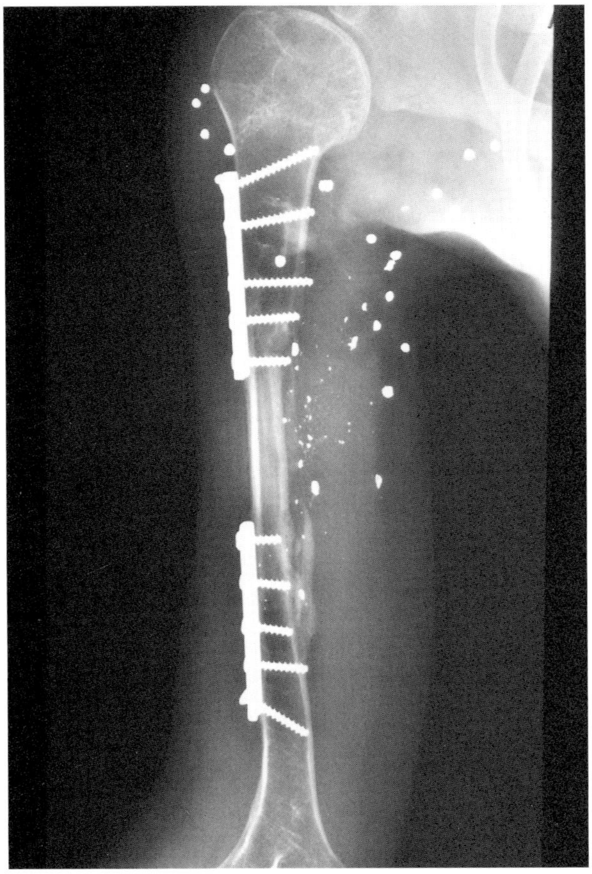

Fig. 21 *AP radiograph illustrating the reconstruction of a humeral diaphyseal defect by vascularized fibula transfer and plate/transcortical screw fixation.*

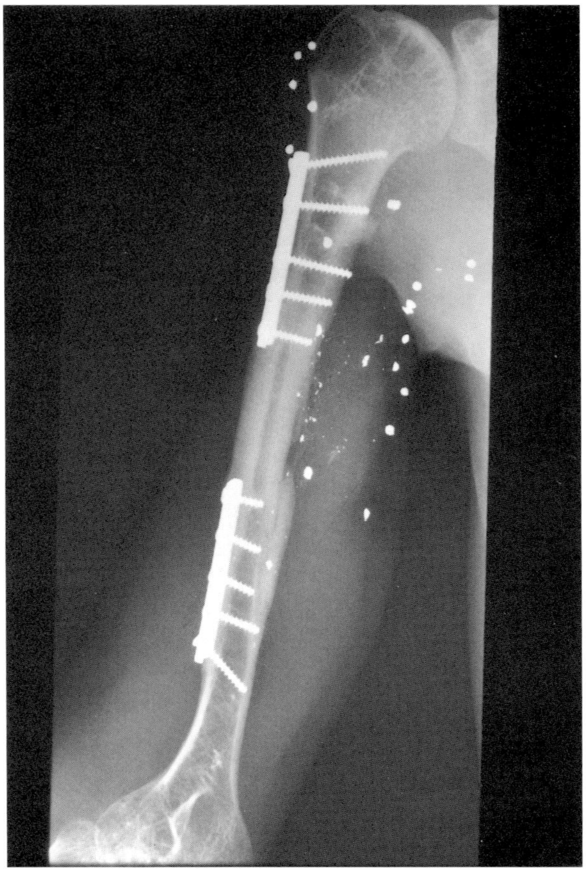

Fig. 22 *AP radiograph of the humerus of the patient depicted in Fig. 21, illustrating union and hypertrophy 14 months after surgery.*

Following fibula fixation within the humeral defect, exposure of the brachial vessels at a level consistent with the position of the fibula vascular pedicle is carried out. If, during the course of exposure of the humeral defect, the brachial vessels are not identified, they may be exposed in the interval between the biceps and brachial muscle. If the humeral defect bed is heavily scarred, exposure of the brachial artery and veins may be more easily and safely accomplished through a separate medial incision over the vessels. If this is the case, then once the vessels and the accompanying median and ulnar nerves are isolated, the medial and lateral wounds are connected by incising the intervening soft tissue just deep to the vessels, in the manner described for the femur.

At times, because of shoulder capsular contracture or other considerations, placement and fixation of the fibula within the humeral defect will impede access to the brachial vessels for anastomosis. Should this be the case, only distal fibular placement and fixation is initially carried out. Then, after completing the microvascular anastomoses, the proximal end of the fibular graft is placed within the medullary canal of the proximal humerus, with care to avoid excessive traction on the vascular pedicle. As with shaft defects of the tibia or femur, the fibular osteosynthesis sites are augmented with a cocoon of cancellous iliac autograft. Suction drains are placed in the depths of the lateral wound and a layered subcutaneous tissue and skin closure is carried out in a manner of the surgeon's preference. Except in patients where stable internal

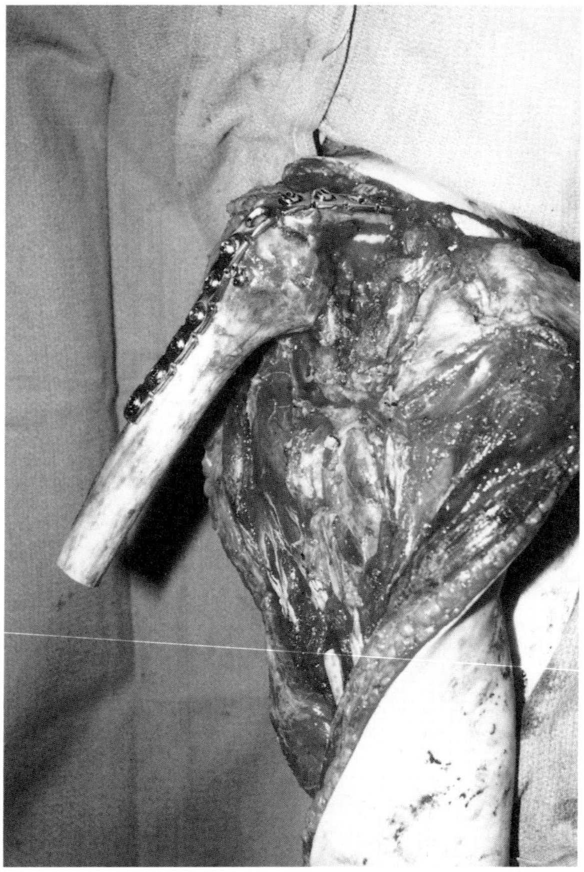

Fig. 23 *A photograph illustrating the fixation of humerus allograft to a scapula with a compression plate prior to distal allograft fixation and vascularized fibula transfer.*

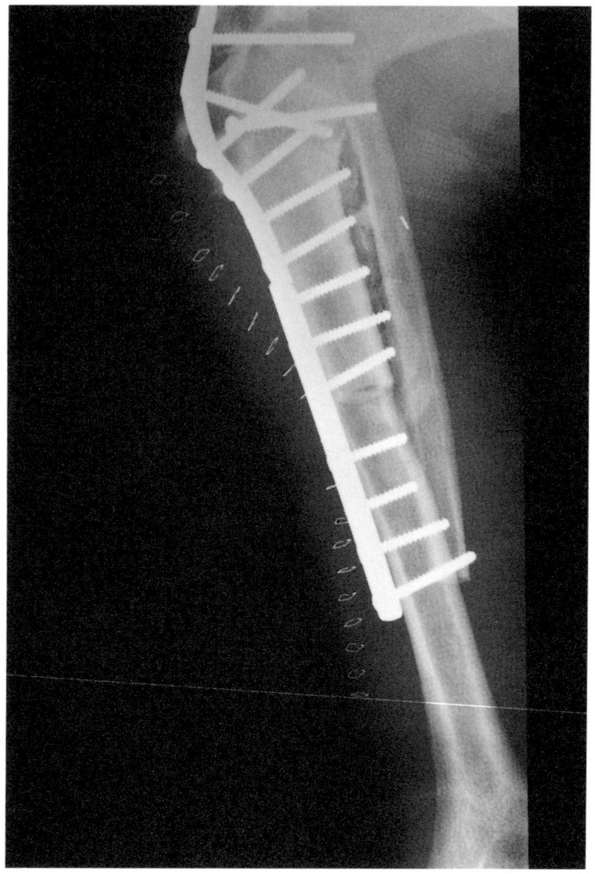

Fig. 24 *AP radiograph illustrating a shoulder arthrodesis with combined allograft and vascularized fibula transfer. Note the fibula spanning the defect from scapula to distal humerus segment.*

fixation is achieved by a locked intramedullary nail, a shoulder spica case is advisable to provide secure limb immobilization for 2–3 months. After 6 weeks the elbow of the cast may be hinged to permit elbow motion. The cast is discontinued when there is radiographic evidence of proximal and distal union of the fibular segment. Continued sling support and limitation of limb function is recommended until there is clear radiographic evidence of adequate fibular hypertrophy.

Proximal humerus reconstruction with shoulder arthrodesis

In patients with either absence of the humeral head or destruction of the shoulder articular surface, upper limb function is best restored by scapulohumeral fusion. In such patients stable internal fixation of the fibular segment to the scapula may be difficult to achieve. Therefore, in this situation a combined whole-bone allograft and vascularized fibula construct is recommended. The allograft is used to provide early and intermediate internal stabilization, while the fibula provides long-term bone union. The allograft is fixed proximally to the glenoid with a stout compression plate coursing along the spine of the scapula (Fig. 23). Distally, a separate plate is used to fix the allograft to the distal humerus (Fig. 24). The fibular segment must span from the scapula well on to the distal humerus. Preferably it should also maximally contact the length of the allograft. The fibula should be doweled into the neck of the scapula as far as the limited amount of scapula in this region will permit. It may be secured by either press-fit or a single screw. Distally it is fixed to the distal humerus by lag screw fixation. Iliac bone autograft should be placed not only about the fibula osteosynthesis sites but also along the length of the interval between the fibula and allograft. This surgical technique and postoperative management is otherwise identical to that described for humeral shaft reconstructions.

When using a massive allograft, wound closure must ensure healthy soft tissue coverage. Therefore one should be prepared to augment the closure in the proximal aspect of the wound with either a latissimus dorsi or pectoralis major musculocutaneous pedicle flap if soft tissues are deficient. Radiographic monitoring during the postoperative course may be difficult because of the size of the allograft. Evidence of union between the fibula and the distal humeral segment may be confirmed using the criteria described for tibial onlay graft union in section A of this chapter.

G. CLAVICLE

Vascularized bone transfer for clavicular reconstruction is rarely required. To the authors' knowledge it has only been used for the management of surgically created clavicular defects in patients with significant symptoms related to scapulothoracic instability. At least theoretically is may be indicated for certain patients with congenital clavicular pseudarthrosis or a resistant post-traumatic clavicular nonunion with a history of prior failed nonvascularized bone grafting. Because of its similar size and shape, the fibula is the donor bone of choice for clavicle reconstruction. Revascularization of the fibula segment may be readily accomplished by end-to-end anastomosis of the transverse cervical vessels coursing through the supraclavicular fossa to the peroneal artery and vein supplying the fibula. The major technical difficulty for clavicular reconstruction is stabilization of the fibula to the short medial and lateral clavicular remnants. Typically the clavicle is chiefly composed of cancellous bone at both its ends, and thus it is difficult to secure the screws tightly in the bone. Because of this, a small neutralization plate is used at each end of the fibula for fixation (Fig. 25), and a shoulder spica cast is additionally used for a 3-month period of time. The elbow of the cast may be hinged to allow elbow motion. Radiographic assessment of union during the postoperative period is difficult using standard X-rays, and therefore tomography may be necessary.

H. MANDIBULAR RECONSTRUCTION

Bruno Coessens

The goal for mandibular reconstruction is a rapid and safe return to normal appearance and function. Facial

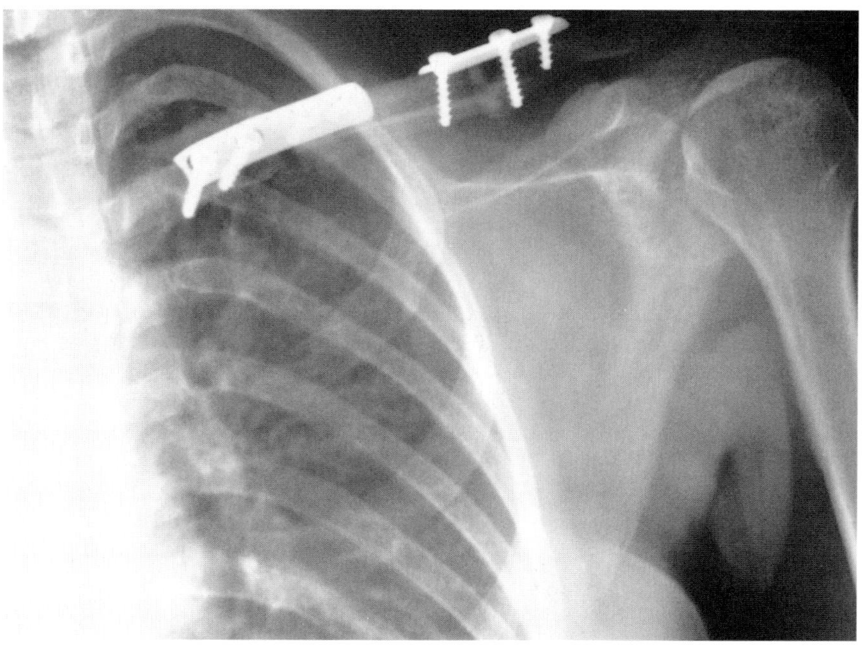

Fig. 25 *AP radiograph illustrating vascularized fibula reconstruction of a clavicle defect with a short neutralization plate at each end.*

contour and oral function are highly dependent on the adequate support provided by the mandible. The deformity caused by mandibulectomy varies greatly depending on the anatomical location and the length of the removed bone segment. Bone loss that includes the anterior part of the mandible causes the most severe disability; its reconstruction is therefore mandatory. Limited defects posterior to the canine tooth are less symptomatic, and their reconstruction more controversial. Most attention to the mandibulectomized patient has placed emphasis on the amount of bony resection; but equally important is the amount of soft tissue that needs to be replaced. The disabilities encountered as a result of both soft and hard tissue loss will be detrimental to speech, articulation, swallowing, and mastication; continuous salivary drooling will impair social life (Beumer et al 1979). Moreover, the remaining portion of the mandible will deviate both at rest and during functional movements. This is particularly true in patients where the missing segment includes the symphysis. The removal of even a small segment of the symphysis dramatically impairs both function and appearance, because of the lack of adequate suspension of the larynx and the lack of adequate support of the tongue, lips, and chin (Coleman and Wooden 1990). Conventional bone grafting techniques have significant limitations for mandible reconstruction. The intraoral mucosa should not be breached, the surrounding tissues have to be healthy to assure good survival, the bony defect should be limited, and no radiotherapy should be used postoperatively. These make conventional bone grafting less than optimal after tumor excision or severe trauma.

Bridging mandibular defects with a reconstruction plate without additional bone graft is advocated for the reconstruction of lateral defects in cancer patients, along with simultaneous provision of soft tissue cover (Davidson et al 1991). The high complication rate observed when plates alone are used for anterior defects precludes their use in that situation (Schusterman et al 1991). Reconstruction plates undoubtedly represent a second choice: with them dental rehabilitation and definitive bone healing cannot be achieved. They should be reserved only for patients with a short life expectancy or with a poor general condition that will make the extra time needed for vascularized bone replacement (on average 90 minutes more than a standard free flap) inappropriate. Microsurgery gives the surgeon the opportunity to replace simultaneously bone segments of various length together with oral cavity lining and even additional soft tissue for the reconstruction of composite facial defects (Sadove and Powell 1993).

The history of microsurgical reconstruction of the mandible starts in 1977 with Ariyan (1980), who described the use of the vascularized rib. Vascularized bone for mandibular reconstruction became so appealing that soon many composite free flaps were used for that purpose. Among the most popular we can find the dorsalis pedis flap with the second metatarsal bone (MacLeod and Robinson 1982; Bell and Barron 1980), the rib based on the periosteal blood supply derived from the subscapular pedicle (Richards et al 1985; Maruyama et al 1985), the iliac crest (Taylor 1982; David et al 1988), the osteocutaneous radial forearm flap (Soutar and McGregor 1986), the scapular flap (Swartz et al 1986; Granick et al 1986), the osteocutaneous lateral arm flap (Martin et al 1988; Matloub et al 1989), and the fibula (Wei et al 1986; Hidalgo 1989).

12. Flap selection for mandibular reconstruction

Flap selection is often influenced by the surgeon's familiarity with a particular technique. However, optimal results can only be accomplished if the donor site is chosen on the basis of the defect, rather than repair of the defect being adapted to a particular donor site. There is no single flap that can be used for all situations, but certain generalizations can be made regarding the quality and the relative amount of bone, muscle, and skin provided.

The ideal vascularized bone composite free flap contains bone of sufficient size and stock to accommodate endosteal implants; therefore a vertical bone height of 7–10 mm is frequently taken as a minimum (Branemark 1985; Frodel et al 1993). The soft tissue component of the flap may need to replace intraoral lining or facial skin, and must provide coverage of the neo-mandible. It is essential that the soft tissue preserves the mobility of the tongue. If total or near-total glossectomy is performed, reconstruction will then require sufficient tissue volume to maintain neo-tongue contact with the palate for articulation and swallowing. In addition to the quality of the bone and skin components, one should take into account the donor site morbidity, and donor site accessibility. A two-team approach permits a dramatic reduction in the overall operative time. This approach is found to be more beneficial to the quality of the results and to allow more time and energy to be focused on proper flap contouring and insetting.

The second metatarsal osteocutaneous flap and the rib are now somewhat obsolete and will not be discussed. They have been replaced by other flaps with less donor site morbidity (in the case of the second metatarsal) or with better bone stock (in the case of the rib).

Donor site review

The iliac crest

The large amount of bone available from the ilium has made it a popular donor site. This bone can be contoured to reconstruct the anterior mandibular arch with osteotomies through the outer cortex, leaving the inner periosteum and blood supply intact. The ramus and the condyle can be sculptured, and only the inner table can be harvested, thus decreasing both the volume of the reconstruction and the donor site morbidity (David et al 1988). The most severe limitation to the use of the iliac crest lies with its skin paddle, which is bulky and poorly pliable. The intimate spatial relationship of the skin flap with the bone component further limits its use in oral reconstruction. The description by Ramasastry et al (1986) of the ascending branch of the deep circumflex iliac artery as the dominant pedicle for the internal oblique muscle has promoted its application to resurface the oral cavity (Urken et al 1989). However the lesser quality of the soft tissue, particularly if it is utilized externally on the face, has not widely promoted its use. The iliac crest advantages include an excellent bone stock and shape that make it useful for posterior reconstruction when bone reconstruction alone without soft tissue replacement is needed.

The scapula

The interest in the subscapular vascular network for mandibular reconstruction depends on the maneuverability of the cutaneous and myocutaneous flaps relative to the bone, which gives great insetting flexibility. The size and thickness of the bone make it suitable for reconstruction of medium-sized defects, with the potential for dental restoration. Moreover, the bone can safely be osteotomized to create a customized contour. This flap can provide enough soft tissue to reconstruct even the largest intraoral soft tissue defect, together with a parascapular skin paddle for additional external soft tissue coverage when needed. The skin, however, is often thick, making subsequent defatting and sulcusplasty procedures necessary for dental appliance fitting. Its major drawback lies in the fact that simultaneous dissections of both recipient and donor sites are impossible, which will significantly prolong the operative time. We therefore limit its use to through and through defects or to cases showing extensive soft tissue loss with more limited bone damage.

The radius

The radial forearm osteocutaneous free flap incorporates the skin on the flexor aspect of the forearm with up to 10–12 cm of the radius bone, which will tolerate up to three osteotomies. The major advantage of this flap is the large area of thin, pliable skin, which makes it possible to reconstruct large, convoluted, and irregular surfaces of the oral cavity. The major drawbacks are the limited vertical height of the bone, the virtual absence of cancellous bone stock, and the risk of radius bone fracture (Boorman et al 1987). Nevertheless, the quality of the skin paddle and the straightforward dissection do much to recommend its use in cases of predominant oral mucosal loss and accessory bone replacement, as, for example, in lateral defects.

The humerus

The major advantage of this flap compared to the radial forearm flap is the potential for primary closure of the donor site if the width of the skin paddle does not exceed 6–7 cm. The thicker humerus bone makes iatrogenic fractures less of a problem. The limited amount of both bone and skin confine its indications to smaller lesions.

The fibula

Up to 25 cm of strong corticocancellous bone with good vertical height can be harvested with minor donor site morbidity (Fig. 1). The rich periosteal blood supply permits multiple osteotomies that will

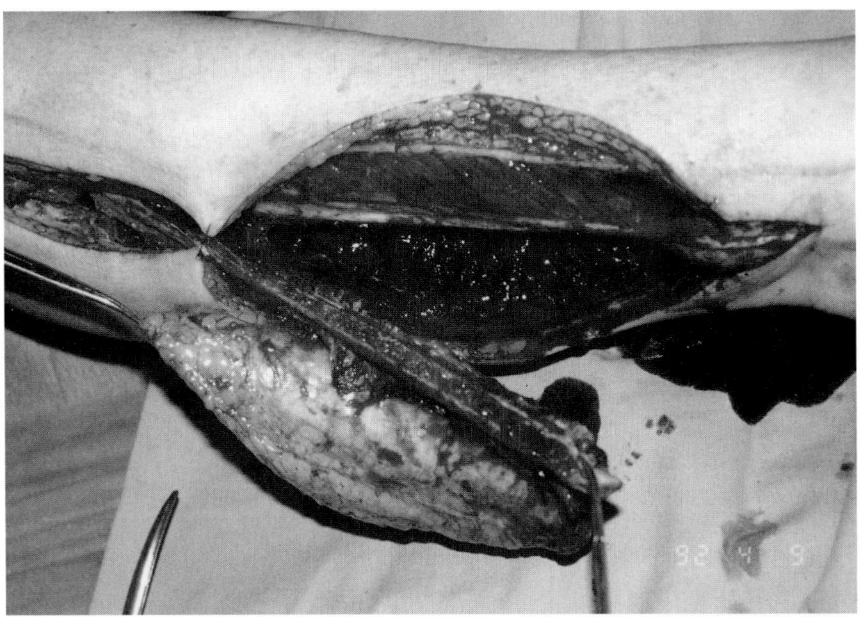

Fig. 1 *An intraoperative photograph of an isolated fibula osteocutaneous flap for mandible reconstruction.*

provide the desired shape to reconstruct, whenever necessary, most of the mandible. The reliability of the skin component has been recently emphasized (Wei et al 1986; Hidalgo 1991; Monstrey and Jones 1992). Its long septal attachment to the bone greatly facilitates skin paddle insetting. This flap is particularly recommended for extensive bone loss or for anterior defects, where its ability to match the initial mandibular contour will produce a fine cosmetic result. The skin component can safely be used to restore large soft tissue defects. The reliability decreases with a small skin paddle that is less likely to incorporate a septocutaneous perforator. The presence of these perforators can be assessed preoperatively by Doppler sound examination (Cariou and LeGall 1991).

Fixation and shaping of the bone

Kirschner wires, miniplates, and reconstruction plates have been used to secure the vascularized bone graft in place (Hidalgo 1991; Boyd and Mulholland 1993; Schusterman et al 1991). All these methods have proved to procure enough stabilization for adequate bone healing without the need for additional intermaxillary fixation. Moreover, intermaxillary fixation, preventing early mobilization, has been incriminated in a higher incidence of postoperative trismus (Coleman and Wooden 1990). The use of bulkier hardware, such as the reconstruction plate, has not been associated with a higher infection rate when used in conjunction with a free vascularized bone graft (Boyd and Mulholland 1993; Schusterman et al 1991). We found reconstruction plates of great value in mandibular reconstruction, not so much because of their better rigidity, but mostly because they greatly facilitate the reconstruction. The plate can be shaped prior to bone excision and used at the same time as a template and a fixation device (Fig. 2). Drill holes are made in the prospective remnants before tumor removal, assuring accurate positioning of the vascularized bone (Boyd and Mulholland 1993). In cases of voluminous tumors, preshaping can be done on a transverse CT scan image reproduced at a 1:1 scale (Hidalgo 1991). When dealing with secondary reconstruction Brough et al have described the use of three-dimensional imaging and software-generated templates to help recreate the contour of the missing part (1993). Having no personal experience with this technique, we rely on the remnants of the mandible, some sculptural skill, and temporary intermaxillary fixation when teeth are present to bend the reconstruction plate. The plate is placed on the inferior border of the mandible (Figs 3, 4), and whenever

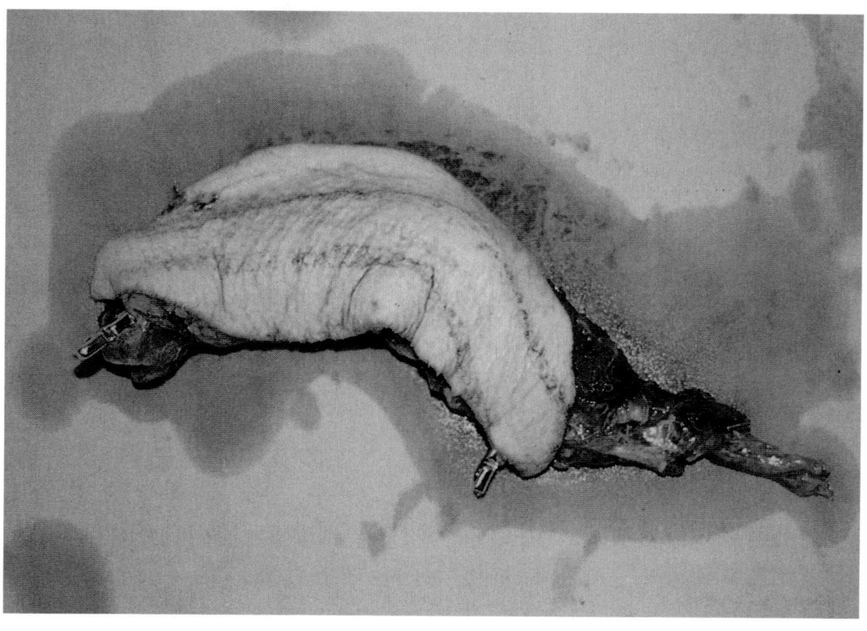

Fig. 2 *An intraoperative photograph of a fibula osteocutaneous flap following multiple osteotomies, with preservation of periosteal continuity and application of a malleable plate (concealed by the overlying skin flap).*

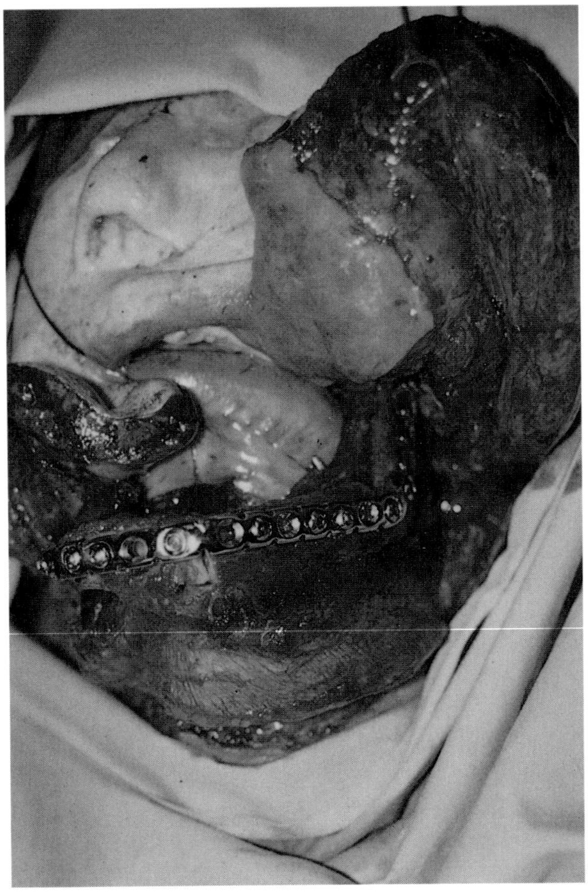

Fig. 3 *An intraoperative photograph of a fibula osteocutaneous construct fixed to a mandibular defect with a malleable plate prior to revascularization.*

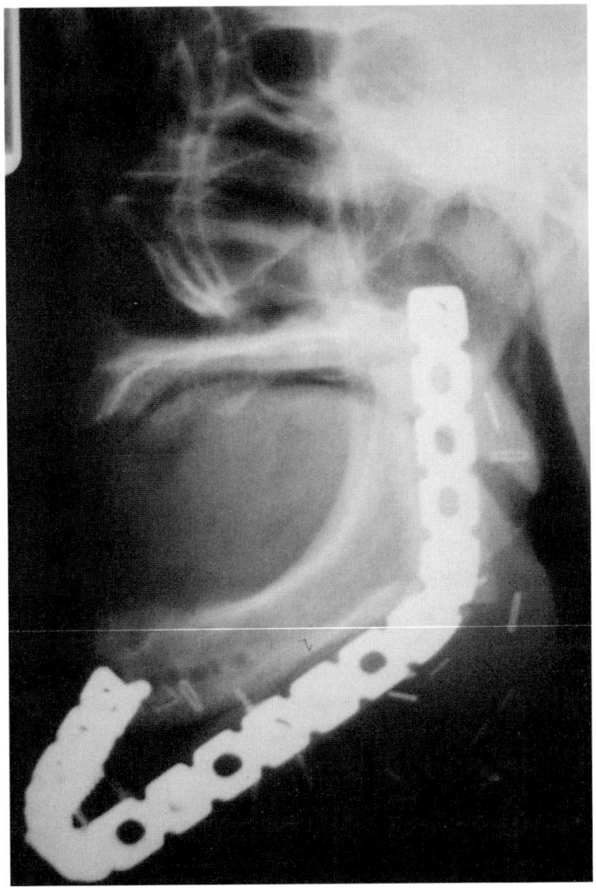

Fig. 4 *Lateral radiograph of a reconstructed mandible (the same patient as is illustrated in Fig. 3).*

possible four screws should be placed on each side of the remaining mandible (Spiessl 1989).

Immediate reconstruction, whenever possible, is always recommended: adequate surgical margins can be reliably obtained (Schusterman et al 1993), the resected segment is available as a template, no scar tissue is present, and overall hospital stay and costs are significantly reduced (Kroll et al 1992).

Conclusion

The use of free vascularized bone grafts has dramatically changed the outcome of mandibular resection; near to normal function and appearance can be achieved in numerous cases. The choice of donor sites enables the surgeon to address reconstruction requirements optimally.

13. Bone fixation

It is established that the rate of union of the osteosynthesis site using a vascularized bone segment transfer is improved by rigid fixation of the bone ends (DeBoer et al 1990). Thus stable fixation should be a goal in all patients. At the same time it is necessary to recognize that the purpose and value of a vascularized bone graft is the preservation of a physiologic blood flow to the bone. Thus any instrumentation of the vascularized bone segment should also have as a goal the preservation of maximal bone blood flow. One then must balance these two somewhat opposing considerations when selecting the most appropriate means of bone fixation. Experience and skill in using external fixators, plating techniques, lag screw application, cerclage wiring, intramedullary nailing, and casting techniques are important prerequisites for the surgeon dealing with bone reconstruction using vascular bone segment transfers. The selection of the most appropriate technique for bone stabilization when using vascularized bone transfers will depend upon a number of variables. These include the age and compliance of the patients, the choice of donor bone graft, the specific recipient bone and site within that bone, the requirement for associated joint arthrodesis, the extent of bony defect, the degree of osteopenia, the use of chemotherapy, and the likely effectiveness of additional external fixation using either external fixators or casts.

Age and compliance of patient

In general, younger patients proceed to more rapid union and hypertrophy. Thus in these cases long-term internal fixation and mechanical protection of the bone construct may be less important. Moreover, in very young patients, internal fixation hardware may be affected by or may affect longitudinal bone growth and remodeling. Thus secondary hardware removal following union is more often necessary. For this reason, external fixation by fixators or casts and minimal internal fixation may be permissible. Of course, in all age groups, patients perceived to be non-compliant more often require rigid and aggressive internal fixation as well as prolonged external casting.

Choice of donor bone graft

Fibula

The fibula as a tubular bone formed by endochondral ossification is composed of dense cortical bone over most of its length. Hence it is well suited to afford purchase to screws, and thus for fixation with either lag or transcortical screws or plate and screws. The vascular anatomy of the fibula is similar to that of all long bones, with a discrete nutrient artery as the chief supply to the endosteal circulation. As is true with all long bones, the endosteal circulation is the most important contribution to the physiologic bone blood flow, with the periosteal supply being of secondary importance. Therefore maintenance of the nutrient artery and preservation of the integrity of the endosteal circulation is essential. If a 'double-barrel' fibula is to be utilized (Jones et al 1988), the nutrient artery requires localization and preservation to the major bone segment. The second bone segment of the 'double barrel' is based only on the periosteal blood supply, and should be recognized as a more poorly vascularized

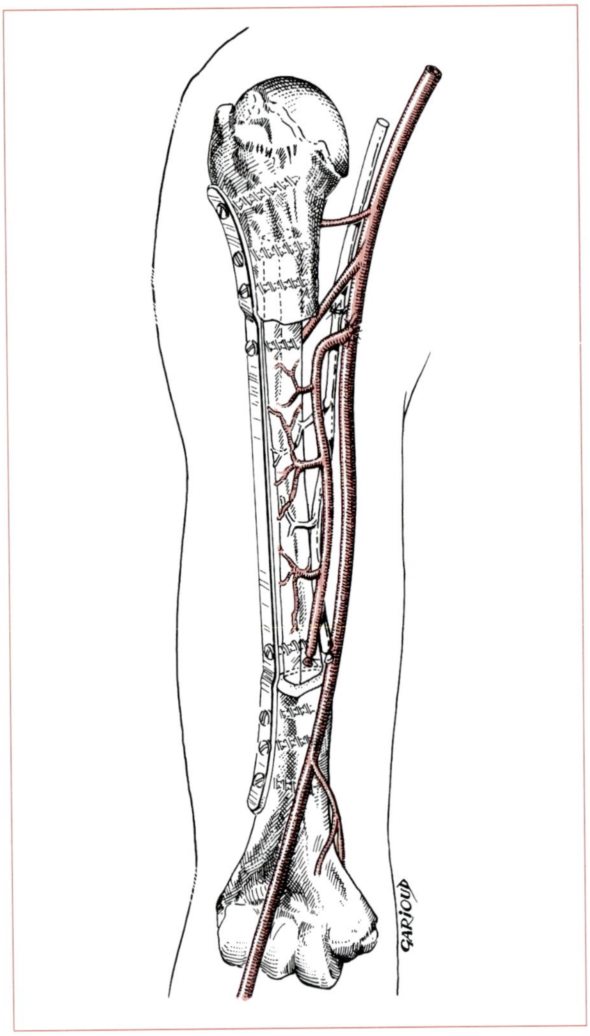

Fig. 1 *Artist's schematic drawing illustrating the use of a single plate spanning the length of the transferred fibula.*

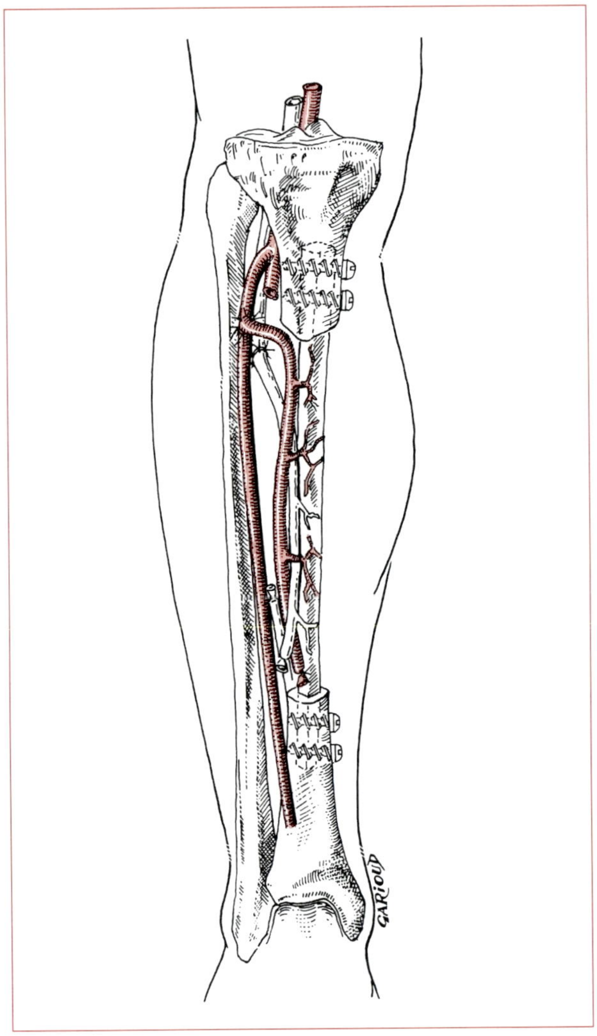

Fig. 2 *Artist's schematic drawing illustrating transcortical screw fixation after intramedullary placement of the fibula within the recipient bone ends. This technique is preferable in a relatively stable bone construct situation in conjunction with cast support.*

bone segment. Because the endosteal blood supply of the fibula is important to maintain, intramedullary fixation of the fibula throughout its length is contraindicated. Likewise, screw holes placed in the fibula can be expected to damage the endosteal blood supply. Thus screw holes placed in the fibula segment should be minimized in number, and placed only in the extreme proximal and distal bone ends. Screws placed in the central portion of the fibula may directly damage the nutrient artery or its ascending and descending branch near its origin. In general, at least half the length of the transferred fibula segment centered over the endosteal nutrient artery foramen should be left undisturbed by transmedullary instrumentation with screws. When plates are used, short stout compression plates at each end are preferred. If the length of the fibula permits, three screws engaging the fibula at each end, which purchase on six cortical surfaces, are recommended. In the recipient bone, at each end at least three screws, purchasing on six cortical surfaces, are also advised. If the length of fibula is too short to permit three screws to be utilized at each end, with at least half the length of the fibula segment left undisturbed, then two- or even single-screw purchase is recommended. In exceptional

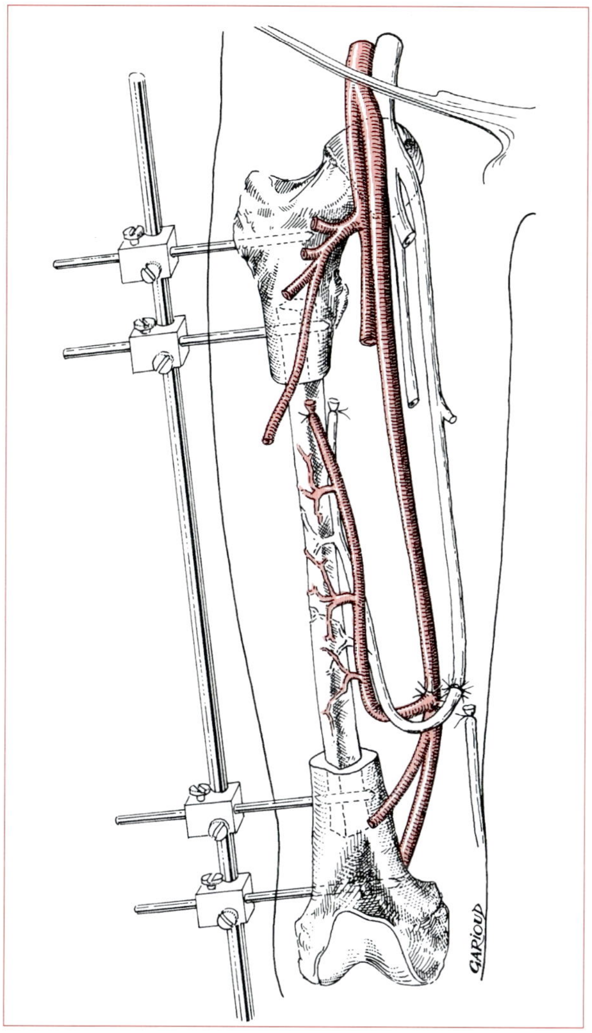

Fig. 3 *Artist's schematic drawing illustrating a 'press fit' of the transferred fibula within the intramedullary canal of the recipient bone. Note the supplementation of fixation by the use of an external fixator.*

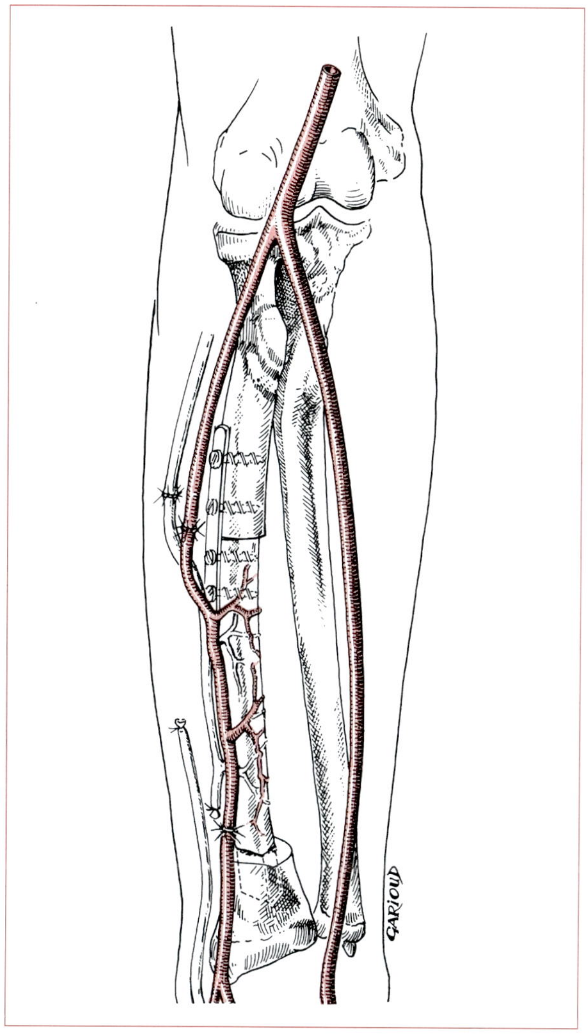

Fig. 4 *Artist's schematic drawing illustrating compression plate fixation of the proximal end of the fibula where intramedullary placement is not possible, and 'press fit' intramedullary placement of the fibula at its distal end.*

cases, a long plate spanning the entire bone defect may be necessary (Fig. 1). In such cases, screws should not be placed in the central portion of the underlying fibula. A long side plate of this type should be used only in patients where effective external support cannot be utilized, because such a construct stress-shields the fibula and impedes bony hypertrophy.

Because of considerations related to screw damage to the endosteal blood supply, intramedullary fibula placement and transcortical screw fixation is the preferred stabilization technique when the anatomic situation will permit, and when this will result in a rigid construct (Fig. 2). This technique allows maximal bone surface coaptation, and presumably preserves a physiologic blood supply to the fibula ends in contact with the recipient site bone. Usually when this method of fibula internal fixation is used, additional external fixation with either a cast or an external fixator is recommended.

If intramedullary impaction of the fibula within the recipient bone produces rigid immobilization as a result of a so-called 'press-fit', then additional transcortical screw fixation is not required and should be avoided (Figs 3, 4). Finally, if a lag screw is placed

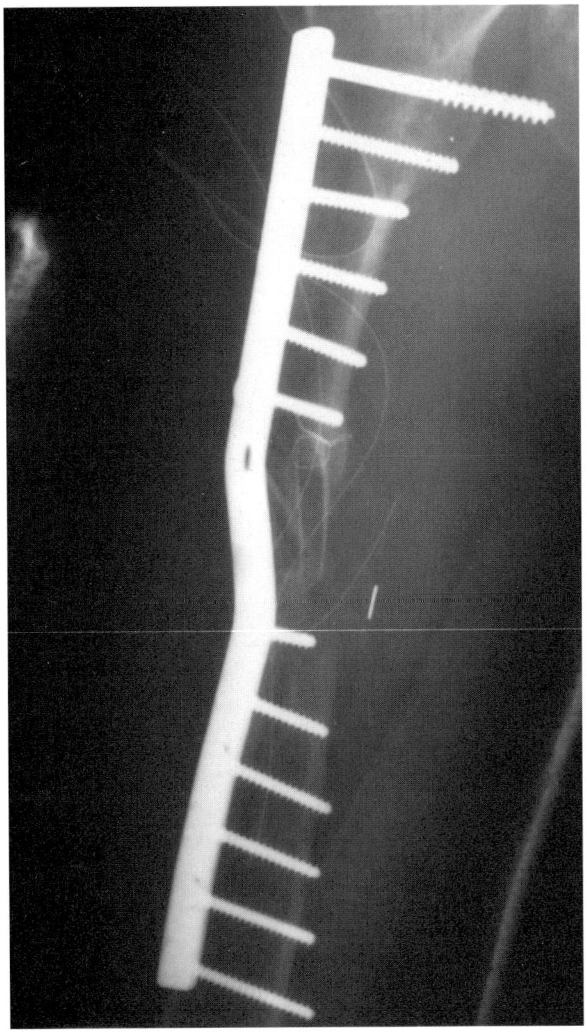

Fig. *5 AP radiograph illustrating plate and screw fixation along the length of a vascularized iliac bone segment.*

across the fibula at either end in a situation involving an onlay or an inlay application, care should be taken to avoid fracture of the fibula as it compresses against the recipient bone with tightening of the screws.

Iliac crest

The iliac crest, in contrast to the fibula, is a flat bone formed by intramembranous ossification, and is composed chiefly of cancellous bone. As a consequence, it may allow rapid bone union and the potential to sculpture the bone ends for maximal bone surface contact, but does not permit ideal mechanical screw purchase. The vascular supply to the iliac crest is not dependent on a single dominant nutrient artery, but rather multiple perforating vessels entering the inner table along its entire length. Thus the iliac crest can be osteotomized in one or several sites or engaged by screws along its length without appreciable damage to its blood supply, provided the soft tissue and periosteum along its inner table are left intact. Because of these characteristics, rigid internal fixation of the iliac crest is difficult to achieve. Rather, rigid external fixation is more reliable, and emphasis should be placed on appropriate bone shaping to accommodate the recipient defect and provide for maximal bone surface contact. To prevent dislodgement of the iliac bone segment, minimal fixation by either a single screw, or Kirschner wire, or cerclage wiring may be used. In nonweightbearing situations where bone hypertrophy is not an important issue, fixation of the iliac crest by a plate spanning the defect may be an appropriate means of internal fixation (Fig. 5). Screws through the plate may engage the iliac crest along its length without significant risk of damage to its blood supply.

Other donor bones

The most appropriate means of internal fixation of other donor bones will depend upon a wide variety of factors. Thus techniques should be individualized, but the vascular anatomy and structure of the bone should be taken into consideration, using similar principles to those applied to the fibula and the iliac crest.

Recipient site

As was discussed in a previous section, reconstruction of bony defects involving the radius, ulna, or clavicle preferentially utilize the fibula because of its similar size and shape (Fig. 4), Thus, for all practical purposes, in these locations bone fixation requires the use of plates and screws at each end of the fibula in accordance with the principles of screw placement discussed earlier. Diaphyseal defects of tibia (Fig. 2), femur (Fig. 3), and humerus (Fig. 1) are also preferentially reconstructed using intramedullary fibula placement and rigid fixation as discussed earlier. Occasionally, intramedullary fibula placement is inappropriate for these diaphyseal defects, because of a poor likelihood of satisfactory stabilization of the

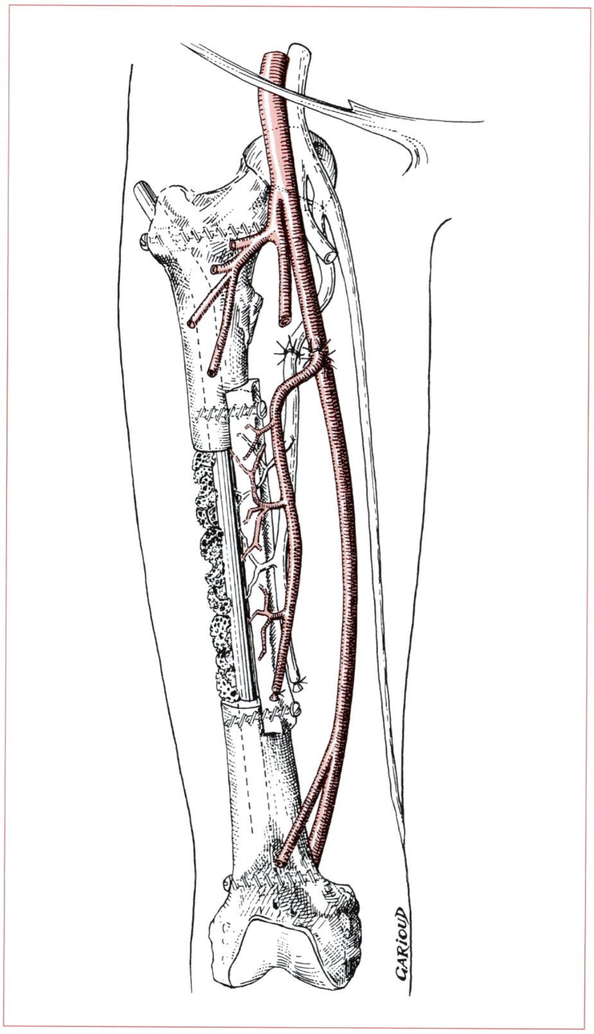

Fig. 6 *Artist's schematic drawing illustrating use of a locked intramedullary nail to provide internal fixation, with a vascularized fibula segment placed as an inlay graft adjacent to the nail. Note the supplemental use of cancellous autograft along the length of the construct.*

bony construct. This is especially true in a patient with poor-quality osteopenic bone or with very obese or non-compliant patients. In such cases, locked intramedullary nail fixation with inlay placement of the fibula may warrant consideration (Fig. 6). Reconstruction of long bone metaphyseal defects or of defects of the pelvis may utilize either fibula or iliac crest. The iliac crest is preferred for shorter defects, and fibula either as a single- or double-barrel construct for longer defects (see Chapter 11 Fig. 19). Fixation techniques appropriate to either fibula or iliac crest as previously described should be utilized.

Requirement for associated joint arthrodesis

The most common sites involving joint arthrodesis in association with a bony defect requiring vascularized bone transfers are the shoulder, knee, ankle, and wrist. The shoulder presents significant fixation difficulties when using fusion of fibula to scapula. In this situation, the use of a nonvascularized bone construct to provide fixation side-by-side with a vascularized fibula segment is recommended. The use of a proximal humerus allograft as described earlier allows sufficient bone mass to permit rigid internal fixation with a plate and screws (see Chapter 11 Fig. 24). In such a case, an eight- to twelve-hole plate is used proximally. The plate is bent to extend along the spine of the scapula, and then distally along the lateral surface of the allograft. At least three screws should engage the scapular spine. Distally the allograft is fixed to the humerus by a six- to eight-hole plate applied along the lateral surface. The parallel vascularized fibula segment requires only minimal fixation with a single lag screw distally, and proximally either a 'press-fit' placement into the neck of the scapula or a single transcortical screw.

Arthrodesis of the knee in conjunction with reconstruction of the distal femoral defect is most commonly indicated for extra-articular tumor resection or following the removal and debridement of an infected knee endoprosthesis. In the former instance, fixation is preferentially achieved by a long, locked intramedullary nail extending from the greater trochanter to the distal tibia. The fibula as a single bone or as a 'double-barrel' construct is placed as an inlay graft adjacent to the rod (see Chapter 11 Fig. 16). Fixation of the fibula in such a case is by a single lag screw at each end. For reconstruction of septic defects, the use of an external fixator may be preferred (Fig. 7). However, if the defect is related to removal of an infected cemented total knee arthroplasty, firm pin fixation in the tibia or femur may not be possible. In such a case, the previously described technique of intramedullary nail fixation after adequate debridement and control of local sepsis may be more effective. If an external fixator is elected, the fibula should be placed within the medullary canal of the femur and tibia using either 'press-fit' or transcortical screw fixation.

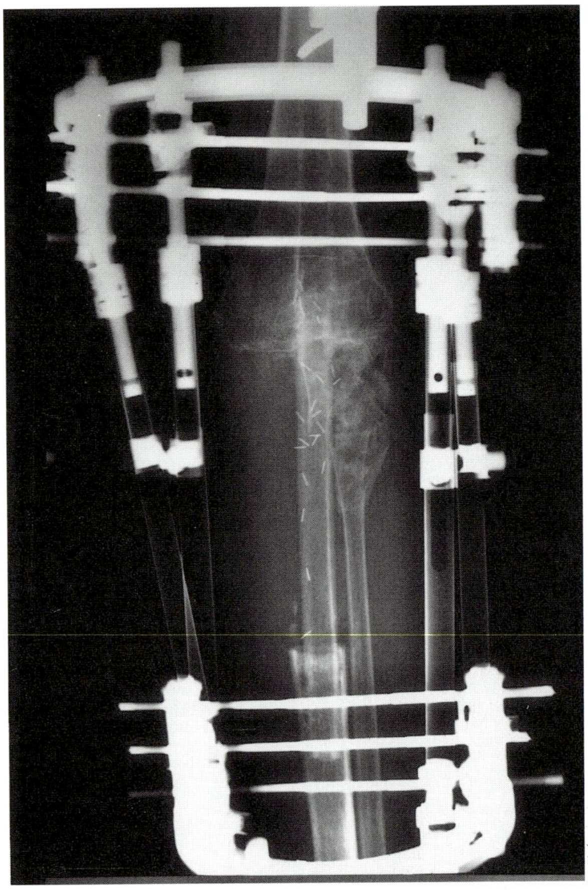

Fig. 7 *AP radiograph illustrating the use of an external fixator for the stabilization of a vascularized fibula segment for reconstruction of an infected extra-articular knee resection previously treated by an allograft.*

Ankle fusion with an associated distal tibia bone defect is usually best suited to stabilization with an external fixator. Depending upon the geometry of the bony defect and the need for soft tissue replacement as well, either iliac crest or fibula may be utilized. Fibula fixation using either 'press-fit' or transcortical screws, or iliac crest fixation using either a screw or cerclage wire, is recommended in conjunction with the fixator. If the fusion extends between the calcaneus and tibia, the iliac crest maybe fixed by a 'kebab technique' using a Steinmann pin passed through the heel pad, calcaneus, iliac bone segment, and tibia intramedullary canal.

Wrist fusion in association with a defect of the distal radius may occasionally be required. Depending upon the geometry of the defect and the need for additional soft tissue, either iliac crest or fibula may be utilized. Fixation in this location is probably most effectively achieved using a plate and screw construct spanning the defect. The plate and screws should engage the third metacarpal distally and the radius proximally. As was previously mentioned, all screw holes along the length of the plate may be engaged by screws passing into the bone segment if iliac crest is used; but if fibula is selected all plate holes overlying the middle half of the bone segment should be left vacant.

Extent of bone defect

In general, extensive long bone defects of more than 15 cm require the use of fibula. Thus the

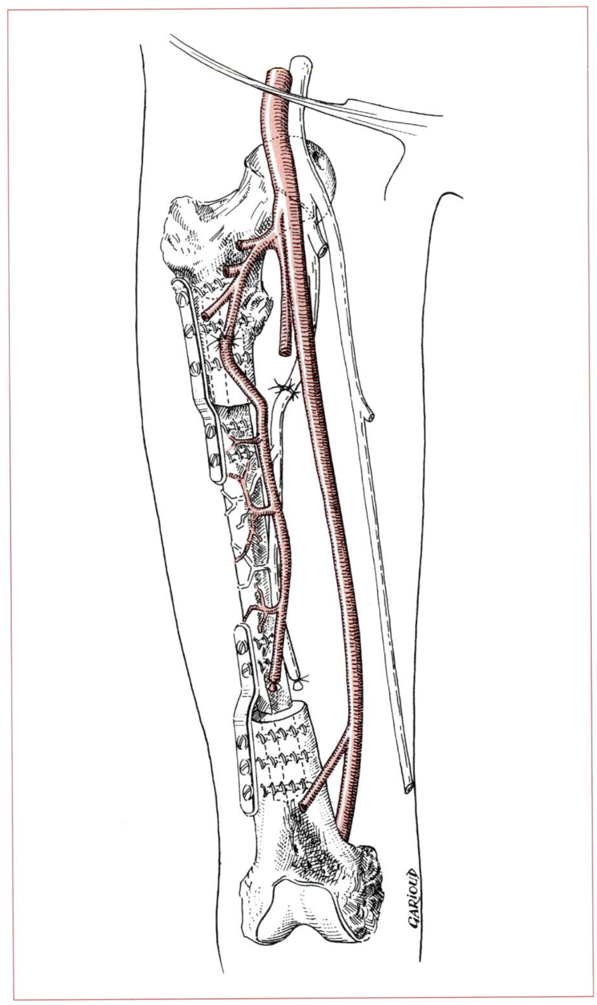

Fig. 8 *Artist's schematic drawing illustrating the use of a compression plate at each end of the bony construct, with intramedullary placement of vascularized fibula. For femoral reconstruction additional external fixation with either an external fixator or a spica cast is advised.*

fixation methods described for the fibula should be selected. For the longer fibula segments, compression plates at each end may be particularly well suited in conjunction with some means of external fixation (Fig. 8). Alternatively, locked intramedullary nail fixation across the defect site with inlay placement of the fibula segment is satisfactory (Fig. 6). For shorter fibular defects, insufficient length of the fibula may exist to allow adequate compression plate fixation at each end. Hence placement of the fibula within the recipient bone medullary canal and 'press-fit' or transcortical screw fixation may be best. If iliac crest is used for a shorter bone defect, the optimal techniques of fixation are as described for this bone.

Degree of osteopenia

If the recipient bone ends are markedly osteopenic as a result of disuse, prior surgery, or infection, the bone may be inadequate for firm screw or pin purchase. In such patients the use of external fixators or internal fixation plates may be much less effective for rigid fixation over a sustained period of time. Preferentially in such patients the use of locked intramedullary nail fixation should be considered, if appropriate to the specific bone defect.

Chemotherapy

Chemotherapy as adjuvant treatment following malignant tumor resection delays bone union for the duration of its administration. Thus in patients in whom postoperative chemotherapy is planned, the selection of technique of bone fixation should take this fact into account. Patients undergoing postoperative chemotherapy will require a longer period of external support and a choice of internal fixation that will impart rigidity for a sustained period of time.

Effectiveness of external fixation

With the exception of intramedullary nail fixation, almost all other internal fixation constructs require additional external fixation. In some cases, external fixation may be sufficiently rigid to permit minimal internal stabilization. This is especially true for the use of external fixators in the femur or tibia of non-obese patients who have normal bone density. Cast support may also be quite effective for the forearm or tibia in these same patients. However, in the obese or poorly compliant patient, with significant bone osteopenia and defects involving the femur or humerus, the surgeon must place a greater degree of dependence on stable internal fixation that is capable of providing rigidity for a sustained period of time.

14. Postoperative monitoring

Following vascularized bone transfer, the management of each patient requires individual assessment and consideration. During the postoperative period the clinical course will require regular and consistent evaluations, which will guide and direct decisions related to further surgery, continued immobilizaton, and progression of activities. Postoperative monitoring may be categorized into early, intermediate, and late phases.

Early-phase monitoring

In the early postoperative period, monitoring is chiefly focused on assessment of sustained patency of the microvascular anastomoses. The simplest means of determining if the arterial and venous anastomoses have remained patent is to include a skin flap with the bone segment that permits continuous visual assessment. A contiguous flap may be readily harvested with either fibula or iliac crest. Both have been described earlier. The skin flap may be directly visualized for signs of capillary refill and turgor (Yashimura et al 1983). Alternatively a laser Doppler probe or pulse oximeter may be continuously used to assess circulation quantitatively and objectively. If visual capillary refill within the flap should suddenly cease, or if cutaneous flow as measured by a laser Doppler probe precipitously declines, arterial obstruction should be respected. In such a case reoperation may be warranted, in order to revise the arterial anastomosis. If the cutaneous flap should show evidence of congestion, with abnormally rapid visual capillary refill and bluish discoloration with swelling, venous obstruction should be suspected. This may be a result of venous thrombosis or compression resulting from swelling or wound hematoma. In such a case, release of skin sutures, evacuation of hematoma, or re-exploration of the venous anastomosis with revision may be required. In some cases venous insufficiency may be managed nonoperatively by elevation and periodic application of medicinal leeches to the congested skin flap. However, in most patients, venous anastomosis site revision is preferred, since it results in a more physiologic venous return for the bone, leads to less tissue loss and, if successful, facilitates ease of subsequent patient and wound management.

If a skin flap or exteriorized muscle flap is not employed with the bone, timely and reliable postoperative monitoring is more difficult. Although the use of invasive angiography for this purpose has been reported (Lau and Leung 1982), its use cannot be recommended, because of the risk of procedure-related complications and cost factors. A variety of semi-invasive methods are available to monitor either blood flow through the pedicle vessels or perfusion from the surface of the bone. These include implantable flowmeters or thermocouples on the pedicle vessels, or a laser Doppler probe (Schuurman and Bos 1991) implanted through a small drill hole into the bone. Although these techniques have been shown to be capable of monitoring flow with a high degree of accuracy, the semi-invasive nature of the techniques and the expense related to instrumentation have resulted in relatively infrequent clinical applications. As a result, the use of the cutaneous skin flap monitor is probably preferable to semi-invasive measuring techniques in almost all situations.

If some means to monitor bone vascular perfusion is not employed, postoperative bone scanning with Tc-99 diphosphonate during the first postoperative week correlates with the vascular status of the transferred bone. There is ample evidence that a clearly positive bone scan on delayed image localized over the transferred bone segment is indicative of sustained blood flow to the bone (Bos 1979; Berggren et al 1982b; Zinberg et al 1985; Takato et al 1988; Greenberg et al 1989). The accuracy of this observation declines after the first postoperative week, because even a nonvascularized graft may show increased scan activity with time as the graft revascularizes spontaneously from the recipient bone and the soft tissue bed. The difficulty with interpretation of bone scintigraphy is that the photon activity related to the transferred bone segment may be obscured by adjacent or overlying bone. Thus there are many instances when the interpretation of the bone scan is equivocal. A bone scintigraphy is therefore of value as a monitor only if it is definitely positive in a well-localized pattern corresponding to the position of the transferred bone segment (Fig. 1), or if it is definitely negative with distinct photon deficiency in the region of the transferred bone segment. The second drawback to bone scanning is that it does not permit real-time assessment of patency of the vascular anastomoses. Thus a negative scan does not allow timely notification of anastomosis site thrombosis. The presence or absence of a positive bone scan may be of value in predicting the clinical outcome and prognosis for a specific patient. In a prior study, a distinctly positive bone scan was associated with a 62.5% likelihood of primary union and a 68.5% likelihood of union after a secondary operative intervention. By contrast, a negative or equivocal bone scan correlated with a 14.3% incidence of primary union and a 28.6% likelihood of eventual union after secondary operative intervention Thus the results of bone scan assessment of the transferred bone segment may be useful in planning the timing of cast immobilization, progression of activities, and secondary operative intervention.

A number of additional imaging techniques to assess bone blood flow in the early postoperative period have been investigated. These include high-resolution computerized tomography (Gonzales-del-Pino et al 1990), magnetic resonance imaging (Manaster et al 1990), and single photon emission tomography (Moskovitz and Lukash 1988). These techniques to date do not seem to offer a clear-cut advantage over bone scintigraphy, but do still have obvious disadvantages of limited availability and very high costs.

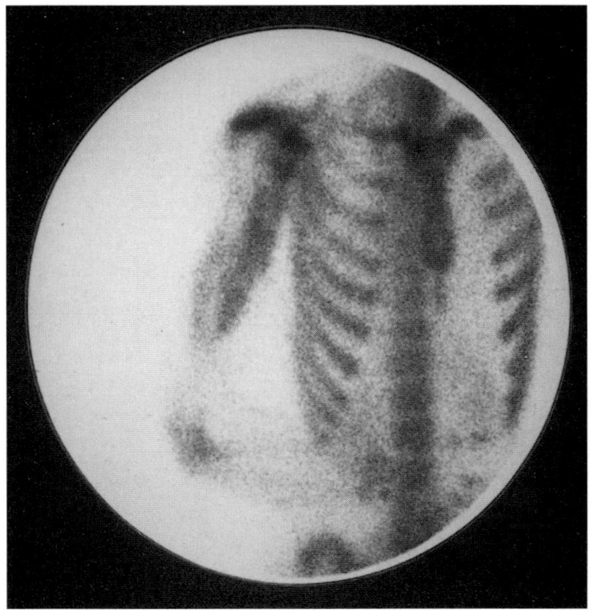

Fig. 1 *Bone scintigraphy at 5 days postoperative of the patient whose radiograph is shown in Chapter 11, Fig. 24. Note the photon-dense collection over the transferred fibula and the photon absence over the proximal humeral allograft.*

Intermediate-phase monitoring

Intermediate-phase monitoring includes the period of 6 weeks to 6 months postoperatively. This phase is focused on assessing bone union at both the proximal and distal ends of the transferred bone segment. In most cases, when union is confirmed, immobilization may be discontinued and cautious progression of activities may be permitted. The most important technique for this phase is standard radiographic evaluation. Signs of radiographic union include obliteration of a space or line at the osteosynthesis site, a continuous cocoon of periosteal callus about the osteosynthesis site, and a progressive confluence of bone formation between the fibula and the recipient site bone. Any or all of these findings may be observed when union is progressing. If plain film radiographs are not diagnostic in this regard, tomograms may provide better detail. Radiographic findings should also be correlated with clinical findings to support a definitive conclusion of bone union. If union is present, there should be, as additional findings, an absence of motion at the osteosynthesis site and an absence of tenderness on palpation over the osteosynthesis site. In very exceptional cases, a definitive conclusion regarding the presence or absence of union may require computerized tomographic scanning or magnetic resonance imaging.

Late-phase monitoring

Late-phase monitoring begins after union is established at both proximal and distal ends of the transferred bone, and may span a period of 3 months to 2 years following surgery. This phase is focused on the assessment of bony hypertrophy. During this phase the patient requires restriction of activities commensurate with the degree of bone hypertrophy. A return to full activity should be prohibited until the bone construct is judged to be able to withstand the anticipated mechanical loads. The progression of hypertrophy is best determined by standardized X-ray radiography. DeBoer has shown that as much as a 15% difference in cross-sectional diameter of the fibula may be attributable to radiographic projection variations (DeBoer and Wood 1989). Thus, to assess hypertrophy, radiographs must be compared using the same projectional view, and ideally should demonstrate at least a 15% difference in cross-sectional diameter to be judged significant. Several patterns of bone hypertrophy may be observed. The most common is that of centrifugal expansion of the bone. There is an increase in cortical thickness and a progressive increase in both bony diameter as well as in the diameter of the medullary canal. This pattern is most characteristic of a weightbearing bone placed in line with the weightbearing axis of the limb that is not subjected to stress shielding by a juxtaposed allograft or metallic implant (Figs 2, 3). The second pattern is that of a parallel

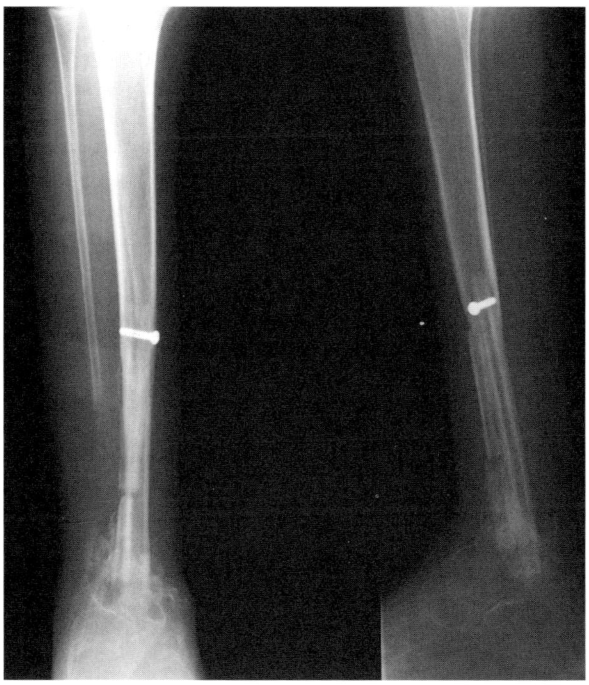

Fig. 2 *Immediately postoperative AP and lateral radiograph of vascularized fibula transfer to resected congenital tibial pseudarthrosis site with tibiotalar fusion (previously destroyed by infection).*

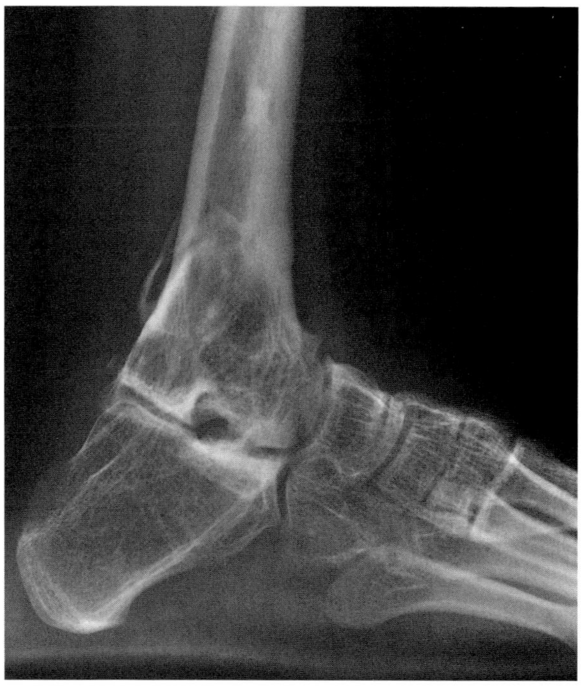

Fig. 3 *Lateral radiograph of the distal tibia following a vascularized fibula transfer for reconstruction of a congenital pseudarthrosis of the tibia. Note the expansion of both the bony diameter and the intramedullary canal.*

ossification adjacent to the transferred bone segment that eventually becomes confluent with its periosteal surface. This pattern may be seen in either a weight-bearing or a nonweightbearing bone. In some cases hypertrophy may not occur. This is particularly true for fibula reconstructions of nonweightbearing bones of similar diameters, i.e. radius, ulna, and clavicle. Hypertrophy may also be less apparent when the vascularized bone transfer is used in conjunction with a massive allograft or with stress-shielding hardware, i.e. a locked intramedullary nail or a large metallic neutralization plate.

15. Indications and results

A. VASCULARIZED BONE TRANSFER VS OTHER TECHNIQUES

The indications for vascularized bone transfer as a reconstructive method for long bone defects following traumatic loss, tumor resection, or debridement for osteomyelitis should be determined by a comparative evaluation of the outcome of this procedure versus that of other reconstructive techniques. Therefore an awareness of the results of long bone reconstruction using alternative techniques is important. Without doubt, the standard of comparison for reconstruction of a bony defect is that of cancellous bone autografting. When placed within a healthy soft tissue bed, cancellous autografting of small (up to 2.5 cm) bony defects may be expected to result in union in approximately 90% of patients (Bieber and Wood 1986). Union rates for cancellous bone grafting of medium-sized defects (2.5–6.0 cm) have not been specifically reported to the authors' knowledge. However, there is consensus that union rates are markedly less and complications are higher in these intermediate-sized defects. For larger bone gaps cancellous autografts are less useful, because it is difficult to obtain enough bone graft material to fill the bony defect completely, and sufficient graft structural remodeling to be consistent with full weight-bearing and functional activities requires a prolonged period of time. Hence stress fractures may occur that complicate and prolong the postoperative course.

Cortical autografts offer the advantage of structural support of a bony defect but require a prolonged period for revascularization, incorporation, and remodeling (Burchardt 1983). Even years after grafting there may be incomplete replacement of cortical autografts, resulting in the potential for late stress fractures. Moreover, when such stress fractures occur there is limited intrinsic healing potential, so that nonunion may occur. Nonetheless, the union and clinical success rates of nonvascularized cortical autografts are such that these are justifiable for certain reconstructions. Using chiefly a post-bone tumor resection population with dual onlay nonvascularized fibula reconstruction, Enneking correlated the outcome with the length of bony defect (Enneking et al 1980). For long bone defects ranging between 7.5 and 12.0 cm a union rate of 67% occurred. A stress fracture rate of 17% was seen in this patient cohort. The result of healing with nonvascularized cortical autografts for defects measuring between 12.0 and 25 cm was an eventual union rate of 68%. However, 30% of these patients required a secondary procedure to achieve this result. In this group there was a stress fracture rate of 58%. The subsequent union rate for stress fractures of a nonvascularized cortical autograft with or without secondary operative intervention has not been reported.

Massive whole bone allografts either as intercalary diaphyseal constructs or as osteoarticular segments have gained considerable contemporary acceptance as a useful reconstructive technique (Parish 1973; Mankin et al 1983). They have been especially utilized for limb salvage following bone resection for malignant or aggressive tumors. Massive bone allografts have the obvious advantage of virtually unlimited size, the potential to preserve major joint motion, cortical structure to permit rigid stable internal fixation, and the lack of donor site morbidity to the recipient patient. However, obvious drawbacks to the use of massive cadaveric allografts include costs related to bone harvest and preservation, the limited source of material, the potential for disease transmission, and the unpredictability of the allograft antigen–host antibody reaction. A variety of measures are available to diminish the antigenicity of the allograft, which include radiation, freezing and freeze-drying (Friedlaender 1991, 1983). None of these, however, can totally eliminate the antigenicity of the allograft. Thus unfortuitous mismatches between host antibodies and donor tissue may result in varying degrees of an immune response. This response may be made manifest in a range of outcomes, from rapid dissolution of the graft to simple nonunion or delayed union at the allograft–host bone osteosynthesis site. Burchardt et al (Burchardt 1987), in the laboratory setting, characterized three mechanisms of allograft incorporation in the dog. The first, observed in a minority of specimens, resulted in bone graft incorporation and eventual replacement by a 'creeping substitution' mechanism indistinguishable from autograft incorporation. This mechanism presumably was indicative of a particularly favorable tissue match between host and donor. A second mechanism also seen in a minority of specimens was one of an aggressive osteoclastic resorption of the allograft. This response was presumably indicative of an extreme mismatch between host and donor. Finally, in the majority of specimens an intermediate healing mechanism was observed, with a slower than normally expected union rate and incomplete allograft revascularization and bony replacement.

Limited data regarding the mechanism of healing of massive allografts in human clinical situations are available. Enneking, in a human allograft retrieval study, demonstrated healing and revascularization to a more limited degree than had been suggested by animal studies (Enneking and Mindell 1991). In these retrieved specimens revascularization to a depth of only 25 mm at a maximum occurred at the bone union sites, and peripheral vascular penetration to a maximal depth of only 4 mm at the bone soft tissue interface was observed. The remaining portions of the allograft, some of which had been implanted for as long as 65 months, were totally devoid of viable tissue in most instances. Overall, in the specimens with the longest duration of implantation, only 20% of the grafts demonstrated repair. Thus, except for surface viability and a very limited replacement with host tissue by 'creeping substitution', massive allografts may be considered in large part as inert endoprostheses. Because of this allografts have a definite potential for late failure related to stress fracture or a singular excessive load or injury.

The success rate reported in clinical series using massive allografts is somewhat checkered. The most extensive study reported is that of Mankin et al (1987): 314 whole bone cadaveric allografts were carried out from 1971 to 1986, 233 of which had follow-up of more than 2 years. Of this group with adequate follow-up, satisfactory results were reported in 76% of patients. However, it should be recognized that 42.5% of these patients experienced some form of significant complication, including infection in 14%, fracture in 19%, and nonunion in 14%. Infection led to failure in 87% of their patients, and fracture resulted in construct failure in 53% of the patients.

Perhaps the greatest volume of contemporary literature on massive bone allografts is that reported at the recent International Society for Limb Salvage Symposium in Montreal in September 1991. At this conference a number of authors emphasized the unpredictability and high complication rates involved in using massive allograft constructs for limb salvage. Zehr and Enneking reported on 138 allografts with a minimum follow-up of 2 years, with specific emphasis on the fate of the fractured allograft (Zehr et al 1981). Of this group a total of 14 (10.1%) allografts fractured. In their series the mean time to fracture was 22.2 months, and therefore these authors felt overall that their series underestimated the true incidence. Only 3 of the 14 fractured allografts healed. The remaining 11 patients either were accepted as a chronic nonunion, went on to amputation, or required revision with the implantation of a second allograft. Clohisy and Mankin concentrated on the long-term outlook of the osteoarticular allograft (1991). They studied 16 patients with tibial bicondylar allograft reconstructions, with a minimum follow-up of 6 years. Overall 50% of their patients went on to good or excellent function. Rock et al (1991) reported on 27 patients with osteoarticular allografts about the knee, involving either tibia or femur. Their follow-up ranged from 4 months to 10 years, with an average of 4 years. For femoral biarticular allografts, 3 of 11 patients had an event-free postoperative course with satisfactory function. For bicondylar tibial allografts 3 of 5 did well at last follow-up, and for hemicondylar allografts 7 of 11 had an event-free postoperative course. Thus these authors suggest that the most predictable outcome of the osteoarticular massive allograft was for hemicondylar reconstruction. McDonald and McGuire (1991) reported on a series of 62 large-fragment allografts, 51 of which were followed up for more than 2 years. In this series they reported frank failure in 32.3% of the patients. This was chiefly related to either infection or nonunion. Moreover, 58.3% of their patient series required some form of reoperation to address complications. Elliott and Simon (Elliott et al 1991) studied 25 patients with cylindrical allografts for femur or tibia reconstruction. Their follow-up ranged from 13 to 57 months. These authors reported some form of significant complication in 14 of their 25 patients, including the usual trinity of infection, nonunion, and fracture. Capanna (Capanna et al 1991) from the Rizzoli Institute reported that only 7 of 22 patients with intercalary allografts achieved union without a significant complication. Clearly, increasing experience with whole bone allografts suggests that, although valuable for limb salvage, these procedures are associated with a very significant complication rate and a potential for late problems.

One of the most contemporary approaches to the management of bony defects is that of distraction osteogenesis as popularized by Ilizarov. Impressively successful applications of this technique for limb lengthening or attempts to gain union with chronic pseudarthrosis and for the management of limited-size bony defects have been reported (Ilizarov et al 1980; Paley et al 1989). However, the limitations of this technique in regard to the size and location of bony defects, presence or absence of infection, adjuvant or neoadjuvant antineoplastic therapy, and economic factors related to duration of treatment are not well clarified. There are relatively few objective clinical series to date that address the expected outcome of this technique.

It is against a background of the above-mentioned alternative techniques that the role of vascularized bone transfer should be determined by critical review of the outcome of this procedure. The largest published clinical series of vascularized bone transfers is that reported by Han et al (1992). This investigation involved the retrospective review of 160 patients, all with 1 year or more follow-up, treated at the Mayo Clinic. The overwhelming majority of patients in this study had major long bone defects, which ranged in size from 4 to 28 cm. The fibula was the transferred bone in 132 patients, and the iliac crest, based in the deep circumflex iliac vessels, in 28 patients. The major indications for the procedure included reconstruction following tumor resection in 69 patients, reconstruction of an infected defect related to chronic osteomyelitis in 60 patients, and a post-traumatic but aseptic defect in 25 patients. Overall these authors reported a 61% rate of primary bony union at an average time of 6 months following the operative procedure. The average interval until full activity (which implies completion of bony hypertrophy) in this group was 16 months. Overall, following secondary surgery, the union rate was 81%. In general these authors noted the highest incidence of primary bone union in those patients undergoing reconstruction of an uninfected bone defect. Conversely, the least satisfactory results regarding primary union were seen in those patients undergoing reconstruction related to chronic osteomyelitis. Ultimate union following secondary operative intervention was not strikingly different between these groups, however.

Weiland (1991) reported on 123 patients undergoing vascularized bone transfer for reconstruction of a long bone defect. These authors reported that ultimately 87% of patients went on to union and adequate bone hypertrophy. A primary rate of 76% in this series was reported. They found the average time to bone union was 6.5 months in the lower limb and 5.5 months in the upper limb.

Gilbert (1982a) reported on 58 patients undergoing vascularized fibula transfer for the treatment of congenital pseudarthrosis of a long bone. A primary union rate of 57% and an ultimate union rate of 90% following secondary operative intervention were found. Minami et al (1989) have investigated a series of 21 vascularized fibula transfers for a variety of indications. Their results are strikingly similar to those of the series already cited, with primary union and overall union rates of 57% and 86% respectively. Yajima et al (1993) reported a series of 20 patients undergoing femoral reconstruction for established nonunion. Half the patients had infected defects. Overall union was achieved in 19 of the 20 patients. Smaller series addressing the outcome of vascularized bone transfer have also been reported (Pho et al 1985; Jupiter et al 1987; Leung and Hung 1989; Newington and Sykes 1991; Simonis et al 1991). Moran and Wood collated the available literature reporting the results of vascularized bone grafting and combined all series, including those cited above, into a total of 411 patients (1993). These included both fibula and iliac crest transfers for reconstruction of bone defects, as well as chronic nonunions without a defect, for a variety of recipient sites and indications. Overall these authors calculated a combined primary union rate of 66% and a final union rate following secondary operative treatment of 85%. Although many factors may influence the results of long bone reconstruction by vascularized bone transfer, most authors suggest that the specific indication for the procedure is an important consideration.

B. CONGENITAL PSEUDARTHROSIS OF THE LEG

This condition (Fig. 1) is one of the most difficult to treat, and in the past a large number of the patients have finally undergone amputation, according to the various series in the literature.

The problem lies in the poor knowledge that we have of the disease, its relationship with neurofibromatosis, and its development. Many of the severe complications of its treatment, such as shortening, ankle valgus, atrophy, and stiffness are due to iatrogenic lesions.

It is a rare disease and large series with adequate follow-up are scarce (Sofield 1971; Andersen 1976; Morrissy et al 1981). The rate of success with various types of bone grafts has been low (10% to 25%). Morrissy finds that the only encouraging results were given by Farmer's procedure (1952). This procedure of vascularized cross leg flap from the opposite tibia was revived from the original ideas of Reichel (1903), Codivilla (1906) and Nove-Josserant (1908). In fact, although the idea was a brilliant breakthrough in the use of bone grafts, the technical execution was a major challenge. Nove Josserand, for instance, cut the pedicle at 8 days, with a subsequent necrosis of the flap; and the final healing was probably due to factors other than the vascularized bone. Farmer, more realistically, cut the pedicle at 3 weeks, and only then inserted the graft. The question is, whether the bone was still alive or not? The application of microvascular techniques led to revival of vascularized bone transplantation. In 1975, Taylor et al described the first use of the fibula as a donor bone.

We have studied the vascular anatomy of the fibula (Restrepo et al 1980) and have described a much simpler lateral approach (Gilbert 1979). Since 1976, we have used the vascularized fibula to treat congenital pseudarthrosis. From 1976 to 1992 we treated 49

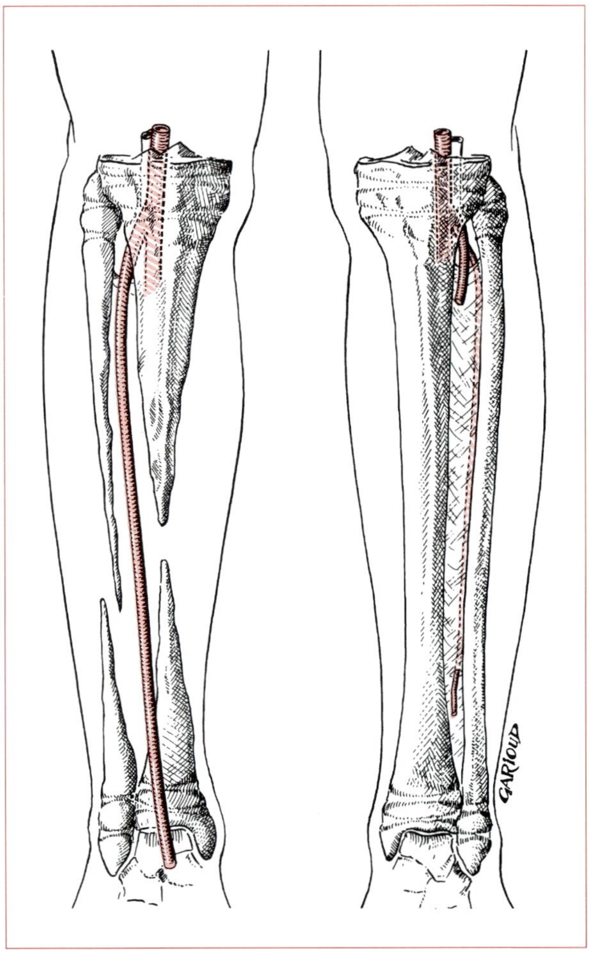

Fig. 1 *Congenital pseudarthrosis often involves both bones, but the vascular axis is intact.*

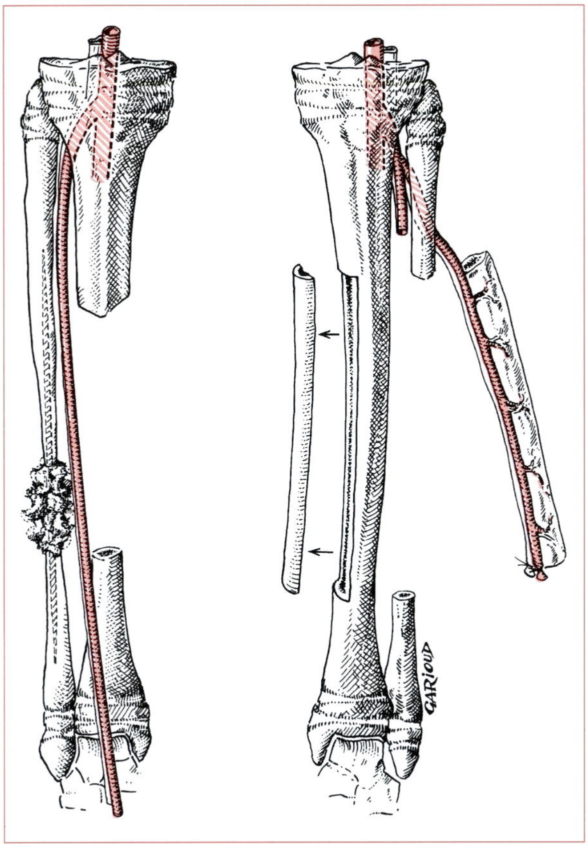

Fig. 2 *On the affected side, the fibula is bone-grafted and stabilized with an intramedullary pin. On the donor side, the fibula is harvested on its pedicle and replaced by a corticoperiosteal bone graft from the tibia.*

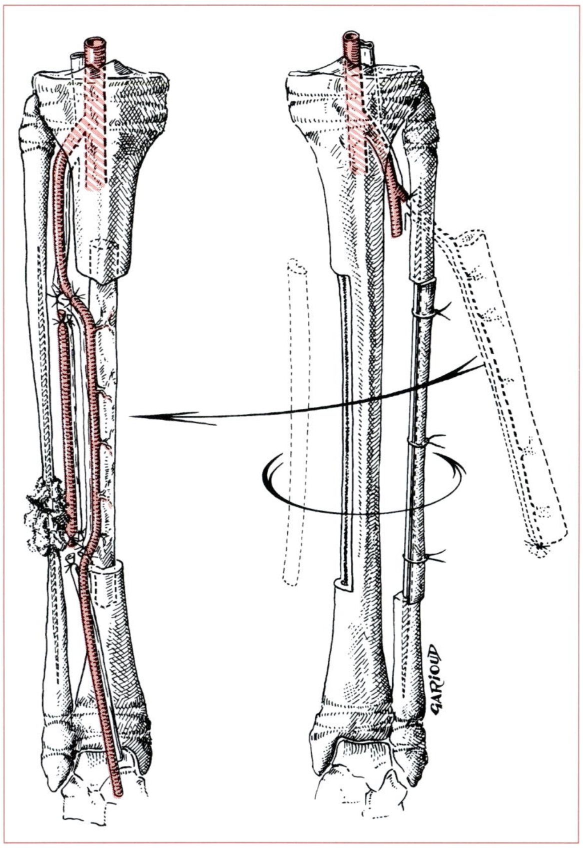

Fig. 3 *The fibular graft is placed between the two extremities of the tibia after resection, and microanastomoses are done under a microscope. The donor fibula is stabilized by a long pin and bone graft.*

congenital pseudarthroses by this method, mostly in the tibia (43 cases).

The method of treatment is based on wide resection of the involved bone and periosteum, and replacement by an contralateral vascularized fibula.

Operative technique (Figs. 2–5)

The patient is supine, with both legs draped. The operation starts with the affected leg. Under tourniquet, an anterior incision allows exposure of the pseudarthrosis and the tibia. The anterior tibial pedicle is dissected and preserved (it is always present except in cases where it was destroyed by previous operations). The pseudarthrosis is widely resected. It is important to resect the periosteum, which is thickened and adherent to other structures, completely – especially posteriorly. The extent of the resection is not easy to determine. There are no particular characteristics of the bone that can testify whether it is still part of the disease. The best way is to follow the radiological limits, and to resect to the limits of abnormal bone morphology. This resection may vary between 6 and 15 cm. The difficulty lies in the distal part of the tibia. In some instances the pseudarthrosis is close to the epiphysis, which has to be respected. This distal fragment is usually small, with soft bone, and is difficult to manipulate and fix.

Fixation is usually, when possible, done with an external fixator. Again, the difficulties lie in the distal fragment. It is sometimes so small that this type of fixation is not possible.

Once stabilized, the defect is measured and the graft is harvested.

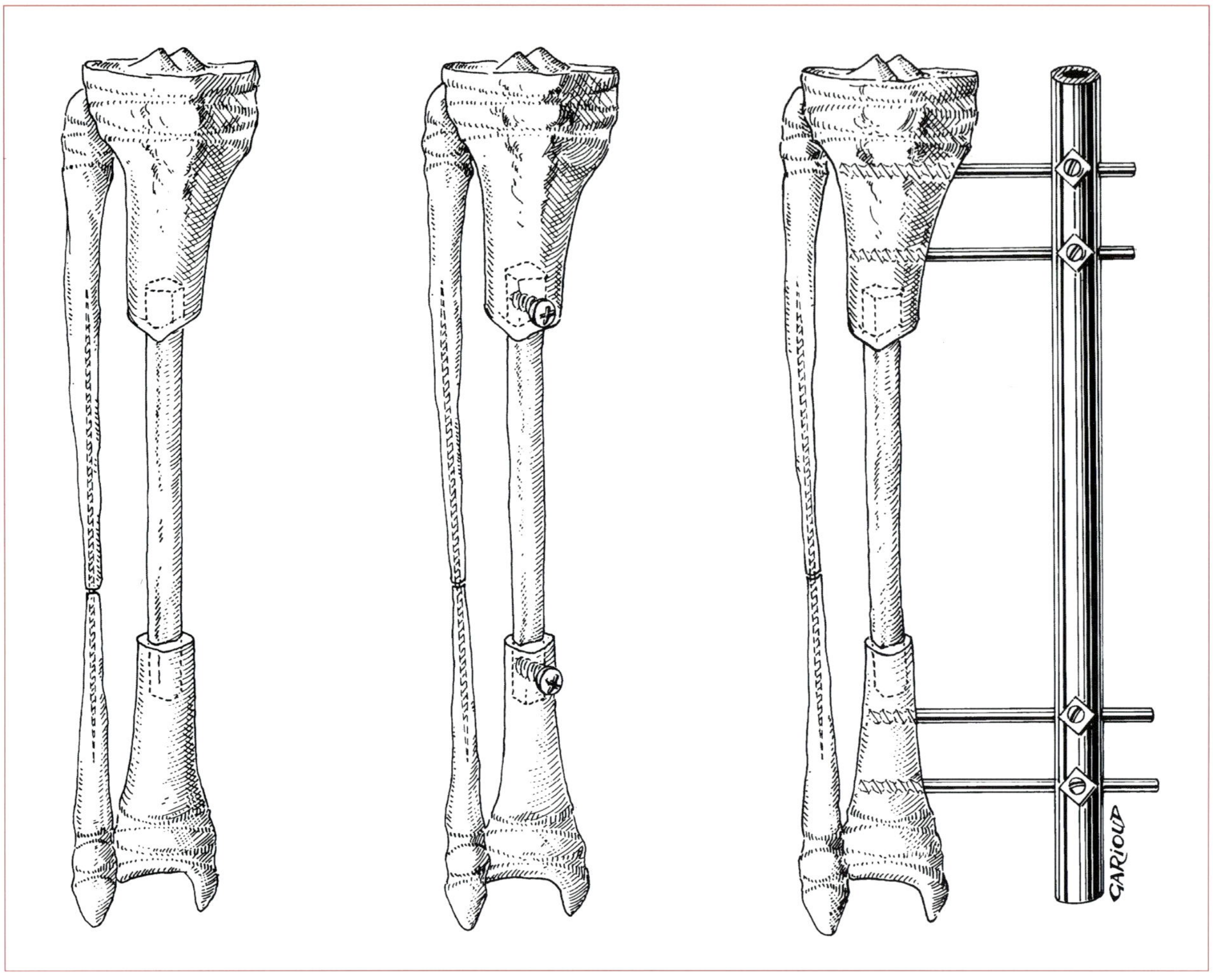

Fig. 4 *Different types of fixation can be used, but the most stable is the external fixator.*

The operation then proceeds to the other leg, and a fibular graft 2–3 cm longer than the defect is harvested. In children a periosteal cuff is dissected 2 cm longer than the graft on each end. This will enhance healing at each point of contact.

The fibular graft is then brought to the defect and positioned. Usually, in the tibia, it is possible to introduce the graft into the medullary canal at each end. The periosteum is wrapped around the junctions.

Stabilization is best made with external fixation, but other types of fixation are possible: either simply two screws at each end and a cast, or in some instances a cast only with no other inernal fixation. When the distal fragment is small, it is sometimes necessary to use transplantar intramedullary pinning. This should be avoided when possible, but in selected cases it has led to a good outcome. The vascular anastomoses are then done using an operating microscope. The peroneal artery is anastomosed at both ends to the anterior tibial artery, creating a bypass. This allows the preservation of good vascularization in a multioperated limb.

The peroneal vein is sutured only proximally, often to the saphenous vein.

If there is a fibular pseudarthrosis on the affected side, it is also treated simply by intramedullary pinning and cancellous bone grafting. The skin is then closed on the recipient side.

On the donor side, it is necessary to reconstruct the fibula in order to avoid a progressive valgus deformity.

A long thin corticoperiosteal graft is harvested from the medial tibial cortex, using a powered saw.

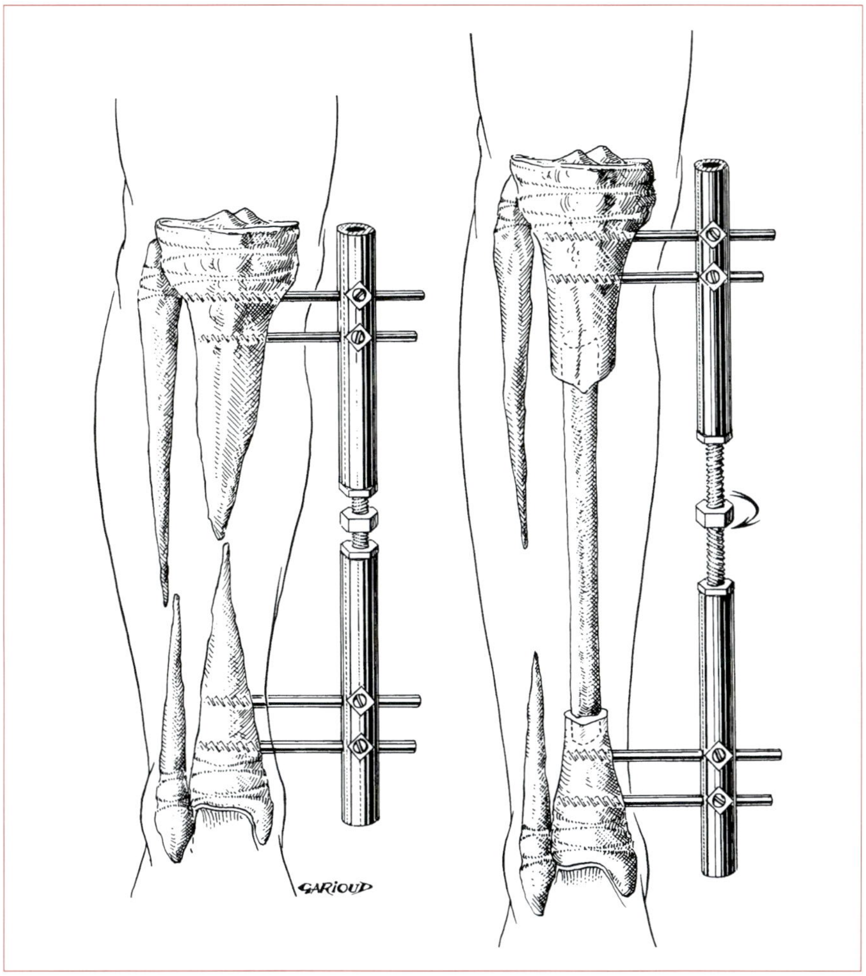

Fig. 5 *In some instances, preoperative progressive lengthening is used. The fibula is transferred in a second stage.*

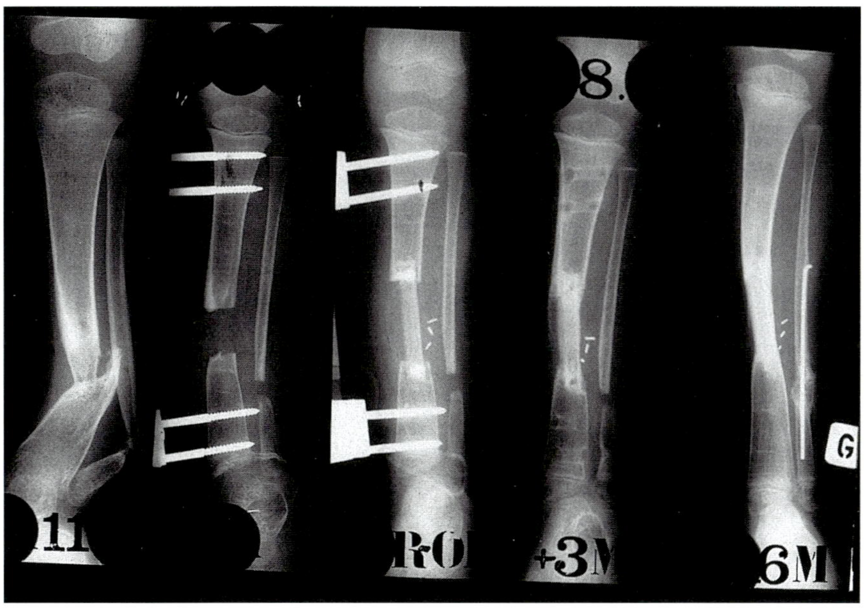

Fig. 6 *Male – 11 months old. Left pseudarthrosis. Uneventful course, with stabilization by external fixation and healing at 3 months postoperative.*

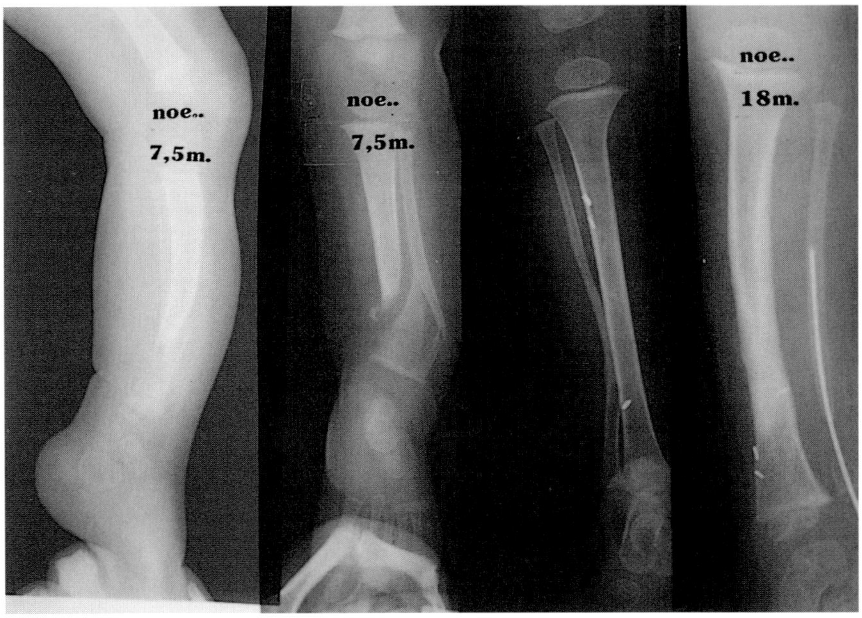

a

Fig. 7 *Girl – 7 months old. Left pseudarthrosis. The youngest case.*
(a) Healing of the lower extremity of the graft was difficult because of fixation. After secondary fixation, healing at 6 months. Osteosynthesis of the fibula was effective.
(b) Bone remodeling 5 years postoperatively.
(c) Clinical result at 10 years.

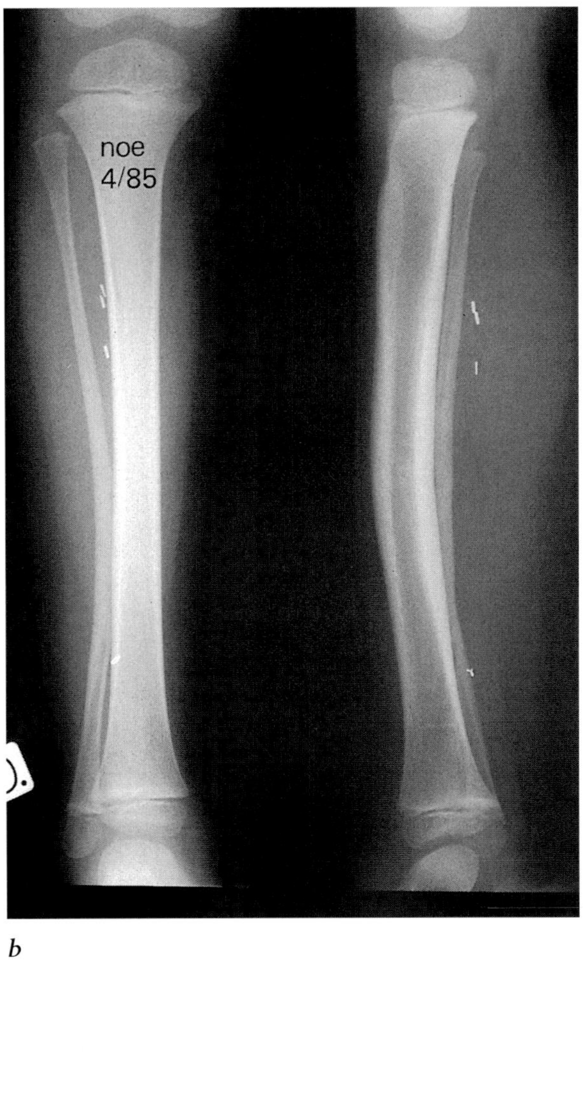

b

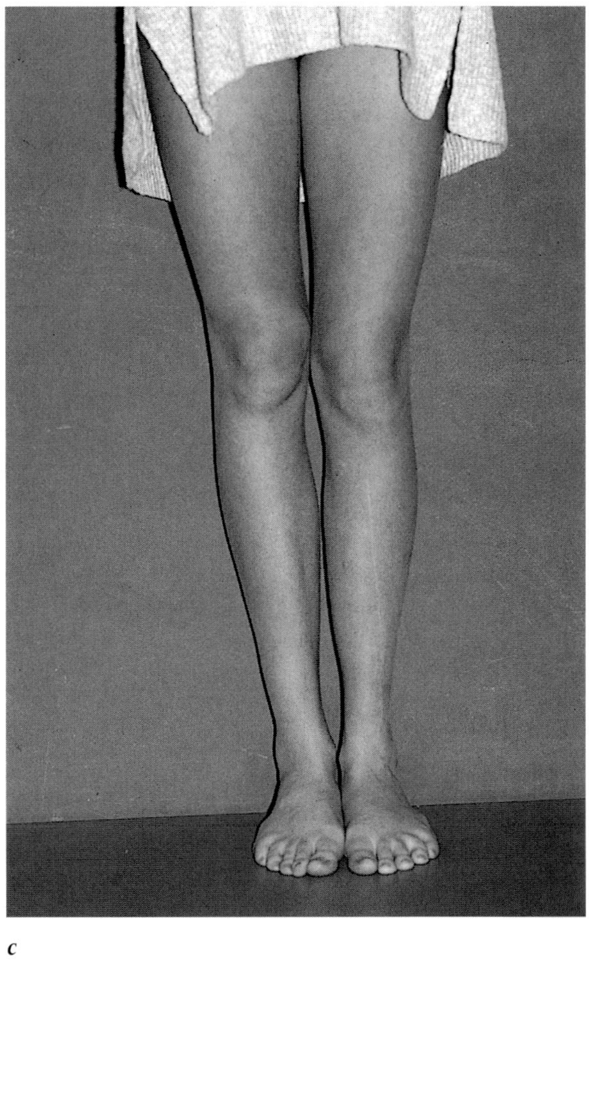

c

Fig. 8 *Girl – 4 years old. Right pseudarthrosis.*
(a) Multioperated pseudarthrosis. Two previous bone graftings unsuccessful.
(b) Fibular transfer stabilized with intramedullary pinning.
(c) Complete healing at 5 months.
(d) Note that the fibula is still not healed 8 years postoperatively.

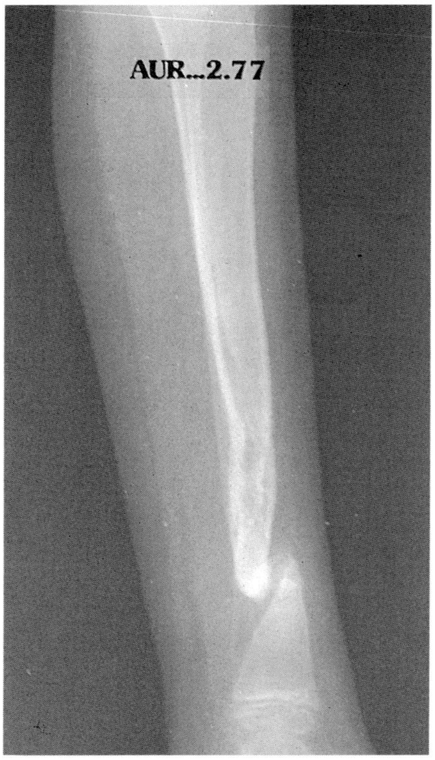

a

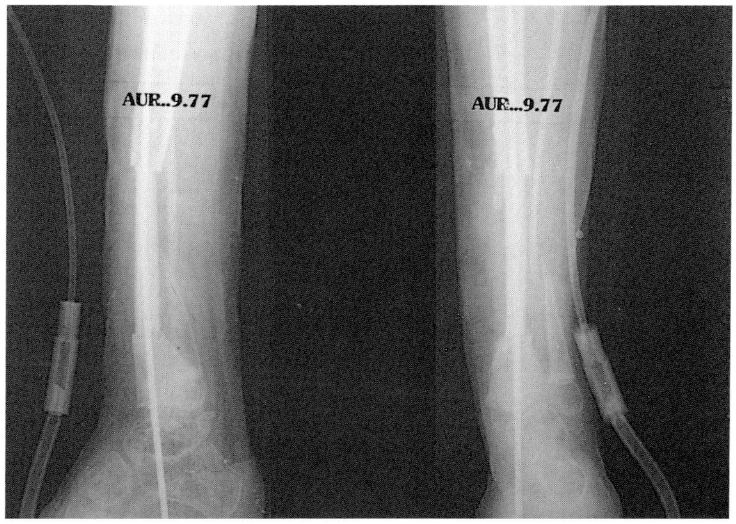

b

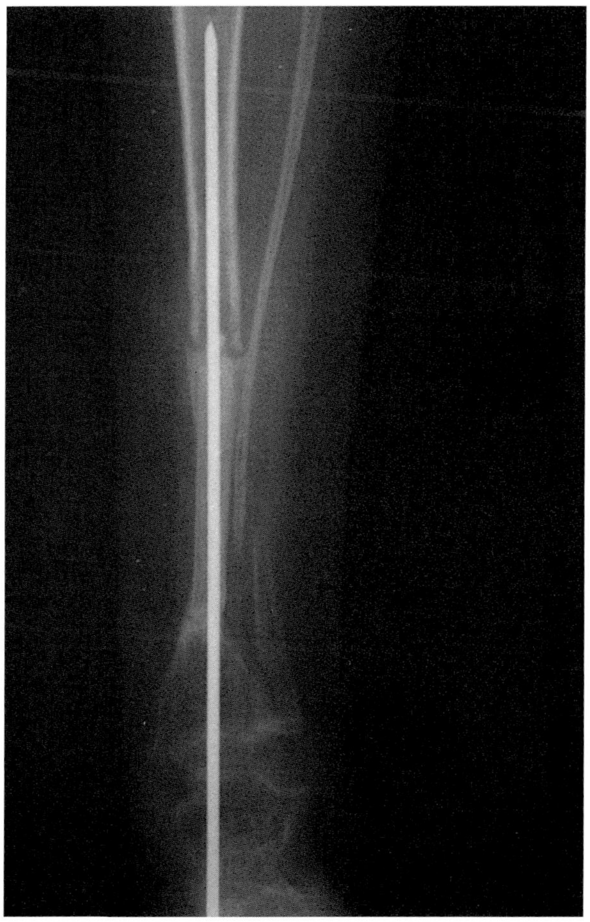

c

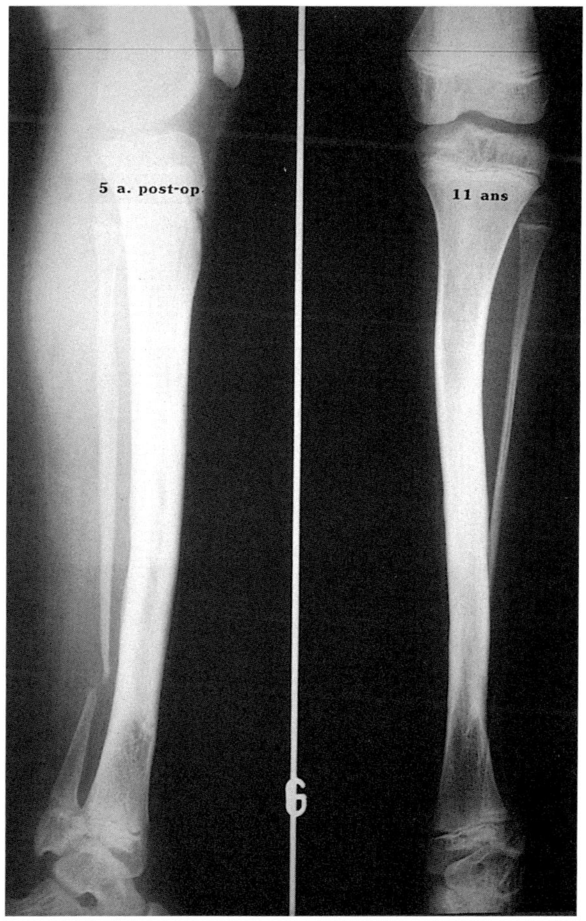

d

Fig. 9 *Girl – 7½ years old. Right pseudarthrosis.*

(a) 11 previous operations. Severe bone loss and shortening (12 cm).

(b) Preoperative lengthening.

(c) Transfer of the ipsilateral fibula. Difficulties of healing of the lower site. Secondary bone grafting.

(d) Final healing after 13 months. The ankle is stiff.

(e) Clinical result after 4 years.

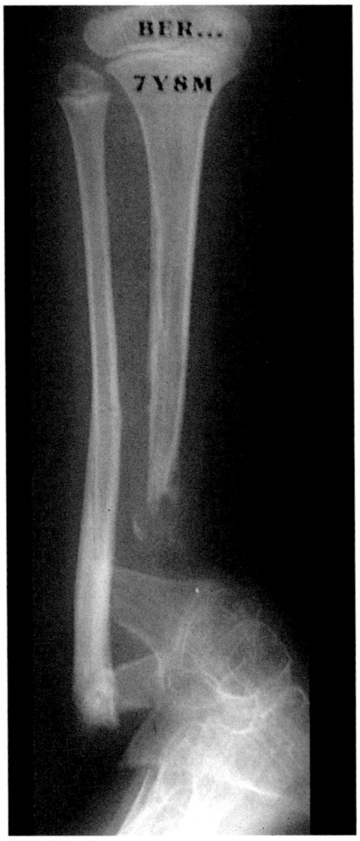

a

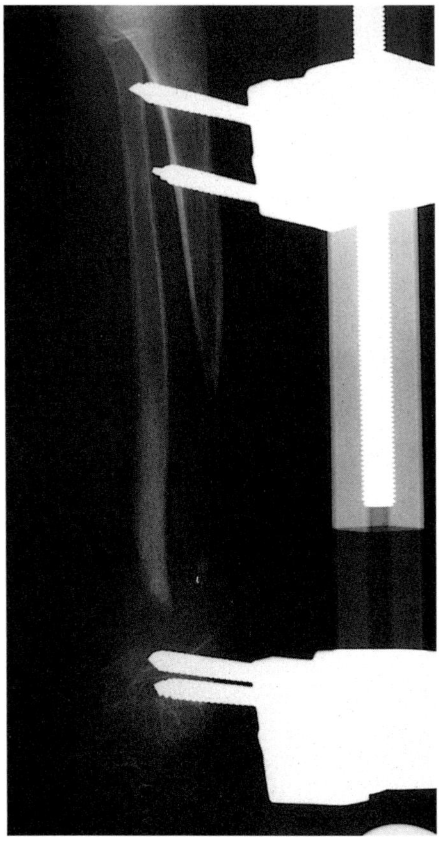

b

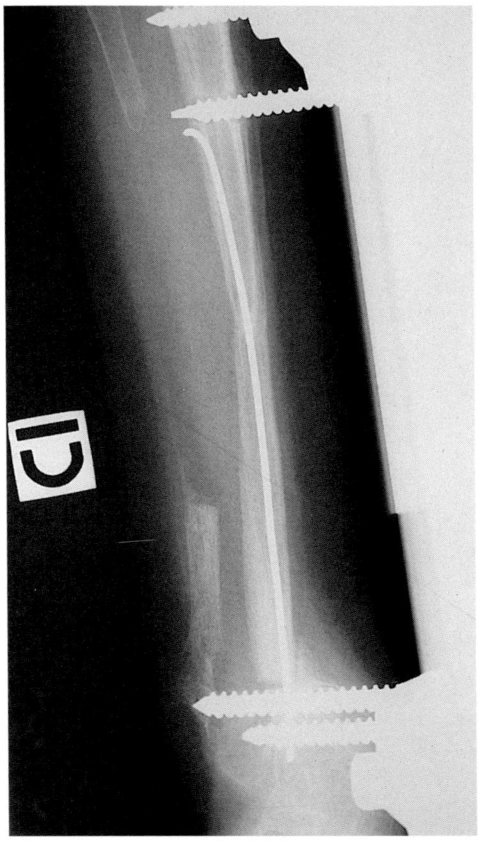

c

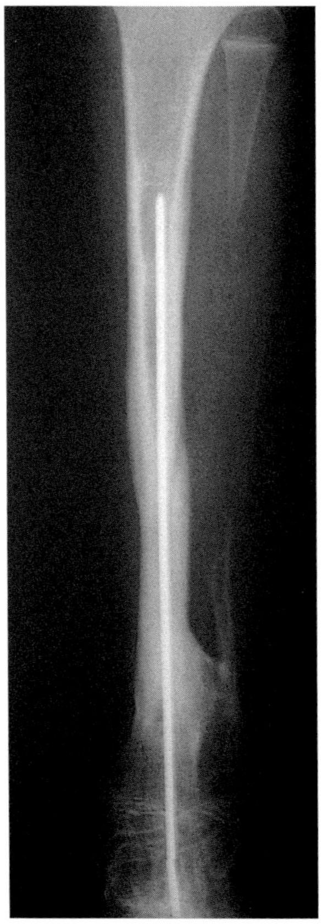

d

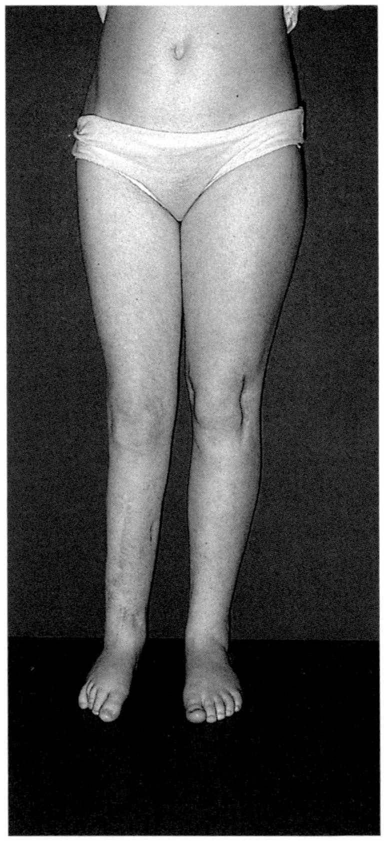

e

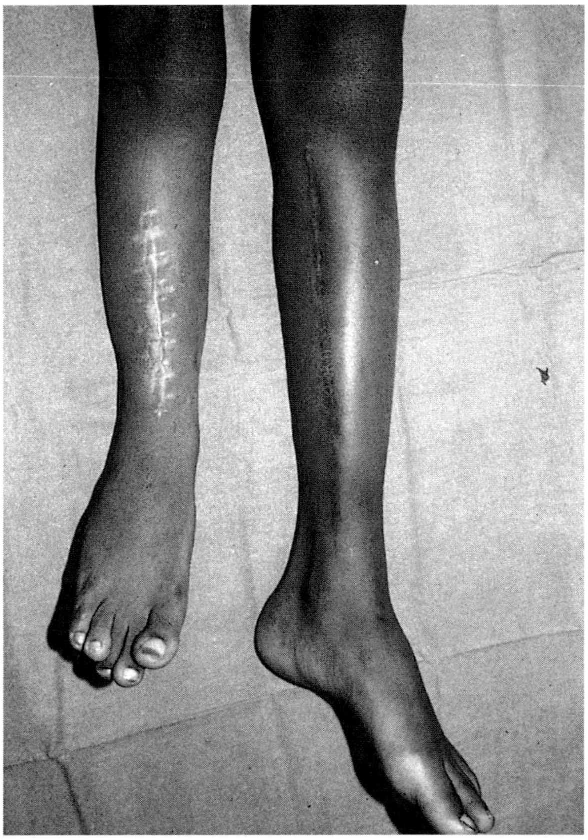

a

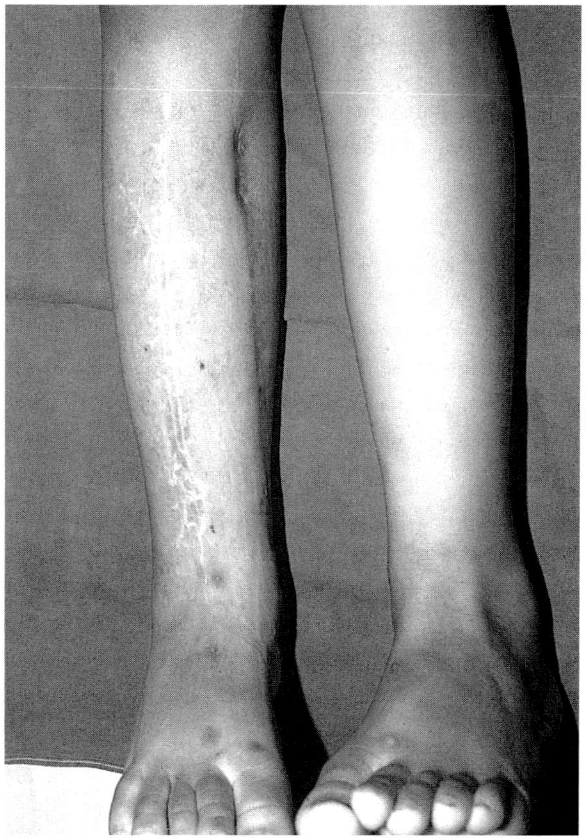

c

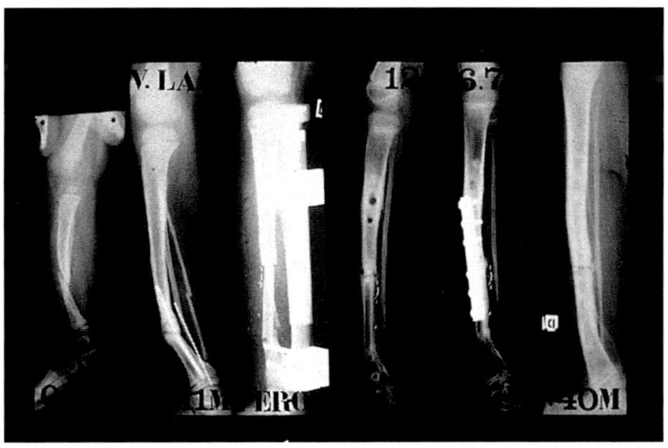

b

Fig. 10 *Girl – 5 years. Right pseudarthrosis.*

(a) Pseudarthrosis with severe shortening.

(b) Preoperative lengthening and fibular grafting. At 3 months, incomplete healing after early removal of the fixator. Plating and healing after another 3 months. Sound bone remodeling at 40 months.

(c) The clinical aspect after lengthening.

This graft is 6–8 mm wide and has the exact length of the fibular defect.

A large (1.8-mm) Kirschner wire is inserted in the medullary canal of both fibula ends, maintaining alignment. The corticoperiosteal graft is then placed and fixed by sutures to the wire. After skin closure, the leg is immobilized by an above-knee cast for 6 weeks.

The affected side is immobilized according to the type of fixation.

Follow-up (Figs. 6–14)

The postoperative care is fundamental to success, as decisions have to be made rapidly and aggressively. Radiographs are taken every month. Usually at 2 months there are signs of healing, and at 3 months

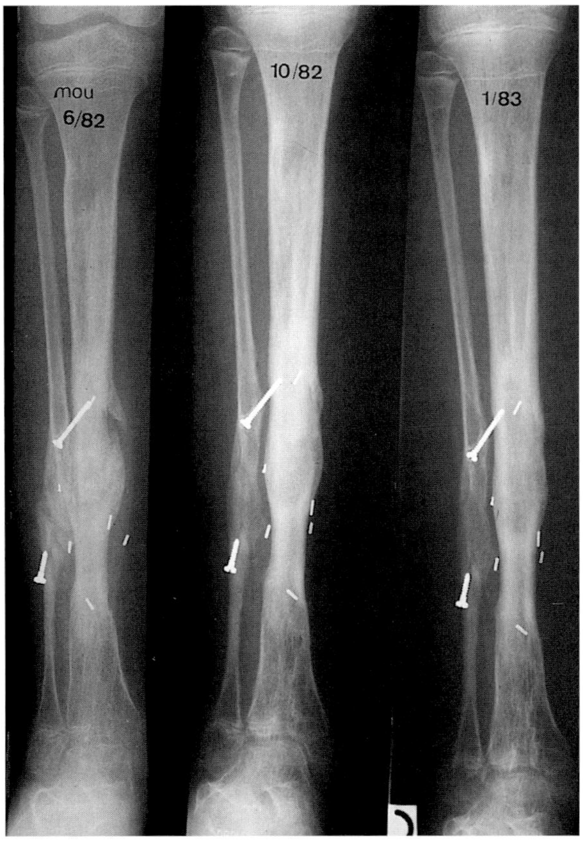

Fig. 11 *Complication – fracture of the transferred fibula. The spontaneous fracture was not painful and was detected late.*
Healing without problems in 3 months, with loss of 8 mm in length.

Fig. 12 *Complication – recurrence.*
(a) Result after uneventful healing (2 years postoperatively).
(b) Recurrence immediately distal to the fibula.
(c) After treatment of the recurvatum and stapling. Quick healing.

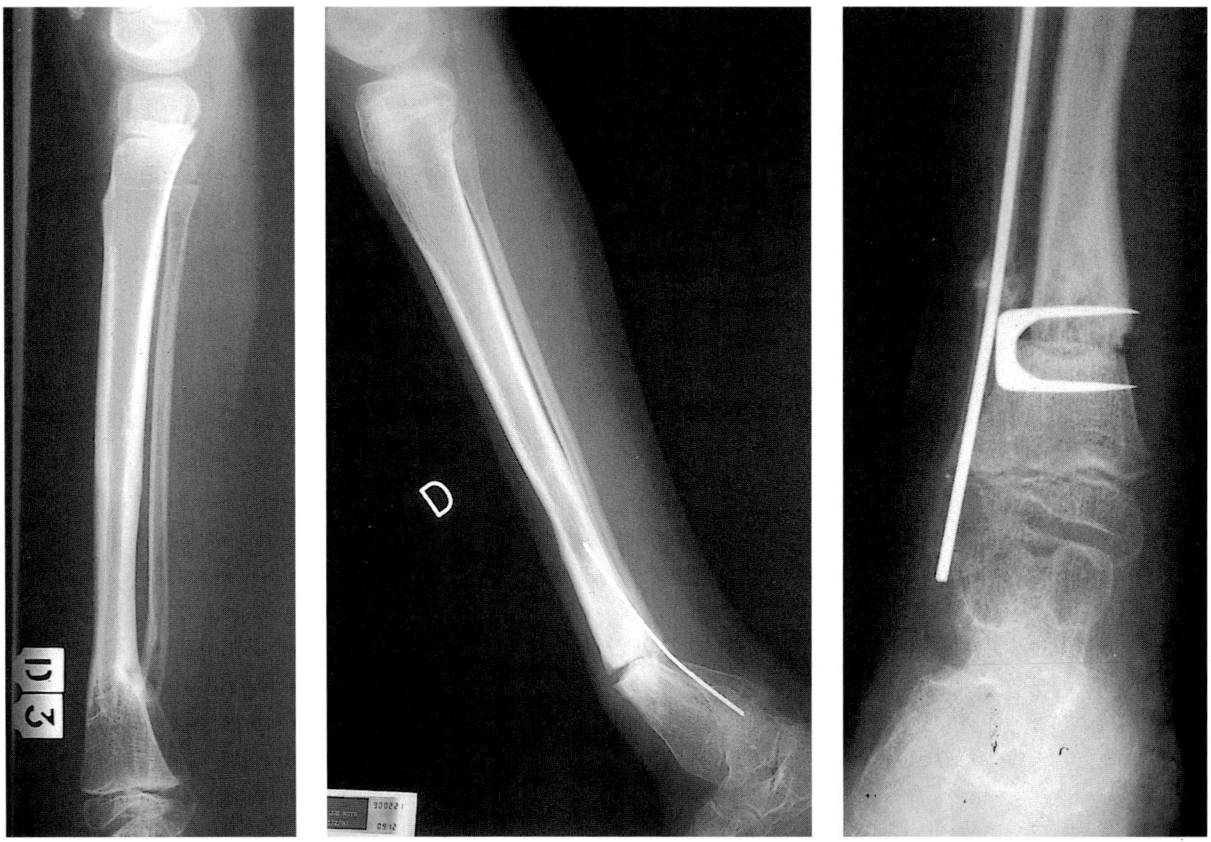

a *b* *c*

some patients are healed. As soon as there are signs of bone union, the fixator should be removed and replaced by a walking cast. In some cases, if healing is not perfect or there are signs of desaxation (if a fixator was not used), one should not hesitate to carry out secondary fixation with plate and screws. This early secondary operation has allowed good healing in most cases. Finally, when the tibia is well healed, it should be protected by an orthosis until approximately the age of 10. There are risks of re-fracture or recurrence of the pseudarthrosis.

Results

Between 1977 and 1992, 43 cases of congenital pseudarthrosis of the leg and 6 cases of congenital pseudarthrosis of the forearm were treated.

Four of the patients, resident in South America or Pakistan, have been lost to follow-up. At last follow-up all were healed, but long-term follow-up is not available. One patient died of an embryonal sarcoma. It was possible to review all the other patients. Two patients were excluded from the review as they were atypical: one case of very late onset (> 9 years old), and one of treatment started after the age of 14 years. One of these patients healed with a contralateral vascularized fibula graft. This healing took almost 1 year, necessitating a secondary plate fixation. The second patient was not healed at age 17, when she was lost to follow-up.

In the 'typical' group there were 20 girls and 16 boys. The right side was more frequently involved (21/15).

Neurofibromatosis was associated in 78% of cases, as well as 3 other tumors:

- 1 nephroblastoma;
- 1 embryonal sarcoma; and
- 1 cerebellar tumor.

The histological findings were positive in 9 cases (32%) at the site of the pseudarthrosis. The average age at surgery was 59 months (5–206 months), reflecting the fact that many of these operations were done as salvage procedures after many other failed operations (average 2.7, with a maximum of 10).

The average follow-up was 59 months (4–111 months), with an average age at last follow-up being 122 months.

At the time of this review 33 out of 36 cases were healed. Two were not healed, despite several operations, and one was too early after operation (4 months) to judge. Average overall healing time was 11 months, reflecting the combination of proximal and distal sites healing. The proximal site healed slightly earlier (7 months) than the distal site (8 months).

In 58% of cases, union was primary, needing no secondary operation, and the average healing time was 4.5 months. In the other cases, the average time to union was 14.6 months.

The average number of reoperations was 1.3, with little difference between proximal site (0.6) and distal site (0.7). Complications were not rare, with two simple pin track infections, but also two deep late infections and one deep early infection. It was never necessary to resect the fibula.

We found three recurrences (two in one patient), which healed quite simply with reoperation and bone grafting.

Fractures were not uncommon (8%–22%). All of these healed with simple immobilization. There was one late graft necrosis after early infection. We feel this is probably due to vascular thrombosis of the graft. This patient is not yet healed.

Factors influencing the results

Neurofibromatosis

The average healing time was 11.4 months in patients with neurofibromatosis, as opposed to 10.3 months in the other patients.

As was claimed by Morrissy et al (1981), we can confirm that neurofibromatosis does not seem to influence the final healing time significantly.

Age at first fracture

We compared the age at first fracture with the healing time.

- When the first fracture appeared at less than 1 year of age average healing time was 12 months.
- When the fracture occurred between 1 and 2 years the average healing time was 9 months.
- When the fracture occurred at over 2 years the average healing time was 11 months.

- When the fracture was secondary to a surgical osteotomy the average healing time was 11.5 months.

There seems to be no correlation between the age at the first fracture and healing time.

Number of previous operations

The results are paradoxical, as the average healing time is 11 months if there have been no previous operations and is also 11 months for up to three prior procedures, but becomes 7.6 months if there have been more than three earlier operations. This may be due to the age of the child, which is 73 months on average in the last group, compared with 27 months and 53 months in the other groups.

Sex

There is a slight difference, as the average healing time is 13 months for boys and 9 months for girls.

Age at surgery

The average time of healing is 15 months in patients operated on up to 39 months of age, 7 months in patients operated between 40 and 89 months of age, and 15 months in patients more than 90 months old. This may be due to the better fixation obtained when the tibia is larger.

Final results

These results are difficult to assess, as operations of this kind are performed on a growing child. Several initially good results have deteriorated with time. The growth potential of the tibia may have been affected by prior operations, especially when using transplantar intramedullary nailing.

It seems, contrary to some suppositions in the past, that there is no natural growth deficiency in congenital pseudarthrosis. Those patients who heal early, with no trauma to the growth plate, do not have leg-length discrepancy. This is why we feel that the end result should be evaluated only in patients who have reached puberty.

In our series, 29 patients have reached 14 years of age or more. They have been reviewed, with an average follow-up of 11.5 years (range 6–16 years). Most of them are now adults (average 17.5 years old).

Neurofibromatosis was present in 22 cases (75%), but was demonstrated histologically only in 6 cases.

The average number of previous operations was 2.9 (0–10). One of these patients still had a nonunion at the proximal site. All other patients healed both proximally and distally. Seventeen of these children healed by primary transfer of the fibula; the others had one to four reoperations:

- 6 had one;
- 4 had two; and
- one had three and one had four.

Residual deformity of the tibia was not uncommon. Nine patients had some kind of valgus between 5° and 25°, and/or some anterior bowing of 15° to 30°. The foot and ankle usually had some limited mobility, involving some pes planus and a valgus deformity of the talus. The size of the foot was usually smaller than that on the other side. Leg length discrepancy was a major preoperative problem, and remained in many instances a post-operative problem.

At the time of operation, the average discrepancy was 3.5 cm, with more than 2.5 cm (max. 9 cm) in 13 patients. At follow-up the average leg length discrepancy was 1.7 cm, with 9 patients having more than 2.5 cm (max. 6.5 cm). In 4 of those patients there was no more discrepancy after operation, but the growth plate injury was responsible for its evolution.

In the case of leg length discrepancy our philosophy is to try to correct it completely at the time of the initial operation. This is possible either during the operation (by an adjustment of less than 2 cm) or by prior progressive lengthening. The length of the graft will be adjusted to the defect.

In cases with growth plate injury it will sometimes be necessary to do a secondary lengthening at puberty. This was done twice with Ilizarov apparatus, and allowed a 7-cm and and a 9-cm lengthening with no special healing problems.

Conclusion

It is difficult to compare this series of patients treated by the same surgeon using one technique with the other series in the literature. In the large series of 40 patients published by Morrissy et al (1981) there were 14 amputations and 8 nonunions.

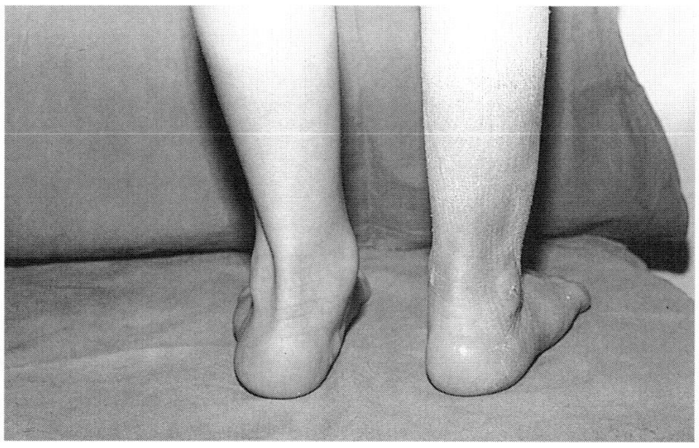

a

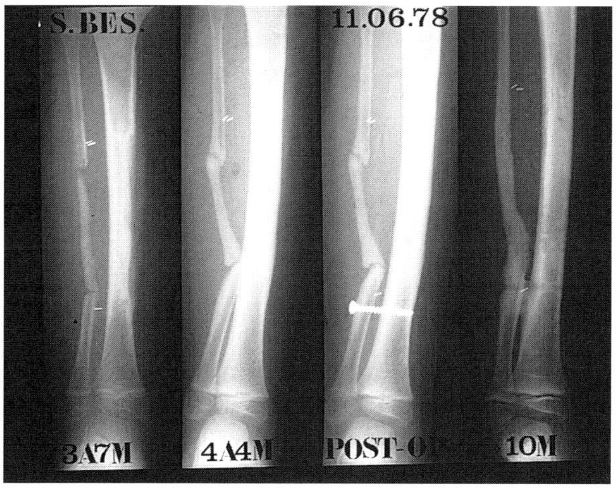

b

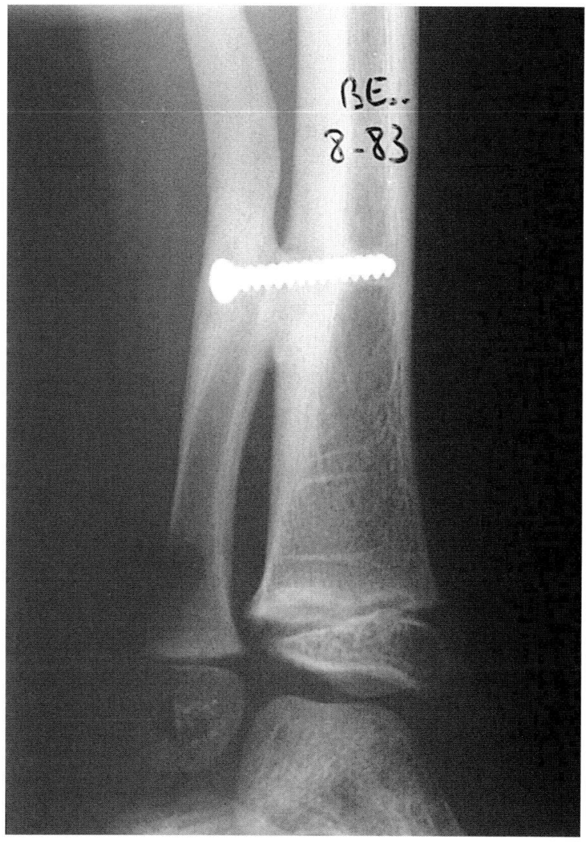

c

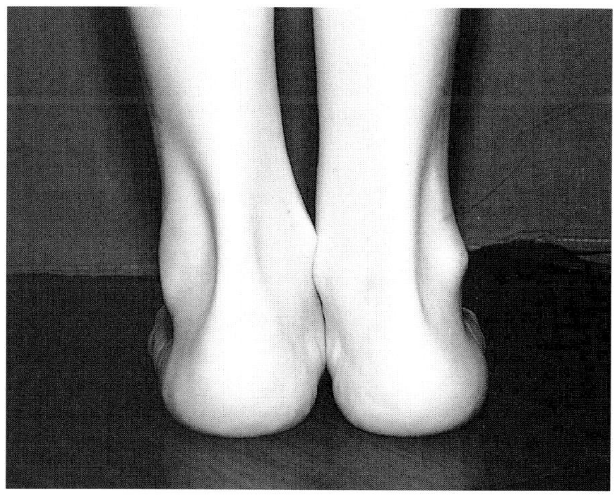

d

Fig. 13 *Complication – valgus of donor ankle.*
(a) Girl – 7 years-old. Four years after fibula transfer, the donor ankle shows a valgus.
(b) The valgus is due to nonunion of the graft. Treatment by stabilization and bone graft of the lower segment. Healing at 10 months.
(c) Progressive correction of the valgus.
(d) Clinical result.

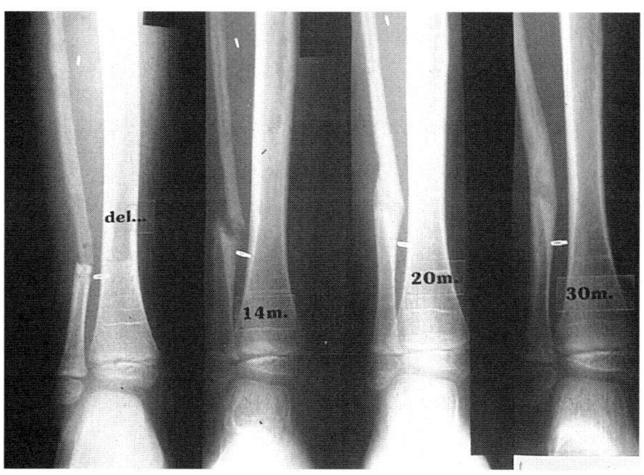

Fig. 14 *Boy – 8 years old. Progressive valgus due to pseudarthrosis of the distal graft. Bone grafting. Healing in 6 months and correction of the valgus.*

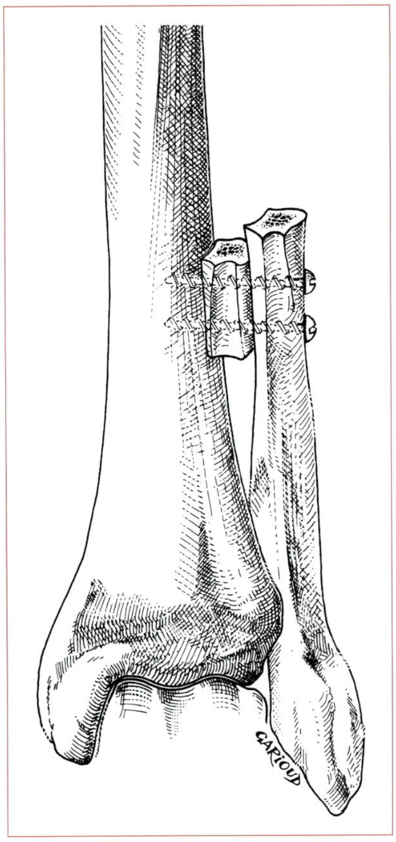

a

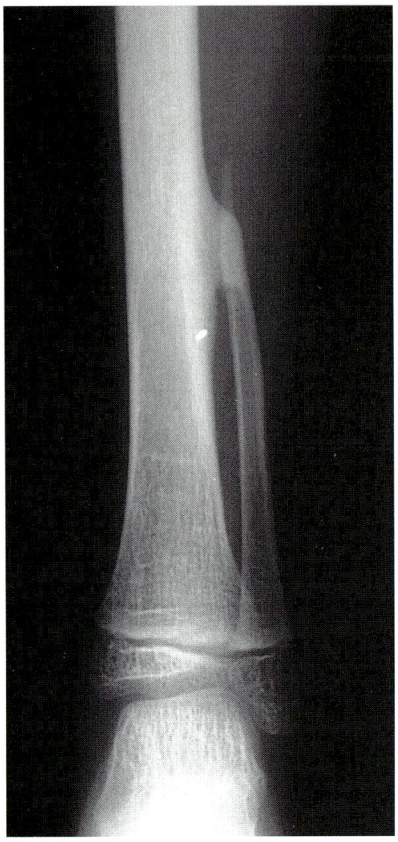

c

Fig. 15

(a) *The valgus may be treated by bone grafting of the distal fragment.*

(b) *Or by the Langenskjold procedure.*

(c) *The Langenskjold procedure after healing.*

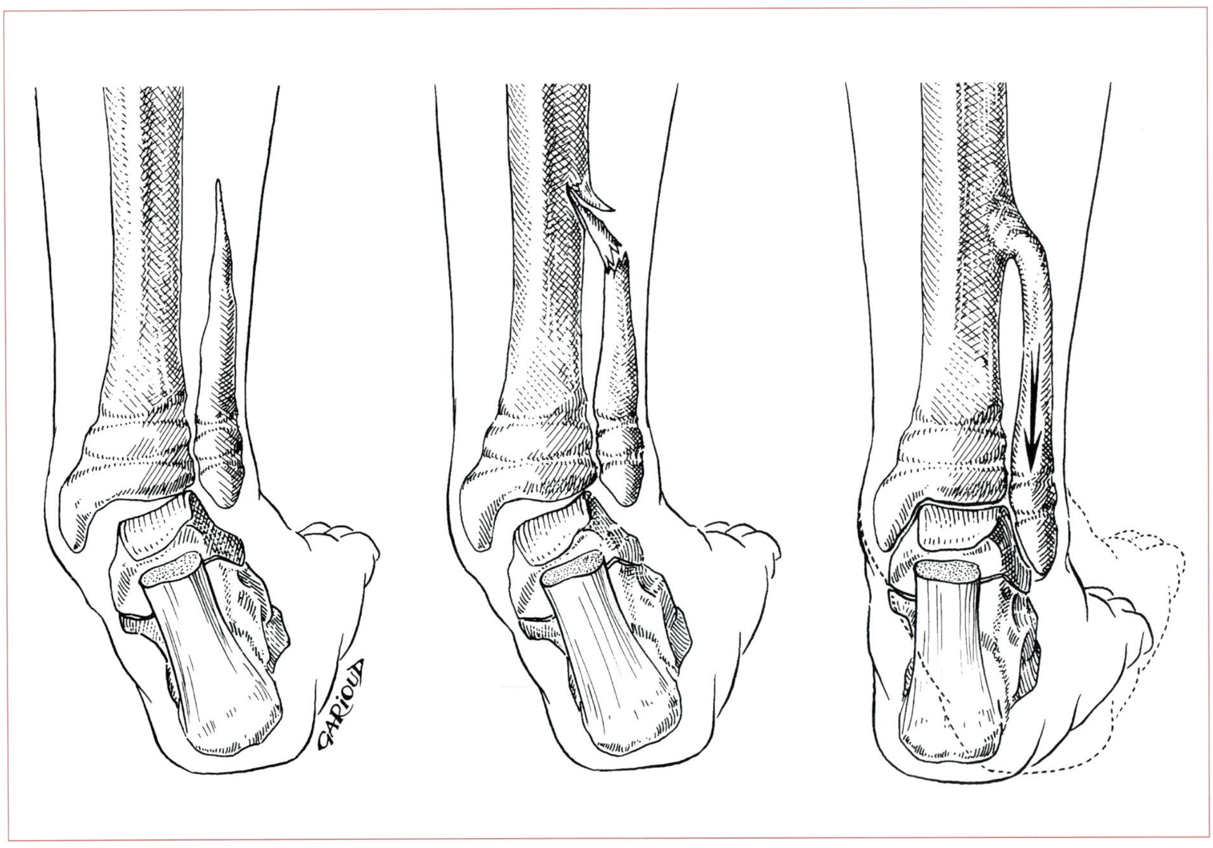

b

The conclusion was that the only predictable method was the Farmer procedure (bone pedicle graft from the other side).

Our experience confirms that vascularized bone transfer seems to be the most reliable method of treating congenital pseudarthrosis, even if the follow-up is difficult and many patients need additional procedures.

C. CONGENITAL PSEUDARTHROSIS OF THE FOREARM

This is a very rare disease, and we have treated only six cases. In the world literature, 26 other cases have been published.

It is unclear why this condition seems more severe and difficult to treat than pseudarthrosis of the tibia? There may be mechanical reasons, as often two bones are involved, with many rotation forces. The destructive nature of the disease then makes reconstruction more difficult.

Since Moore (1949), a variety of treatments have been used, but the outcome remains poor. Of 22 cases treated with classical techniques (bone grafts or cast) only 9 healed, usually after a long period of treatment and with severe stiffness.

Since introduction of the vascularized fibular transfer, several authors and we ourselves have treated 10 cases and reported 10 successes.

In our series the average time for union was 6 months (3–24). When union occurs it proceeds rapidly, initially occurring proximally in our series. One patient had a secondary fracture of the graft 2 years after healing, and this necessitated several reoperations, including a second vascularized fibular transfer.

One-third of the 32 cases in the literature involved pseudarthrosis of both bones. In 4 cases the authors and ourselves tried to reconstruct a one-bone forearm and succeeded.

There was no success in attempts to reconstruct both bones using classical methods. Here again, only the use of vascularized fibula allowed healing in each case. In our series, the mean follow-up was 6 years (2–12), and we found only a slight shortening (average 2 cm) of the forearm.

In those patients who did not have a one-bone forearm, there was only a mild residual loss of supination (av. 25°).

Perhaps for even a greater degree than for tibial pseudarthrosis, the treatment of choice for congenital pseudarthrosis of the forearm is vascularized fibular transfer. Early operation and stable fixation are the bases of the treatment. When the disease is advanced and destruction severe, one should consider the alternative of a one-bone forearm reconstruction between the proximal ulna and distal radius.

D. TRAUMATIC BONE LOSS

Traumatic bone loss uncomplicated by chronic osteomyelitis is usually the result of penetrating trauma or a highly comminuted open fracture. Depending upon the injury mechanism, there may be concomitant severe soft tissue injury. The extent to which soft tissue is lost, devitalized, or directly traumatized will certainly influence the complexity of the reconstructive plan. Most authors agree that in the absence of severe soft tissue loss or fibrosis, the most favorable results for long bone reconstruction by vascularized bone transfer are in this group. In the Mayo Clinic series the best results were seen in the subgroup of 25 patients with this indication (Han et al 1992). Nineteen of these patients went on to primary union (76%), and four of the remaining six patients healed with an onlay cancellous graft at the site of nonunion, resulting in an overall final union rate of 92%. Gilbert in his review of vascularized bone reconstructions of femoral defects also found a difference in outcome between infected bone defects and those without infection (Gilbert et al, in press). At 6 months following bone transfer, 45% of the patients with nonseptic defects, as compared with 18% with previous osteomyelitis, had undergone union. By 18 months the union rates were 100% and 82% respectively. The more favorable result seen in patients with aseptic bone defects probably relates to a number of factors. It is probable that patients in this group are less likely to have severe soft tissue injury than their counterparts who go on to the complication of chronic osteomyelitis. Moreover, in the absence of active or recent infection the surgeon is more likely to employ aggressive internal fixation, resulting in rigid osteosynthesis and supplementary cancellous bone grafting about the osteosynthesis sites.

E. BONE TUMOR RESECTION

Undoubtedly long bone reconstruction by vascularized bone transfer has been a great contribution to limb preservation management of malignant and locally aggressive bone tumors. As a result of improved imaging techniques, accurate preoperative staging of such aggressive bone and juxtaosseous soft tissue tumors is frequently possible (Rock et al 1993). This fact, taken together with an improved understanding of the natural history of many tumors, as well as the recognition of the effectiveness of adjuvant and neoadjuvant chemotherapy and radiotherapy, has lead to an increasing emphasis on limb-sparing radical resections rather than limb ablation. Typically, patients undergoing bone tumor resection will have a massive bone defect, but with supple and adequate surrounding soft tissue, relatively normal tissue planes, and healthy blood vessels for microvascular anastomoses. Thus, from a technical perspective, the management of the bone recipient site is easier than for those patients with chronic or relatively acute traumatic wounds. On the other hand, adjuvant or neoadjuvant chemotherapy or radiotherapy may complicate the postoperative course, particularly in relation to the rapidity of bone union and hypertrophy. It is likely for this reason that the results of vascularized bone transfer for limb-sparing tumor resection are somewhat inferior to those for traumatic bone reconstruction. In the Mayo Clinic series reported by Han et al (1992), the most common indication warranting reconstruction by vascularized bone transfer was tumor resection. Of 69 patients in this group, fibula was utilized in 65 and iliac crest in 4. The most common types of bone tumor among this group included osteogenic sarcoma, chondrosarcoma, giant cell tumor, and adamantinoma. Of these 69 patients, 46 (67%) progressed to primary union. Union occurred in an additional 10 patients after a secondary procedure for ultimate limb salvage, bringing the union rate up to 81%. A number of additional authors have reported the value of vascularized bone transfer for the management of long bone aggressive tumors in the form of small series case reports (Yajima et al 1993; Leung and Hung 1989; Leung and Chan 1986; Watari et al 1978) or as a portion of larger series consisting of fractures in patients with neoplastic conditions (Minami et al 1989; Yajima et al 1992; Weiland et al 1983). From these series it is difficult to extract sufficient data to predict the outcome of post-neoplastic long bone reconstruction in terms of limb salvage, union, hypertrophy, complications, and tumor recurrence.

F. CHRONIC OSTEOMYELITIS

The value of vascularized bone transfer for the management of chronic osteomyelitis is less convincing than that for other indications. Theoretically this procedure may permit the replacement of infected poorly vascularized bone by sterile bone with an intact physiologic blood supply (Wood and Cooney 1984). However, a number of factors associated with chronic osteomyelitis may present difficult challenges for the surgeon contemplating reconstruction by vascularized bone transfer. Not the least of these is the fact that almost all patients in this group have fibrotic and indurated soft tissue about the infected bone site. Thus dead space obliteration and skin closure may be difficult to achieve successfully. Successful vascular anastomoses may also be a challenge as a result of fibrosis about the arteries and veins and of the frequently associated problem of venous hypertension arising from prior deep venous thrombosis. Moreover, rigid internal fixation with large metallic plates and screws and supplementary cancellous bone grafting about the osteosynthesis sites is usually avoided in this setting because it may risk exacerbation or promote persistence of infection. As a result, in the author's experience, the lowest incidence of primary bone union with vascularized bone transfer is in this group of patients. In the Mayo Clinic series reported by Han et al (1992) a total of 60 patients underwent management of chronic osteomyelitis by an aggressive resection of obviously infected bone and soft tissue followed by vascularized bone or osteocutaneous flap transfer. All patients in this series had had multiple prior unsuccessful debridement and reconstruction procedures, and for all practical purposes were considered candidates for amputation. Of the 60 patients, 54 had involvement of either tibia or femur. Of the whole group only 29 of the 60 went on to primary union. Despite this fact, the overall success rate using vascularized bone grafting for osteomyelitis is not strikingly different from that with other indications. Following secondary bone grafting a final union rate of 77% (46 of 60 patients) was reported. Modest results were also reported by Weiland (Weiland et al 1984a) in a series of 13 patients treated by vascularized fibula or osteocutaneous flap transfer for chronic osteomyelitis with 2 or more years follow-up. Thrombosis of the microvascular anastomosis and resultant failure occurred in 23% of patients in the early postoperative period. Of the remainder, 60% of patients experienced union with no evidence of further infection.

G. FEMORAL HEAD OSTEONECROSIS

Aseptic necrosis of the femoral head is a well-defined entity. It is the consequence of ischemia to the bone cells, but the etiology is ill defined. Many factors are involved (alcoholism, tobacco, hyperlipidemia, steroids, etc) but the exact effect and importance of each is unknown.

Although the progression and physiopathology have been well described by Glimcher (1968) and Kenzora there is no preventive or specific treatment. Prosthetic replacement is a standard treatment in older patients, but this alternative is not well accepted in the younger. Several type of osteotomies have been designed, but these treatments are usually limited by the extent of the disease. Drilling has been favored by several authors (Kleinberg, Ficat, Hungerford), but, though it seems to improve the pain in the early stages, it has been criticized from a biomechanical point of view.

Others have added a cortical bone graft to the drilling procedure in the hope of achieving a better mechanical support of the femoral head. Many authors have been disappointed by this procedure, although Bonfiglio et al reported in 1980 on a satisfactory long-term result in 56 patients operated on at an early stage.

In 1962 Judet et al introduced the concept of vascularized bone transplantation for the femoral head. They used a posterior muscle bone pedicle from the posterior part of the greater trochanter. This technique was used initially to prevent necrosis after femoral neck fractures, and was later extended to the treatment of established osteonecrosis. Although an experimental study suggested this possibility in 1966, the clinical results were not satisfactory, as the procedure endangered the posterior circumflex artery. Myers (1978–85) has used this technique and has obtained good results in the early stages (I–II) of disease (Marcus and Enneking 1973). Other authors have also reported on the use of this technique (Baksi 1991; Lee et al 1990).

Another form of vascularized muscle pedicle bone graft was described by Palazzi et al in 1975. It consisted of a piece of ilium attached to the tensor fasciae femoris muscle. These techniques, like that employing iliac crest pedicled on the rectus femoris muscle (Echevarria 1975), are difficult to use owing to the limited length of the pedicle and limited vascularization to the bone.

A significant improvement was offered by Ganz (1983), who designed a vascularized iliac crest segment, pedicled on the deep circumflex iliac vessels. This segment is introduced into the femoral head after excision of necrosis through an anterior approach.

An intertrochanteric flexion osteotomy is associated. Lippuner (1990) presented the results of this team on 45 hips. The results were clinically good or very good in 75% of all cases, and in 90% of those classified as Stage II. A similar technique was used by Leung (1981) and Chen (1983). Hori has designed a technique of direct implantation of the anterior circumflex vessels into the femoral head (1979). In his technique, the necrotic bone is not excised. Various experiments (Boyd, Alnot, Gartsman, Griss), including our own, have shown that it is possible to prevent necrosis in a devascularized piece of bone, but not to revascularize a bone segment with established necrosis. We are not aware of the long-term results of the clinical experience with the Hori technique. In 1978 with H. Judet we decided to attempt to transplant a vascularized fibula into the femoral head. In our first technique we introduced the fibula by an anterior opening of the femoral neck. The necrosis was excised through this approach without hip joint dislocation. We still recommend this approach in early stages, where the cartilage cannot be easily detached from the subchondral bone.

The main disadvantage of this technique is the difficulty of excising the necrotic bone properly. For this reason we modified the technique in 1980 to include dislocating the hip and excising the necrotic bone through a chondral flap (Judet et al 1981). Free fibula transfer has been used by several authors. In 1979 Brunelli presented his technique of transplantation from a trochanteric approach, drilling a large hole, curetting the head and then filling it with cancellous bone. The fibula is then inserted and fixed by a screw. Anastomoses are made with the anterior circumflex artery and vein. Urbaniak has used a very similar technique. Fujimaki (1983) has used a posterior approach to transfer the fibula, but with only early experience. Gonzales del Pino (1986), author of an excellent thesis on femoral head necrosis, proposes a technique of lateral implantation of the fibula, but with an anterior neck approach to resect the necrotic bone.

Preoperative assessment and staging

The precise diagnosis and staging of the disease is paramount. We have routinely used radiographs, CT scans and selective arteriograms.

- *Radiographs:* provide clear delineation of the shape of the femoral head and the quality of the joint, but are sometimes insufficient to determine the extent of the disease.
- *CT scans:* give a good appraisal of the extent of necrosis, especially on horizontal cuts. In early stages they allow density measurements.
- *MRI:* has also been used in some cases. It is useful in early stages for diagnosis.
- *Arteriograms:* are useful for preoperative planning of the operation, and have been used in many cases for clarification of the anastomoses.

Staging is an important step, and we have used the grading system published by Marcus and Enneking (1973) based on the radiographic appearance:

- Stage I : Some increase in density
- Stage II : Sclerosis – Cyst
- Stage III : Crescent sign – Subchondral fracture
- Stage IV : Some collapse – No joint space narrowing

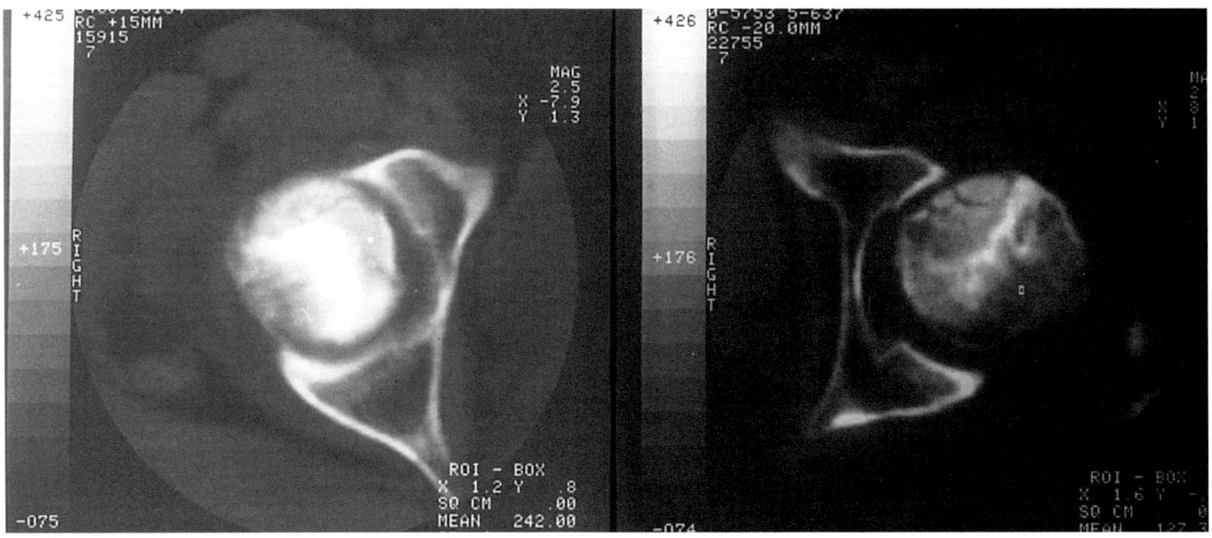

Fig. 16 *Preoperative assessment: the CT scans show the extent of the necrosis.*

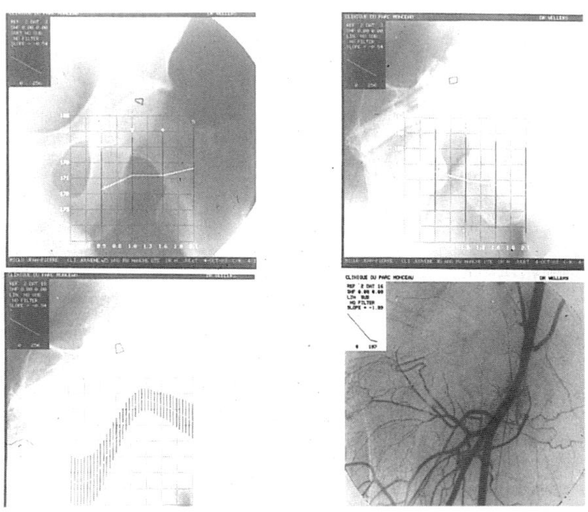

Fig. 17 *Arteriogram with selective injection of the anterior circumflex artery.*

- Stage V : Collapse – Joint space narrowing
- Stage VI : Severe deformation – Advanced arthritis.

Surgical technique

The operation is performed with the patient lying supine on a fracture table. The fibula is harvested from the opposite leg, which is draped, with the knee acutely flexed and with a tourniquet.

Two surgical teams work simultaneously, one on the hip, the other preparing the fibula. This allows the operation not to exceed 2 – 2½ hours.

One team prepares the hip through an anterior Smith–Petersen approach. Immediately after incision of the fascia, the anterior circumflex artery is isolated and dissected as far laterally as possible. The joint capsule is incised and the femoral head is anteriorly dislocated, using the traction of the fracture table.

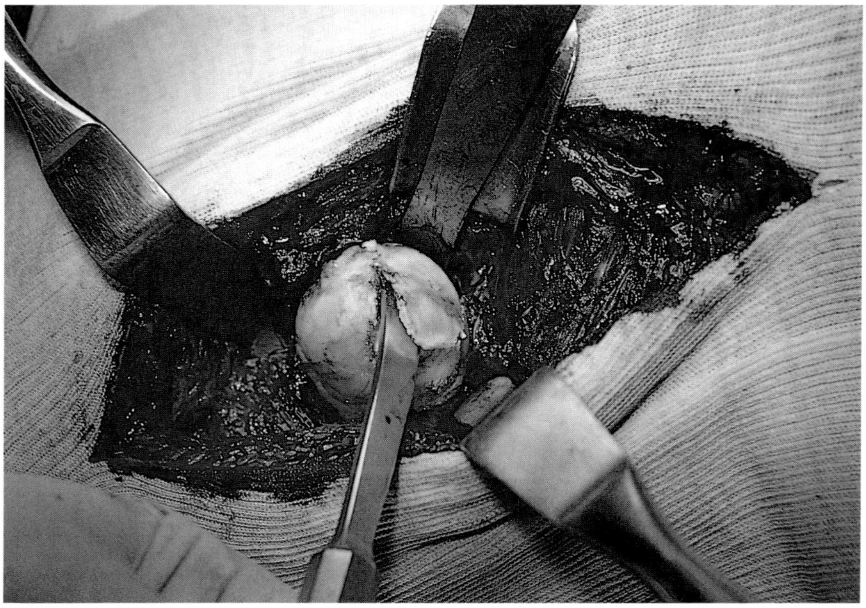

a

***Fig. 18** (a–f) Surgical technique*
(a) Anterior approach with dislocation of the head. Incision on the borders of the cartilage flap.

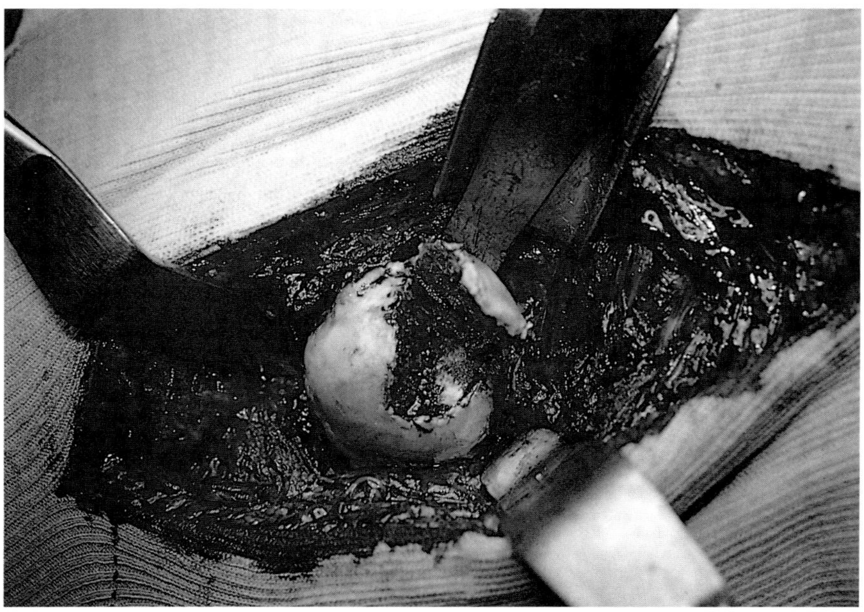

b

(b) The flap is elevated.

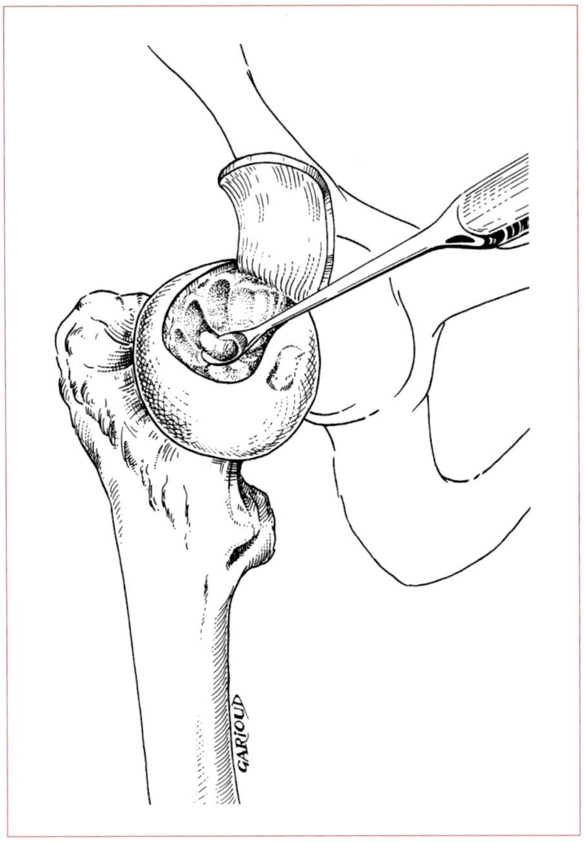

c

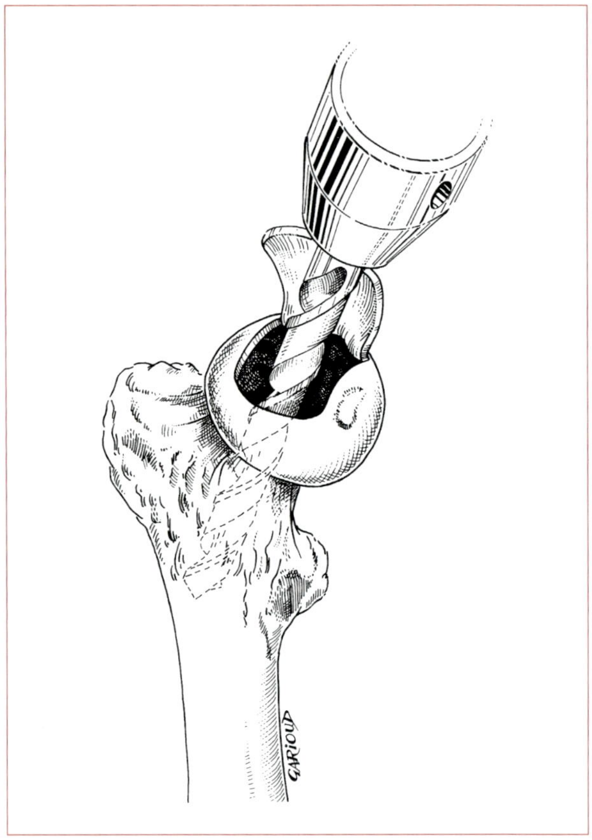

d

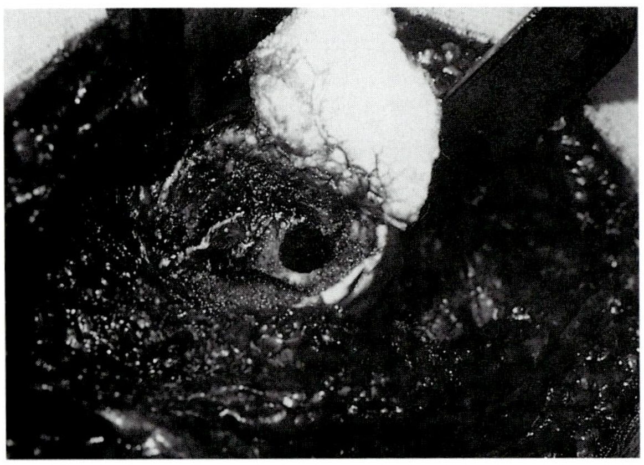

e

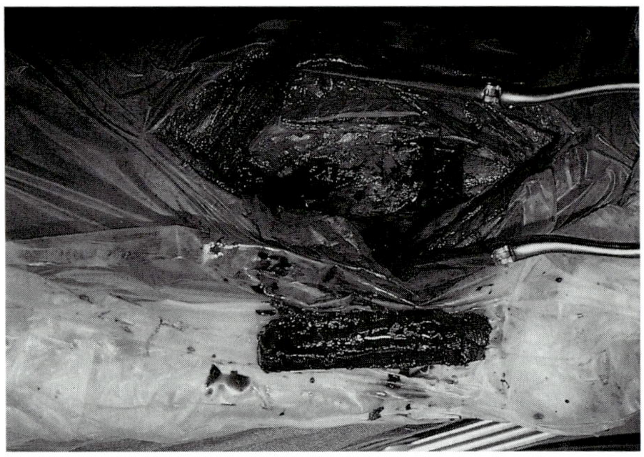

f

Fig. 18 continued

(c) Curettage of necrotic bone.

(d) Drilling of the neck down to the lateral cortex.

(e) The head is evacuated of necrotic bone.

(f) Raising a 9-cm piece of fibula.

A large chondral flap is designed on the head, leaving a wide attachment. This flap is easy to lift in femoral head with Stage III disease, as it is already separated from the subchondral bone. In an early Stage II lesion it may be very difficult to define and elevate this flap. We now tend in those cases to do the operation through the femoral neck, without lifting a flap or even dislocating the hip.

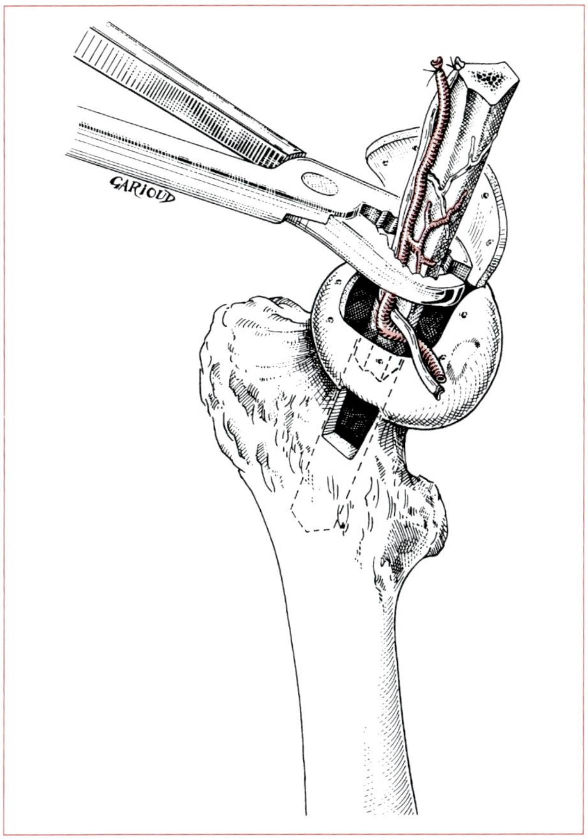

g

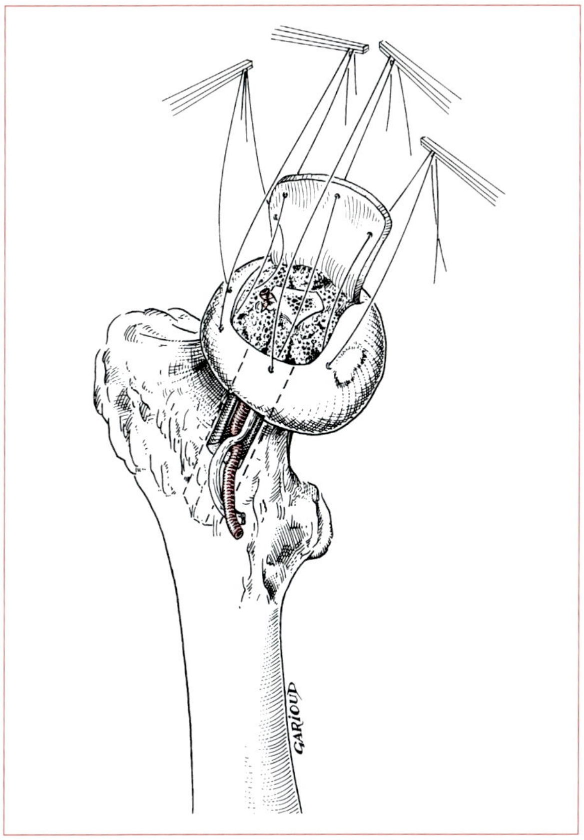

h

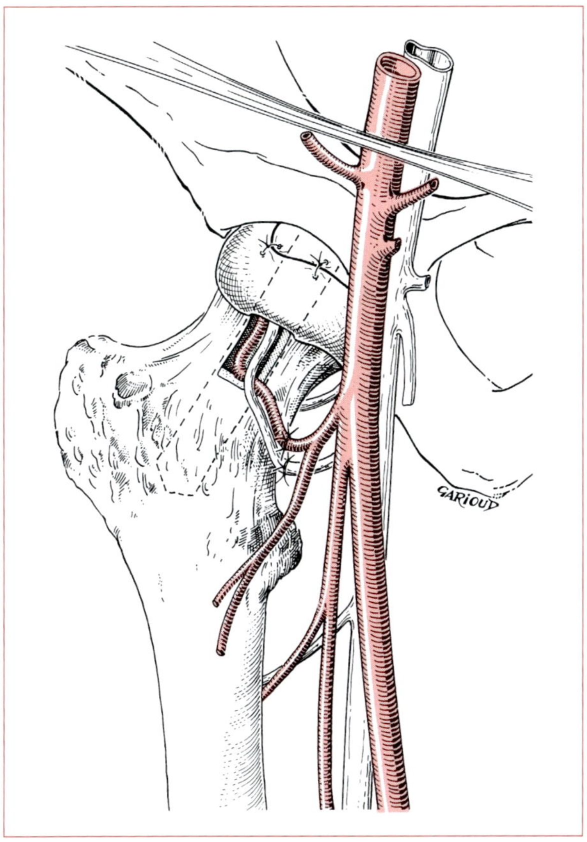

i

Fig. 18 continued

(g) The fibula is introduced into the neck.

(h) The fibula is in place with bone graft around it. The vessels are coming through a hole in the anterior neck cortex.

(i) The flap is sutured back and the head reduced. Microvascular anastomoses are accomplished using the anterior circumflex vessels.

Once the flap is elevated, the sclerotic necrotic bone is obvious. The necrotic area is then excised with chisels and large curets. It is important to remove all necrotic bone and expose the adjacent viable, well vascularized, and softer cancellous bone.

The neck is then drilled to the lateral cortex to provide space for the fibula. A square piece of cortex on the anterior part of the neck is removed, to allow passage for the peroneal vessels.

Simultaneously, the second team harvests the contralateral fibula (see Chapter 13). The length of fibula required is determined by preoperative measurements of the length of the femoral neck and head. Usually the length varies from 6 to 8 cm. The vascular pedicle must be dissected to be as long as possible.

The fibula is then brought to the hip and inserted into the pre-drilled canal. It may be necessary at this stage to widen the canal or reduce the length of the graft in order to permit easy closure of the cartilaginous flap. The vessels are exteriorized through the hole on the femoral neck.

The area within the femoral head around the fibula is then packed with cancellous bone obtained from the femoral neck and the nearby iliac crest.

The osteocartilagenous flap of the femoral head is closed with resorbable sutures, and the head is cautiously reduced into the acetabulum.

It is then time for the vascular anastomoses, done with 10-0 nylon, using an operating microscope. The peroneal artery and one vein are sutured to the anterior circumflex vessels. The diameters are large (1.5–2.0 mm for arteries, 2–2 mm for the veins). Venous back flow is usually slow.

After capsular closures, the wound is closed on suction drainage.

A transtibial pin is placed to allow skeletal traction for 3 weeks. Progressive weightbearing will be allowed after 6 months.

Clinical results

Since 1978 more than 130 hips have been operated on, but it is only since 1979 that we have used the more advanced technique with dislocation of the hip.

C. Mathoulin (1992) has reviewed the cases with more than 5 years of postoperative follow-up. In total 49 patients (59 hips) were operated on during the period 1980–87.

The disease was unilateral in 39 cases and bilateral in 10 cases. The series comprised 39 men and 10 women, with an average age at operation of 35 years old (range 14–51).

The etiologies included:

- Corticosteroid therapy ... 11 hips
- Chronic alcoholism ... 12 hips
- Sequelae of childhood disease ... 2 hips
- Idiopathic ... 34 hips

The preoperative staging (according to Enneking) was:

- Stage II : 13 cases (3 more than ⅔ of femoral head)
- Stage III : 21 cases (12 more than ⅔ of femoral head)
- Stage IV : 23 cases (15 more than ⅔ of femoral head)
- Stage V : 2 cases.

We have been able to review 48 of these hips with a follow-up of more than 5 years (average 7 years 4 months, maximum 13 years). All these patients had preoperative clinical (d'Aubigne) and radiologic (Enneking) examination and staging.

Among these 48 hips the overall results include:

- 20 good or excellent (41.7%), associating good clinical results and radiological improvement or stabilization;
- 5 average (10.3%), where the patients have no pain but some joint stiffness and no radiological improvement; and
- 23 poor (48.0%), with 21 having had a secondary total hip prosthesis.

Altogether 52% of the patients have good or satisfactory results at 5 years, although the potential for late deterioration exists.

When we look at the results according to the preoperative staging the differences are striking.

- Stage II : 72.7% good or excellent results
- Stage III : 88.2% good or excellent results
- Stage IV : 95.0% poor results.

These results show clearly the limitations of this technique. With more than 82% of good and excellent results in Stages II and III, we have defined the exact indications for using the technique. It should not be applied to Stage IV cases, where it seems to accelerate the joint degeneration.

If we evaluate the results according to the age of the patient, it is striking that the excellent and good results

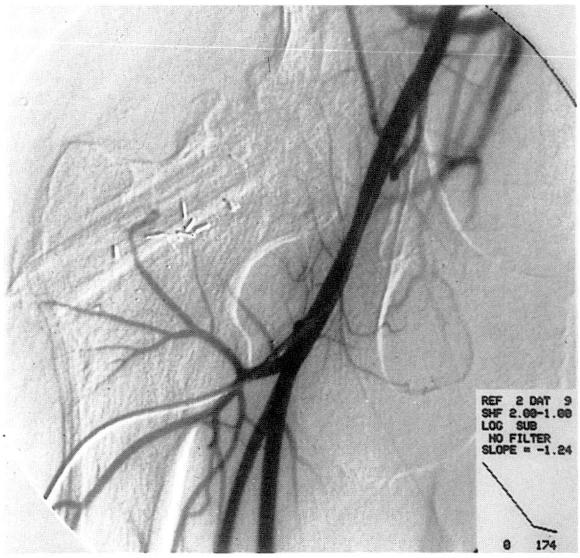

Fig. 19 *Postoperative arteriogram.*

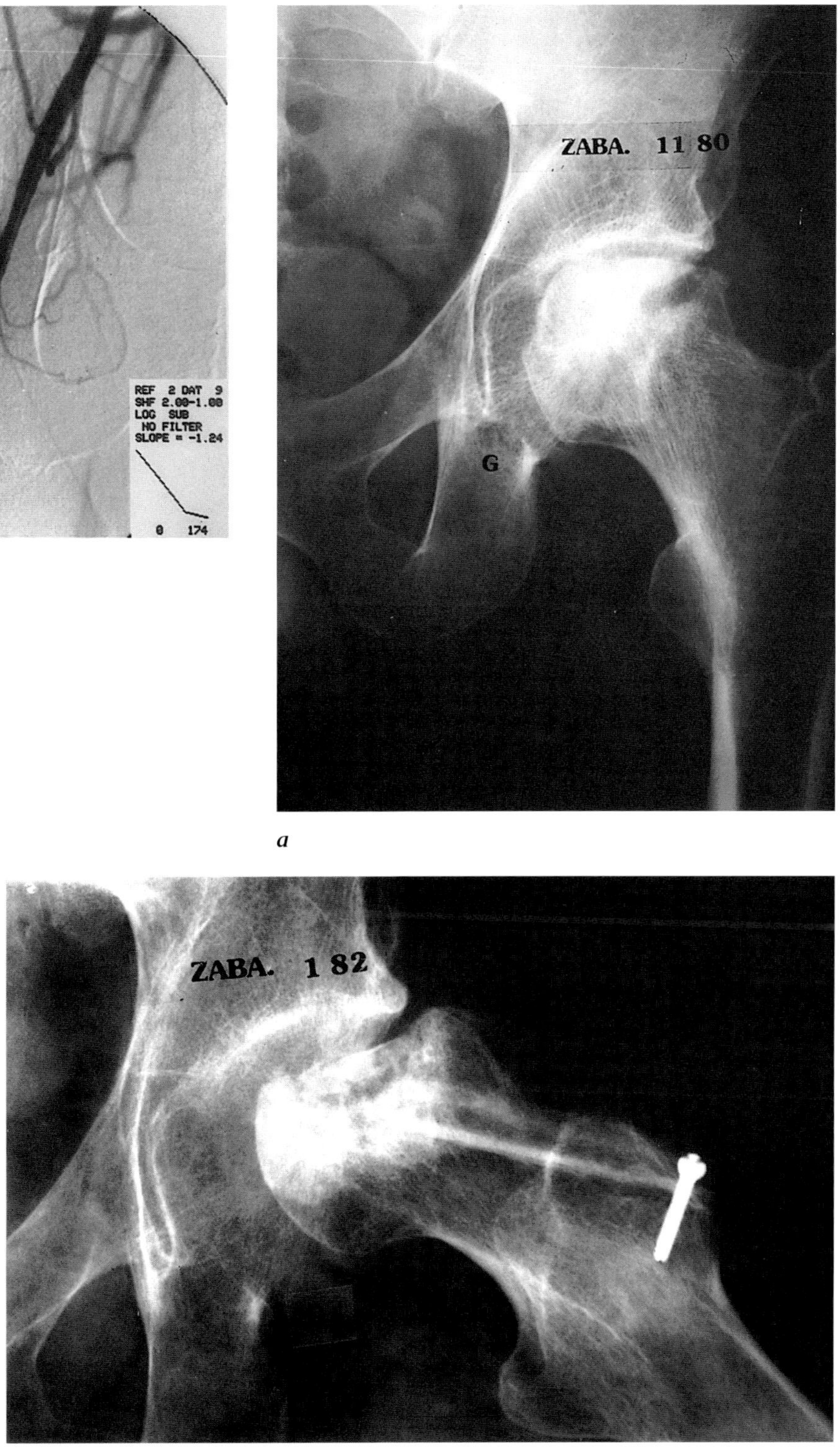

Fig. 20 *Poor result:*
(a) Advanced stage.
(b) Early destruction after transfer.

are seen in 72% of patients aged less than 35 years, and in only 37% of those more than 35 years old.

The ideal indication is represented by:

- a young patient (30 years old);
- an early stage (II and III Enneking); and
- unilateral necrosis.

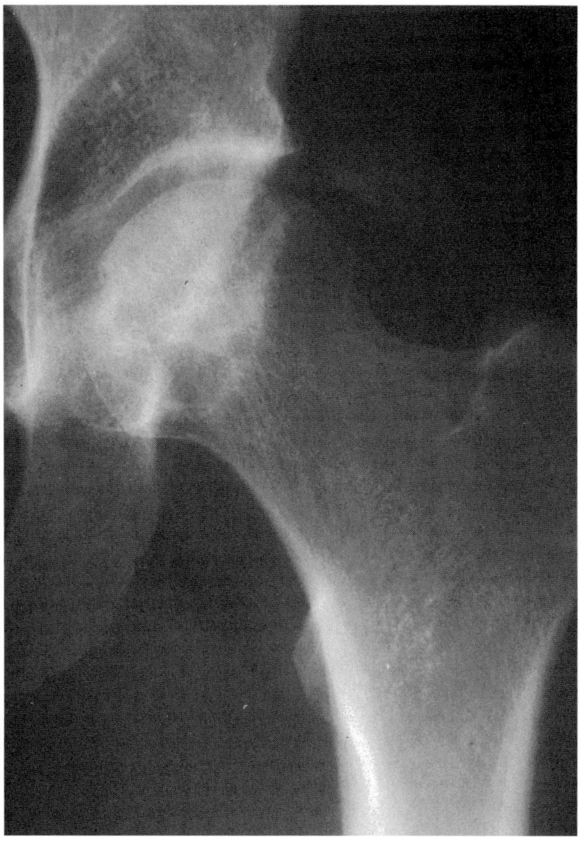

a

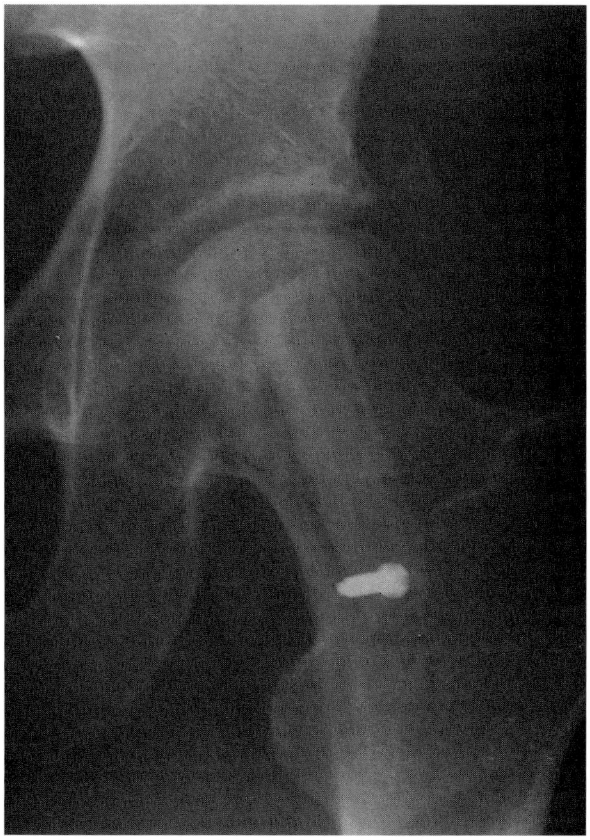

b

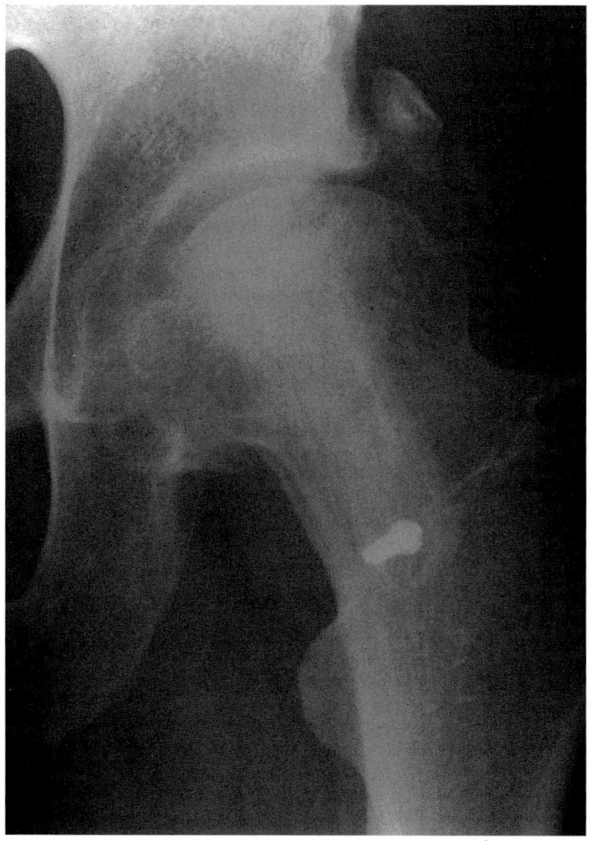

c

Fig. 21 *Good result:*

(a) Extensive necrosis, Stage III, in a 38-year-old male.

(b) Two years postoperative, with a good clinical result.

(c) The clinical results have remained good at 8 years postoperative.

The careful measuring of the extent of the necrosis with radiographs and CT scans will allow refinement of the relative strength of indications for vascularized bone grafting versus rotation osteotomy.

In our series the patients operated on before 1985 had a 49% rate of secondary hip prosthesis, compared with 25% for the patients operated on since 1985. This is as a result of a better assessment of the indications.

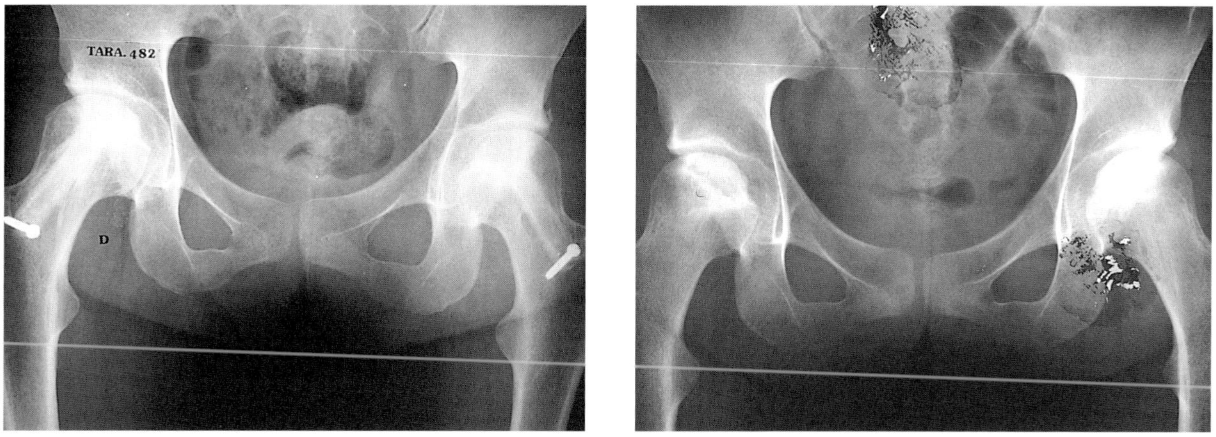

a *b*

Fig. 22
(a) Bilateral necrosis in a 42-year-old woman post-corticotherapy.
(b) A good clinical result 4 years postoperatively.

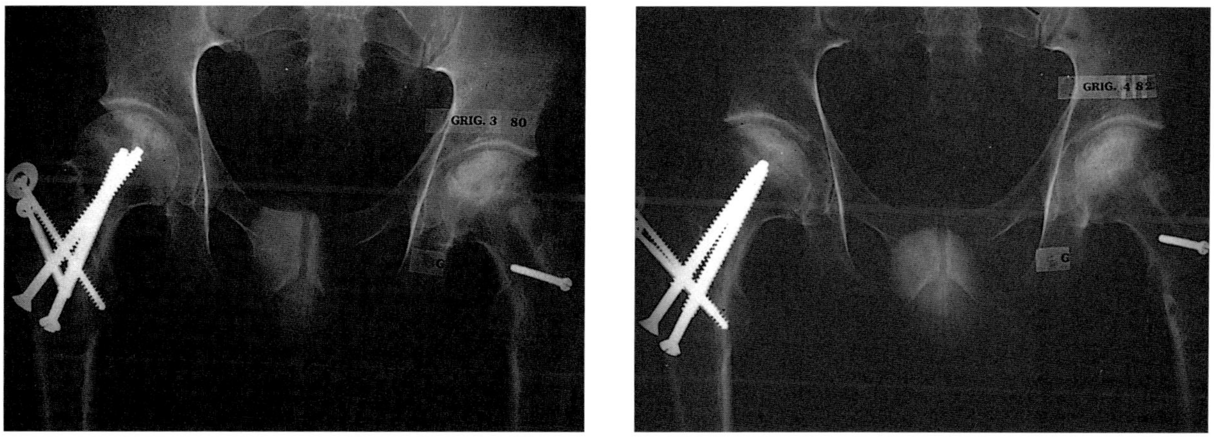

a *b*

Fig. 23 *Bilateral case, treated on the left with a fibular graft, and on the right with a rotational osteotomy:*
(a) After 18 months.
(b) After 5 years.

H. GROWTH ARREST HYPOPLASIA

Luc Téot

Many authors have reported good results concerning the shape, adaptation, and growth of transplanted growth plate areas. With colleagues coming from different teams, we were able to establish more than 20 clinical cases for different indications. In 10 cases, the iliac crest was used as an extra-articular means of enlargement of the acetabulum. These cases were followed up over more than 3 years. Seven cases were operated on for myelomeningocele, one for congenital dysplasia, and two for hemiplegic dysplasia.

In 7 cases, the upper fibula was used to replace an upper extremity epiphysis (radius, humerus, ulna) for a variety of reasons, including trauma or tumor.

The scapular apophysis was used clinically in 3 cases, for:

- radial club hand (enlargement of the lower ulna);
- short stump elongation (used in combination with skin and muscle); and
- lateral apposition on a longitudinal ectromelic tibia.

The surgical technique of harvesting of the scapular apophysis has previously been defined by the authors. The patient is placed in a lateral position. Contours of the body of the scapula on the skin are outlined. The skin is incised longitudinally along the lateral border of the scapula (obliquely), except when a skin flap (scapular flap or parascapular flap) is needed. Muscle insertions on the scapular crest are severed (teres minor and teres major) at a distance of 2 cm from the crest, to protect the nutrient arteries running along the crest. The infraspinatus insertions are separated. The long portion of the triceps muscle is visualized at the upper part of the crest. The circumflex scapular vessels are visualized, including the collateral branch coursing in a caudal direction to the lower apophysis. Dissection must be done carefully until the bifurcation point of the lateral thoracic branch. Osteotomy is done from distal to proximal. The upper end is cut below the insertion of the long head of the triceps muscle. The vascular pedicle must be protected during the osteotomy to prevent any damage, as the vessels run just deep to the osteotomy plane.

Three patients were described, with a mean follow-up of 5 years. In these clinical situations, the most important difficulty is to predict the amount of growth that may occur in both the transplanted epiphysis and the malformed epiphysis. The rate of growth of a malformed epiphysis can be deduced from curves in which the limb discrepancy is proportionately related to normal expected growths. The epiphyseal growth following transplantation will depend on the exact location of the epiphysis in the newly formed structure. In other words, the mechanical situation will influence the growth. It has been observed experimentally that appositional transfer will result in a better mechanical situation than a complete transfer.

The first patient, a 9-year-old child, presented with a short congenital amputation below the knee, secondary to amniotic band syndrome. A combined bone–skin flap, which included a scapular crest and the corresponding apophysis, was transferred to lengthen the short stump, in order to facilitate prosthetic fitting. Growth and remodeling were estimated for a period of 5 years. The total amount of growth was evaluated, clinically and through radiography, at about 5 cm. The most important result was the transverse enlargement of the transplanted epiphysis, which approximated the diameter of the tibial diaphysis. A below-knee prosthesis was fitted 1 year after transfer.

This case was also interesting in terms of donor site morbidity. The difference between the two sides, harvested and not harvested, was estimated on radiographs at about 3 cm in 5 years. This had no apparent effect on the scapular and shoulder functions.

The second patient was a 3-year-old boy, presenting with unilateral ectromelia of the distal right leg. The fibula was absent. A progressive valgus deformity was present. After resection of the fibular band, the distal apophysis of the scapula was transferred and revascularized with the anterior tibial vessels. The scapular apophysis was placed at the same level as the tibial epiphysis. Three years later, the growth was estimated at 2 cm. Radiologically, the scapular growth plate was still open. Gait pattern was nearly normal. Anteroposterior and lateral views on the radiographs confirmed a concomitant growth between the two apposed epiphyses.

In the third patient, a 3-year-old girl presenting with a radial club hand, the transplanted scapular apophysis was positioned laterally to the distal cubital epiphysis. This created a 'V' shaped construct which stabilized the carpal bones. At the age of 4 years, pollicization was performed. Ulnar lengthening was done at the age of 7. Ultimately a satisfactory prehensile function between the pollicized second digit and the third digit was obtained.

Conclusions

Epiphyseal plate vascularized transfer is still a subject of controversy. Most of the experiments carried out during the past 15 years have step by step brought new information concerning the physiology, immunology, and function of the growth area. Recent experimental work has shown that orthotopic transplantations using microsurgical techniques can potentially result in normal growth. Heterotopic vascularized transplantations, however, are associated with less predictable results in term of longitudinal growth. The remaining growth after transfer is difficult to evaluate; it depends on several factors, including the anatomical position of the graft on the recipient bone and the mechanical resistance of the transplanted epiphysis compared to that of the original epiphysis. Only a few autograft donor sites are available in children: the upper fibula, the lower scapula, and the iliac crest. The iliac crest seems, from the short clinical series studied by the authors (25 cases), the most suitable for replacing partial or total epiphysis. The main clinical indications seem to be radial club hand reconstruction (appositional grafts to stabilize the lower epiphysis of the ulna) and acetabular augmentation (enlarging of the acetabular roof by a growing shaft in difficult dysplasias).

I. GROWTH PLATE TRANSPLANTATION

Destruction of growth plate is a major challenge for orthopedic reconstruction in children. As time passes the length discrepancy increases, and may become untreatable.

Transplantation of a growth plate has always been a dream for pediatric orthopedic surgeons, but as a result of lack of knowledge of growth plate physiology and anatomy many attempts have failed (see Chapter 13 Section G).

Nevertheless, several studies have shown that, with proper vascularization and in recipient site locations that mimick physiologic stress loads, epiphyseal transplantation may be of value.

In the limbs, two main donor sites have been used: the proximal fibular epiphysis and the iliac crest apophysis.

Their vascular anatomy and technique of surgical harvest have been described (see Chapter 13).

Fibular epiphysis

The vascular anatomy of this site is complex, arising from three main sources (Restrepo et al 1980).

- The peroneal artery gives off an ascending branch which is responsible for vascularization of the metaphyseal part of the growth plate.
- The inferior genicular artery, a branch of the popliteal artery, penetrates the capsule of the tibiofibular joint and reaches the epiphysis.
- The anterior tibial artery, as it passes from the posterior to the anterior compartment, gives rise to a branch which courses toward the growth plate, and gives off multiple branches to the physis.

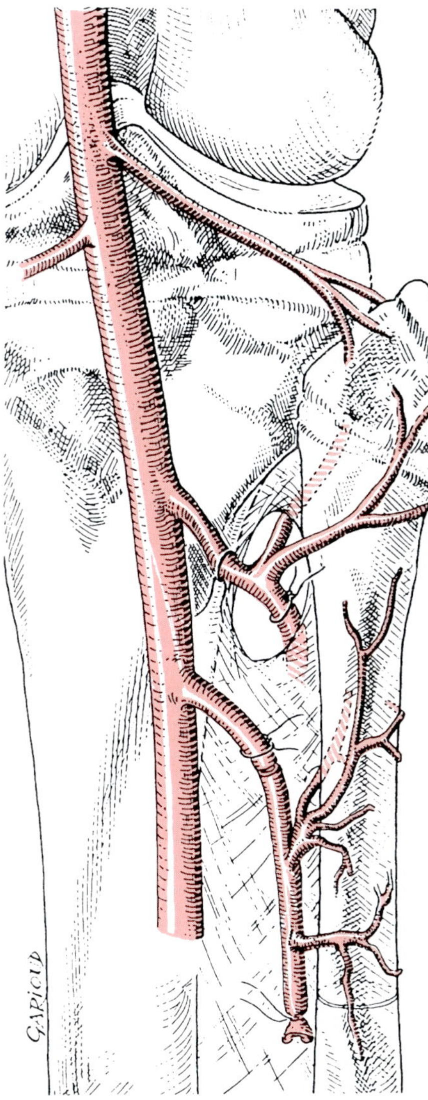

Fig. 24 *The vascular anatomy of the fibular growth plate. The three sources should be preserved. Only a 1-cm piece of anterior tibial artery will be preserved.*

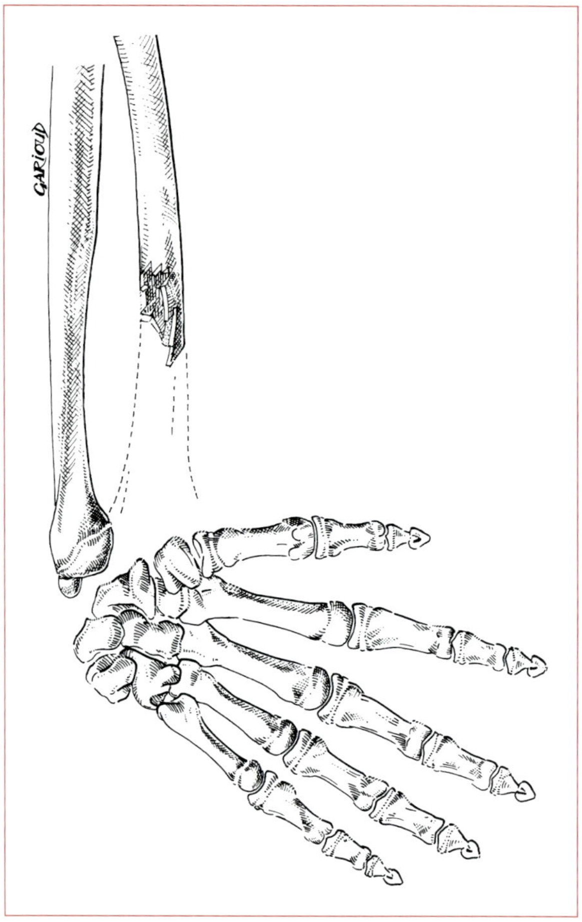

Fig. 25 *After post-traumatic loss of the inferior radius, the wrist has a radial deviation.*

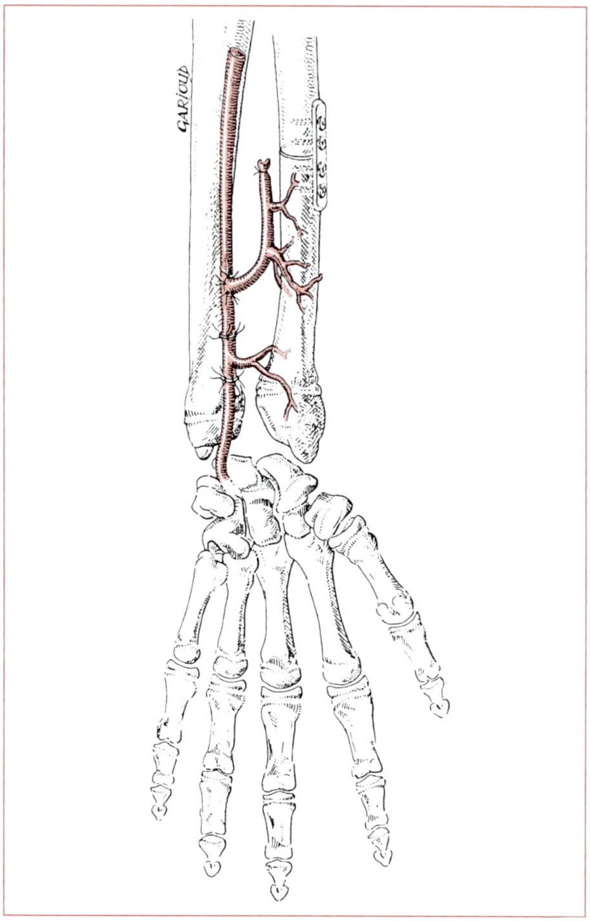

Fig. 26 *Transplantation of the fibular growth plate. The piece of anterior tibial artery has been interposed on the ulnar artery; the peroneal artery is sutured end-to-side.*

An ideal proximal fibular epiphyseal tissue transfer would preserve all three vascular sources. However, it is usually not possible to preserve the inferior genicular artery, as the capsule has to be cut in order to dislocate the fibular head.

It is thus very important to preserve the peroneal and anterior tibial arteries. The anterior tibial artery may be harvested on only a 1 cm leash, which permits both ends being anastomosed to provide a flow-through construct. This little piece of anterior tibial artery can then be sutured to the peroneal artery. Then, with one suture on the recipient site, the fibular head is revascularized.

Iliac crest

The iliac crest apophysis is entirely vascularized by the deep circumflex iliac artery, a branch of the femoral artery. Harvesting can be done as a pedicle flap (Téot) or as a vascularized free flap. There are few indications, but the best one is probably the reconstruction of a destroyed condyle.

Our experience of growth plate transplantations is somewhat disappointing. There are few cases in which subsequent growth is satisfactory, especially in the upper extremities. The best results have been obtained in the lower extremities. Biomechanical conditions, and especially the

Fig. 27 *Clinical case.*

(a,b) Boy – 5 years. Radial club hand after septic destruction of the radial epiphysis.

(c) The fibular epiphysis is ready to be inset.

(d) Immediately postoperative radiograph.

(e) After 2 years. The epiphysis is open, but there is ventrally no growth.

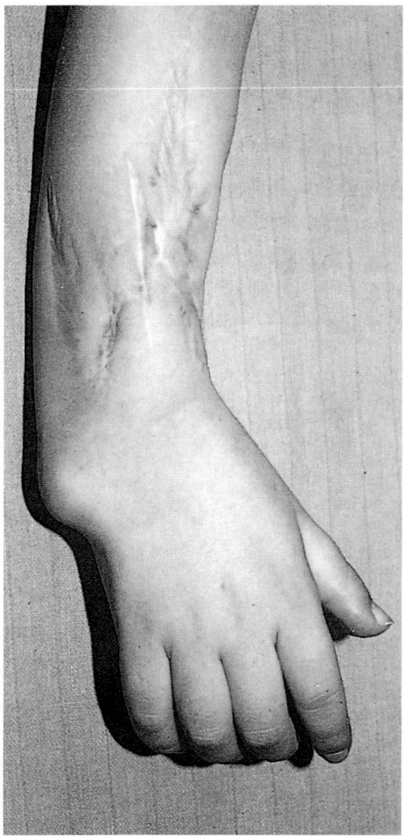

a

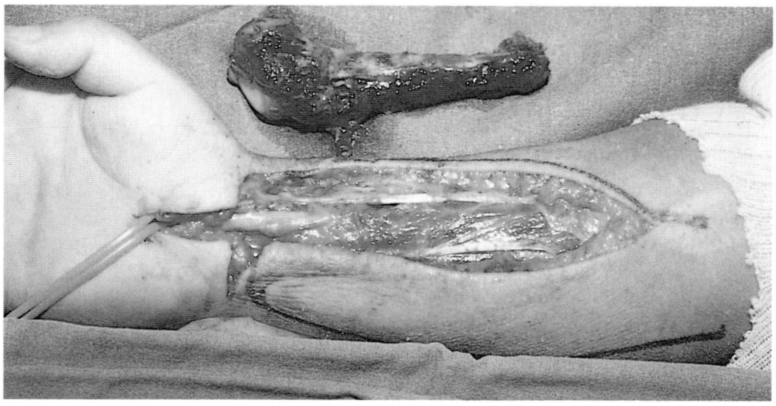

c

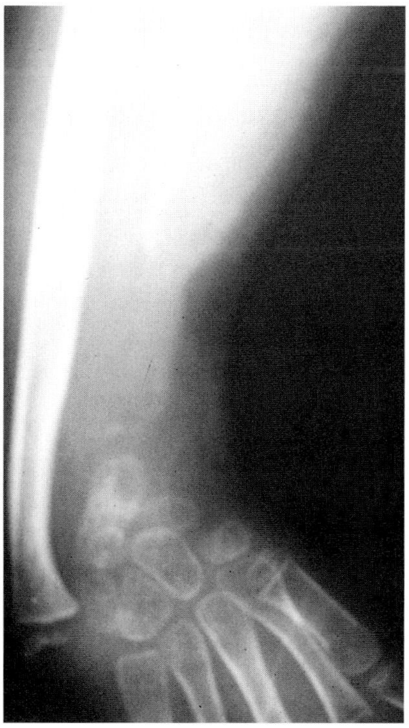

b

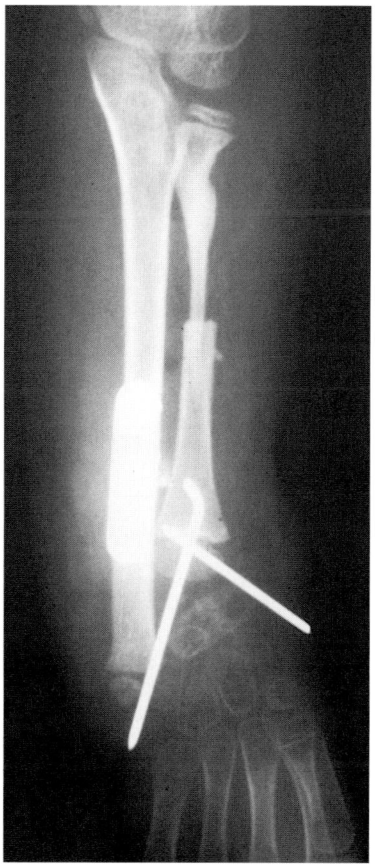

d

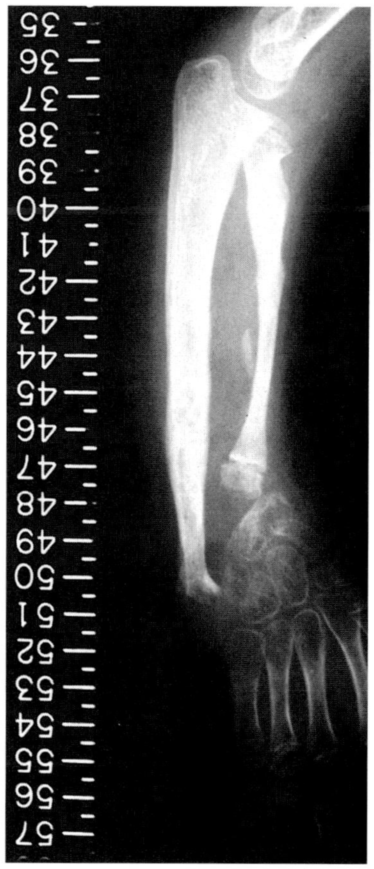

e

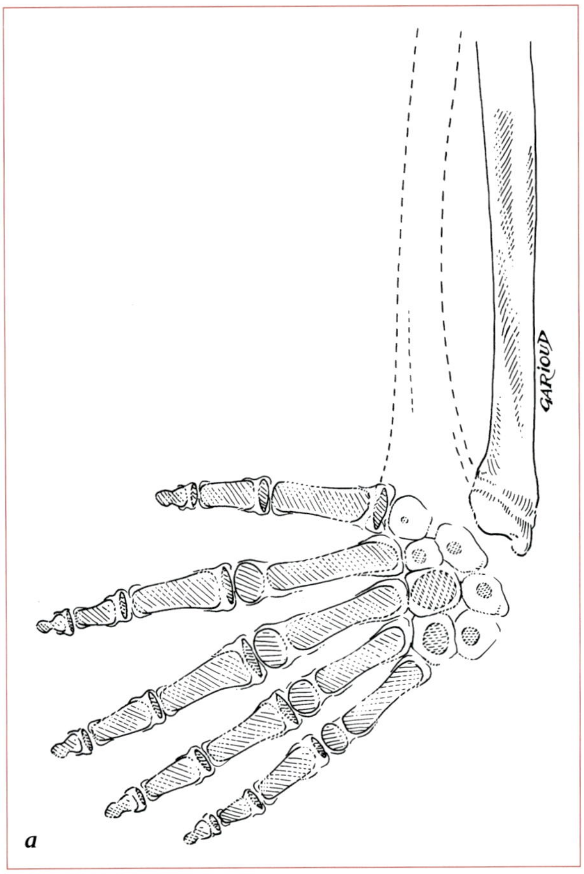

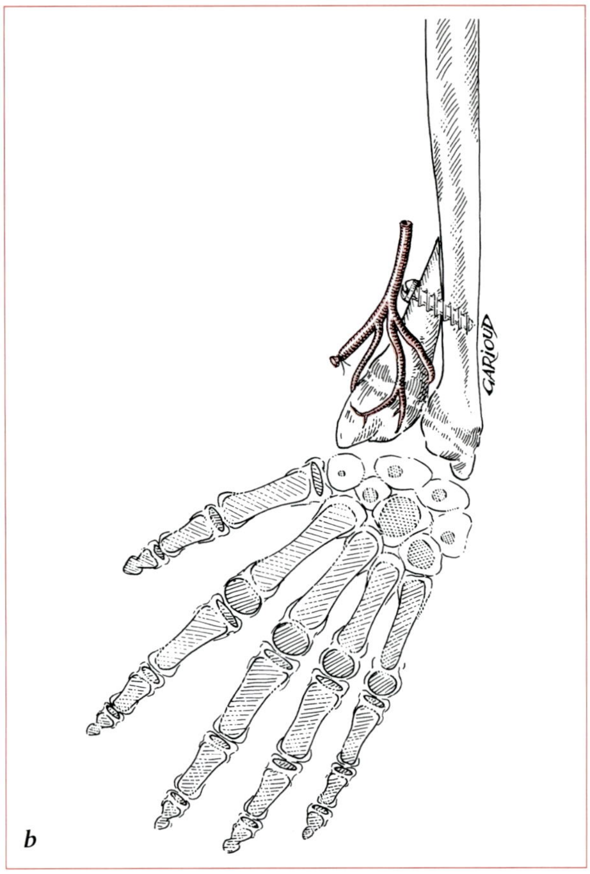

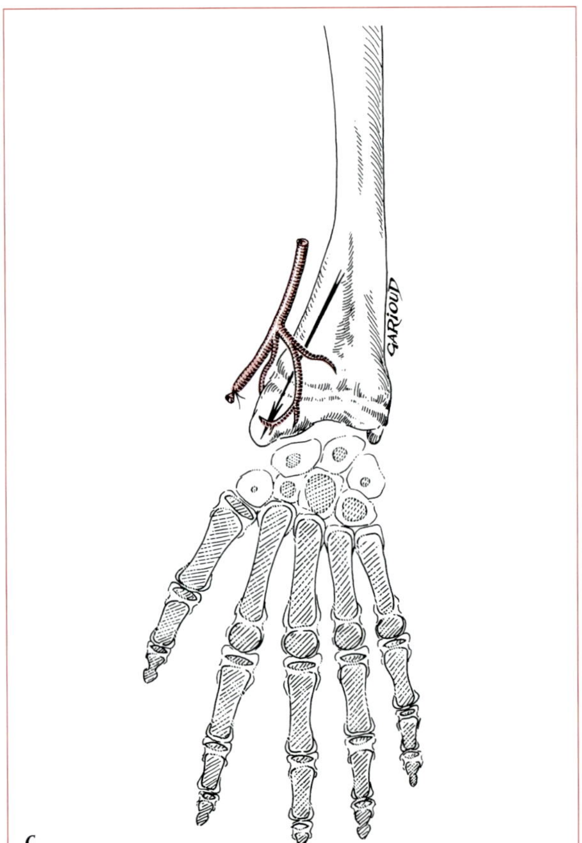

Fig. 28

(a) Radial club hand with absence of the radius.

(b) Transplantation of the fibular epiphysis.

(c) After fusion, reconstruction of a large epiphysis.

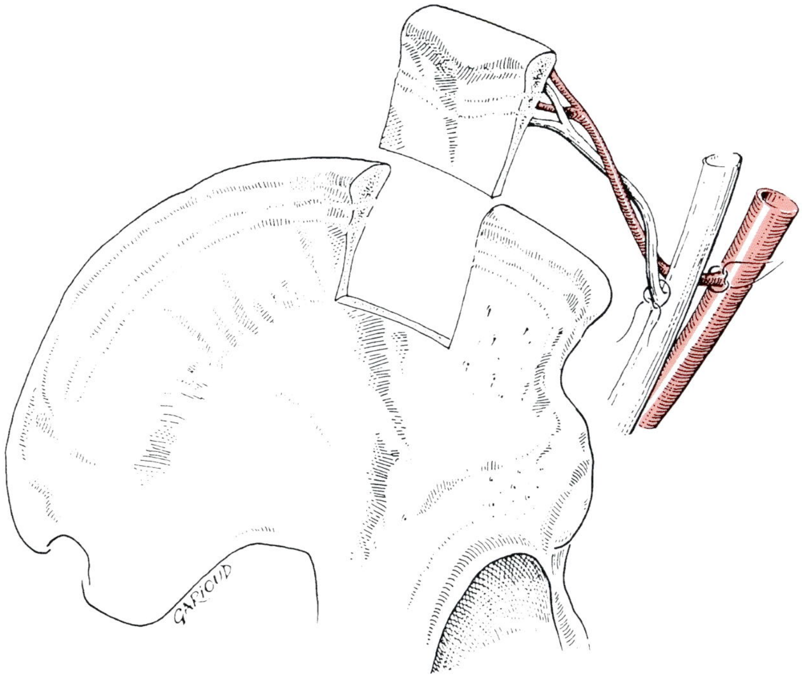

Fig. 29 *Harvesting a piece of iliac crest growth plate with the deep circumflex iliac vessels.*

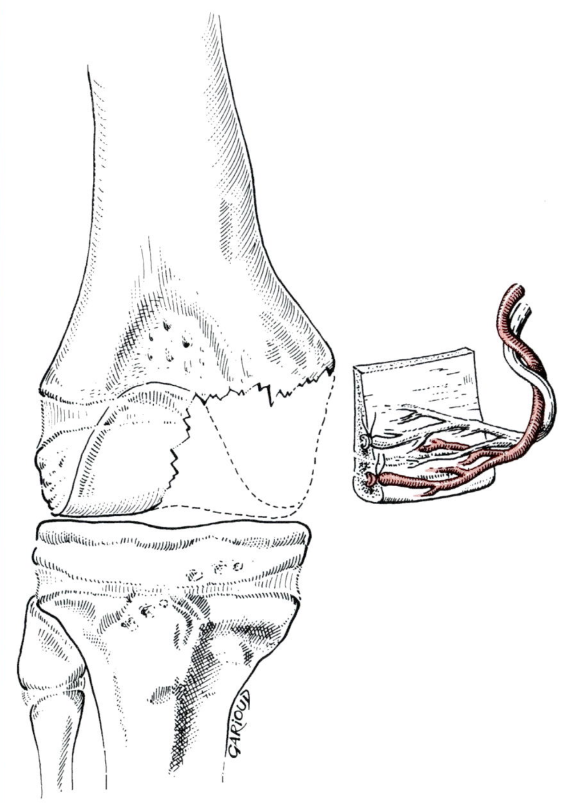

Fig. 30 *In case of traumatic condylar loss, the iliac crest is used to reconstruct the medial condyle.*

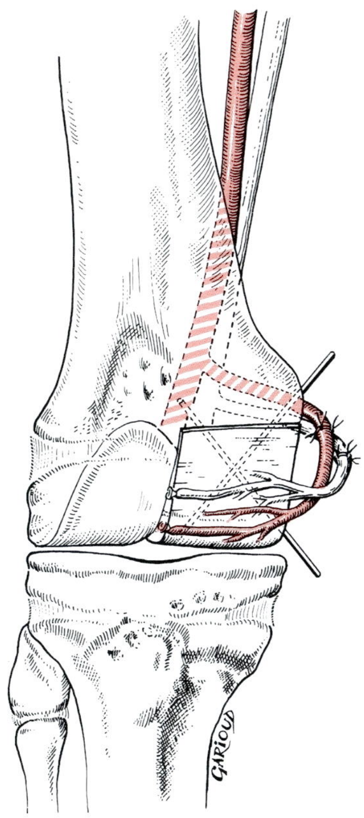

Fig. 31 *The vascular pedicle is anastomosed with the superior genicular pedicle.*

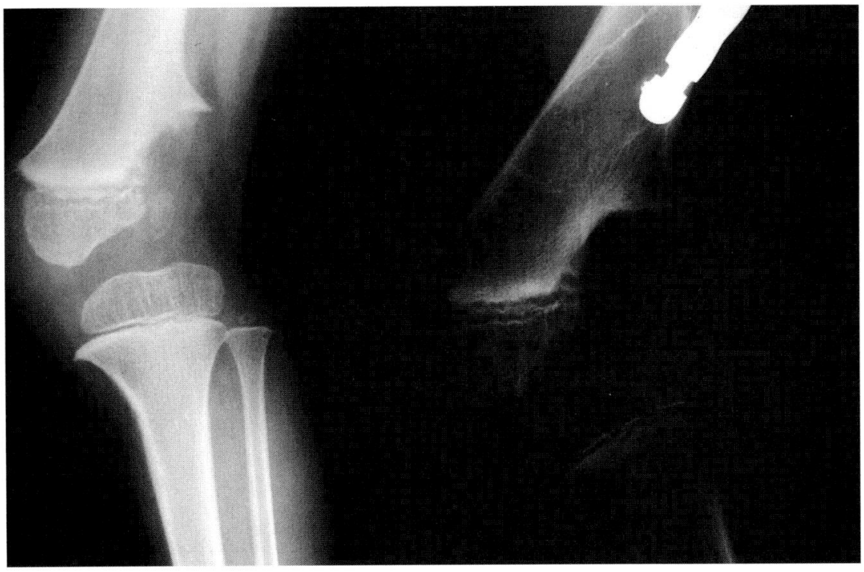

a

Fig. 32 *Clinical case:*
(a,b) Boy – 6. Post-traumatic destruction of the medial knee condyle.

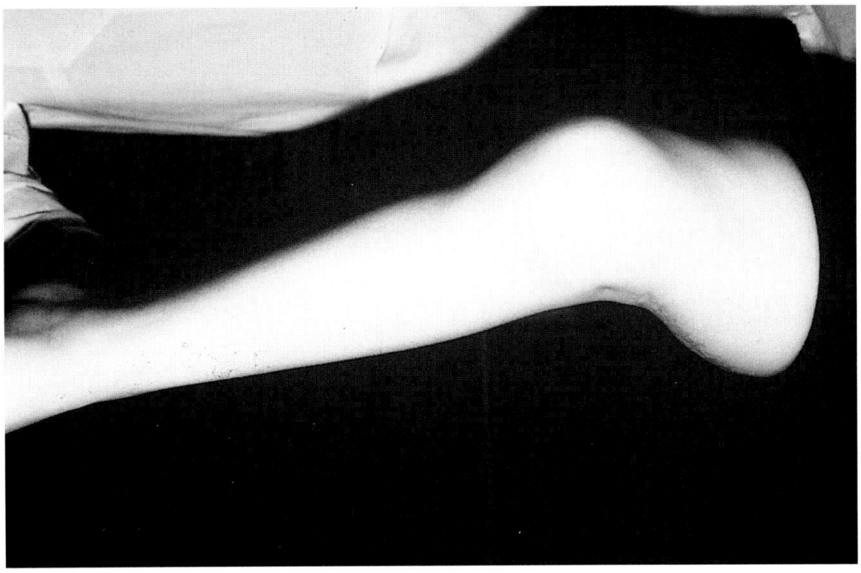

b

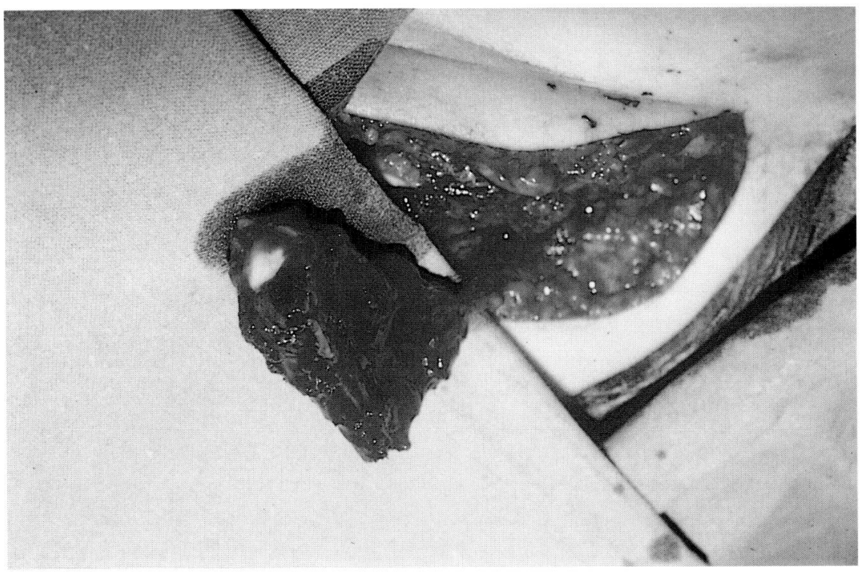

c

(c) Harvesting of a piece of iliac crest and growth plate.

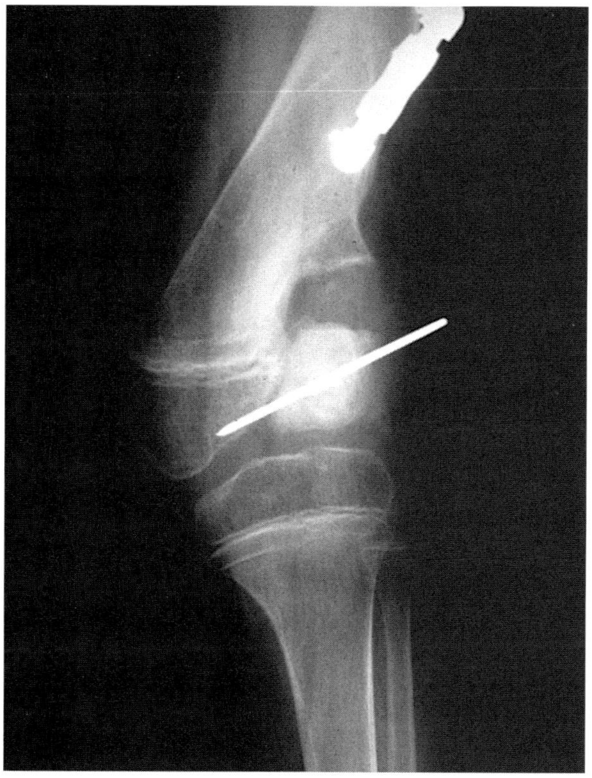

(d) The iliac crest replaces the medial condyle.

d

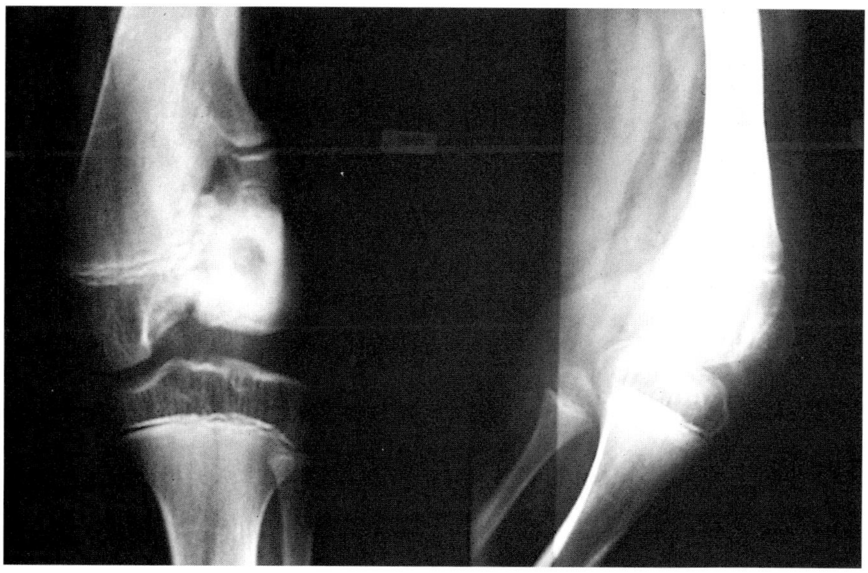

(e) After 6 years. Excellent growth of the transplant.

e

permanent pressure on the growth plate, seem to be important factors.

Experience with large series of epiphysial transfer from the toe suggests that, when the revascularization is adequate, one can expect a reasonable rate of growth from the transferred epiphysis. A study done on the growth of our toe transfers with more than 8 years of follow-up demonstrated a growth loss of 0 to 25%, with an average of 10%. If we can obtain 90% growth with growth plate transplantation, the future of this technique is indeed promising.

16. Complications

A variety of complications may be seen following reconstruction by vascularized bone transfer. These may be systemic or specifically related to either the donor site or the recipient site.

Systemic

Most free tissue transfer procedures are relatively prolonged in duration, and may be associated with significant blood loss and hemodynamic fluxes. Thus the usual myriad of general orthopedic surgical complications may be expected. These include pressure sores and decubitus ulcers, pressure and positional traction neuropathies, hypovolemic hypotension with associated cardiac and renal complications, deep venous thrombosis and pulmonary embolism, adult respiratory distress syndrome, drug allergic reactions, transfusion-related disease transmission, cholecystitis, *Clostridium difficile* colitis, and other conditions. Management of these complications is best addressed by prevention when applicable, or by prompt postoperative recognition and management. Because most of these procedures involve the lower extremities, the most common significant complication is deep venous thrombosis.

Donor site

Any number of donor site complications may occur, but in general most large clinical series conclude that donor site morbidity with the common vascularized bone transfer procedures is indeed minimal. Weiland in his series of 123 free fibula transfers claims no donor site morbidity (Weiland 1991). Han et al (1992) reported an 8% donor site complication rate with 132 vascularized fibula harvests, and a 7% donor site morbidity rate with iliac crest based on the deep circumflex iliac vessels. Moran in his comprehensive literature review (Moran 1993), which included the previously cited series, collected 26 donor site complications from a collated series of 265 different patients. These specific complications are cited in Figure 1.

Youdas et al (1988) conducted a quantitative analysis of donor site morbidity after vascularized fibula transfer, using patients with a comparable normal lower limb who had undergone upper limb reconstruction. These authors did serial studies on these patients, evaluating gait using a three-dimensional electrogoniometer and measuring strength using a modified Cybex II isokinetic dynamometer. Moderate knee and ankle–foot motion changes were observed in patients within 10 months of surgery, but these changes were not noted on longer follow-up testing. Muscle strength, however, particularly in regard to ankle inversion and eversion, was impaired in all patients, even with long-term follow-up, and was correlated to the length of the resected fibula.

Recipient site

Recipient site complications may be seen in approximately 25% of patients undergoing vascularized bone transfer. The most common complication has been earlier discussed, namely failure to progress to bone union. However, the most disastrous complication is acute major vascular thrombosis, leading to

Fig. 1

Donor site complications

Complication	Number	Total patients	Reference
Fibula			
Transient peroneal nerve palsy	5	132	Han et al (1992)
Flexor hallucis longus tenodesis	3	132	Han et al (1992)
Extensor hallucis longus paralysis	5	11	Simonis et al (1991)
Compartment syndrome	1	132	Han et al (1992)
Osteomyelitis	1	21	Minami et al (1989)
Fracture, ipsilateral tibia	1	132	Han et al (1992)
Valgus deformity, ankle (pediatric)	6	58	Gilbert et al (1982)
	2	6	Minami et al (1989)
	1	5	DeBoer (1988)
Motor weakness	3	10	Lee et al (1990)
Iliac crest			
Incisional hernia	2	28	Han et al (1992)

critical limb ischemia and/or a compartment syndrome and myonecrosis. Recipient site infection may be seen in any major procedure, but is particularly prevalent in reconstructions for chronic osteomyelitis. Stress fracture following union is seen in 25% of fibula transfers within the first postoperative year (DeBoer and Wood 1989). It is of course more common following reconstruction of the weightbearing bones of the lower limb. Many stress fractures may be asymptomatic, and are diagnosed retrospectively by the presence of fusiform callus about the fracture site (Fig. 2). Additional complications at the recipient site include malunion, neuropathy, wound dehiscence and hematoma.

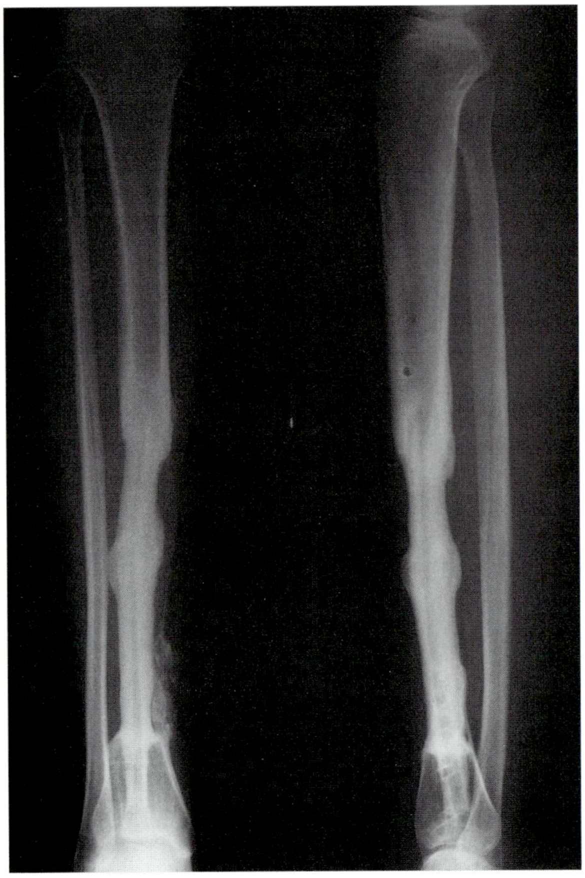

Fig. 2 *AP radiograph of a healed vascularized fibular reconstruction of the tibia. Note the callus at the site of the healed stress fracture in the mid-portion of the fibular segment.*

Bibliography

Acland RD (1978). Caution about clinical use of vascularized periosteal grafts (Letter). *Plast Reconstr Surg* **62**:290.

Albee FH (1915). *Bone Graft Surgery*. Saunders, Phildelphia.

Altierre RJ, Kiritsy-Roy JA, Catravas JD (1986). Acetylcholine-induced contractions in isolated rabbit pulmonary arteries: role of thromboxane A2. *J Pharmacol Exp Ther* **236**:535–41.

Andersen KS (1974). Operative treatment of congenital pseudarthrosis of the tibia. *Acta Orthop Scand* **45**:935–44.

Andersen KS (1976). Congenital pseudarthrosis of the leg: late results. *J Bone Joint Surg* **58A**:657–62.

Ando K, Hirata Y, Shichiri M, Emori T, Maromo F (1989). The presence of immunoreactive endothelin in human plasma. *FEBS Lett* **245**:164–6.

Arai H, Hori S, Aromori I, Ohkubo H, Nakanishi S (1990). Cloning and expression of a cDNA encoding an endothelin receptor. *Nature* **348**:730–2.

Arata MA, Wood MB, Cooney WP III (1984). Revascularized segmental diaphyseal bone transfers in the canine. An analysis of viability. *J Reconstr Microsurg* **1**:11–19.

Ariyan S (1980). The viability of rib grafts transplanted with the periosteal blood supply. *Plast Reconstr Surg* **54**:140–51.

Arora BK, Laskin DM (1964). Sex chromatin as a cellular label of osteogenesis by bone grafts. *J Bone Joint Surg* **46A**:1269–76.

Auguet M, Delaflotte S, Chabrier PE, Pirotzky E, Clostre F, Braquet P (1988). Endothelin and Ca^{2+} agonist Bay K 8644: different vasoconstrictive properties. *Biochem Biophys Res Comm* **156**:186–92.

Axhausen W (1956). The osteogenic phases of regeneration of bone. *J Bone Joint Surg* **38A**:593.

Azuma H (1964). Intraosseous pressure as a measure of hemodynamic changes in bone marrow. *Angiology* **15**:396–406.

Baadsgaard K, Medgyesi S (1965). Muscle pedicle bone grafts. *Acta Orthop Scand* **35**:279–93.

Bakris GL, Fairbanks R, Traish AM, Akerstrom V, Kern S (1991). Arginine vasopressin stimulates human mesangial cell production of endothelin. *J Clin Invest* **87**:1158–64.

Baksi DP (1991). Treatment of osteonecrosis of the femoral head by drilling and muscle-pedicle bone grafting. *J Bone Joint Surg* **73B**:241–5.

Barth A (1894). Ueber histologische Befunde nach Knochenimplantationen. *Arch Klin Chir* **46**:409.

Baselga J (1986). *La vascularisation osseuse tibiale dépendant de l'artère tibiale antérieure. Mémoire d'Anatomie*. UER Biomédicales des Saints Pères, Paris.

Bassett CAL (1972). Current concepts of bone formation. *J Bone Joint Surg* **44A**:1217–29.

Baud CA, Biovin G (1978). Effects of hormones on osteocyte frunction and perilacunar wall structure. *Clin Orthop* **136**:270–81.

Bell M, Barron P (1980). A new method of oral reconstruction using a free composite foot flap. *Ann Plast Surg* **5**:281–7.

Beneux J, Rigault P, Pouliquen JC, et al (1979). Courbures et pseudarthroses congénitales de jambes chex l'enfant. *Chir Pédiatr* **20**:99–113.

Bennett A, Wilson DW, Liu F, et al (1983). Levels of insulin-like growth factors I and II in human cord blood. *J Clin Endocrinol Metab* **57**:609.

Bennett A, Chen T, Feldman D, et al (1984). Characterization of insulin-like growth factor-I receptor on cultured rat bone cells. *Endocrinology* **115**:1577.

Berggren A, Weiland AJ, Dorfman H (1982a). Free vascularized bone grafts: factors affecting their survival and ability to heal recipient bone defects. *Plast Reconstr Surg* **69**:19–29.

Berggren A, Weiland AJ, Östrup LT (1982b). Bone scintigraphy in evaluating the viability of composite bone grafts revascularized by microvascular anastomosis, conventional autogenous bone grafts, and free non-revascularized periosteal grafts. *J Bone Joint Surg* **64A**:799–811.

Beumer J, Curtis T, Firtell D (1979). Acquired defects of the mandible. In: Beumer J, Curtis T, Firtell D (eds) *Maxillofacial Rehabilitation*, pp 90–187. Mosby, St Louis.

Bidder A (1906). Osteobiologie. *Arch Mikrosk Anat* **68**:137–213.

Bieber EJ, Wood MB (1986). Bone reconstruction. *Clin Plast Surg* **13**:645–55.

Bjurholm A, Kreicbergs A, Terenius L, Goldstein M, Schultzberg M (1988a). Neuropeptide Y-, tyrosine hydroxylase- and vasoactive intestine polypeptide in bone and surrounding tissues. *J Auton Nerv Syst* **25**:119–25.

Bjurholm A, Kreicbergs A, Brodin E, Schultzberg M (1988b). Substance P- and CGRP-immunoreactive nerves in bone. *Peptides* **9**:165–71.

Blair VP (1917). *Surgery and Diseases of the Mouth and Jaws. A Practical Treatise on the Surgery and Disease of the Mouth and Allied Structures*, 3rd edn. Mosby, St Louis.

Boettcher WG, Bonfiglio M, Smith K (1970). Non-traumatic necrosis of the femoral head. Part II: Experiences in treatment. *J Bone Joint Surg* **52A**:322–9.

Bolander ME (1991). Inducers of osteogenesis. In: GE Friedlaender and VM Goldberg (eds), *Bone and Cartilage Allografts*, pp 75–83. American Academy of Orthopedic Surgeons, Park Ridge, IL.

Bonfiglio H (1983). The biology of bone graft repair. *Clin Orthop* **174**:28–42.

Bonfiglio M, Voke EM (1968). Aseptic necrosis of the femoral head and non-union of the femoral neck. Effect of treatment by drilling and bone grafting (Phemister technique). *J Bone Joint Surg* **50A**:48–66.

Boorman JG, Brown JA, Sykes PJ (1987). Morbidity in the forearm flap donor arm. *Br J Plast Surg* **40**:207–12.

Bos KE (1979). Bone scintigraphy of experimental composite bone grafts revascularized by microvascular anastomosis. *Plast Reconstr Surg* **64**:353–60.

Bost FC (1947). The evaluation of cortical and cancellous bone as grafting materials. *J Bone Joint Surg* **29**:381–414.

Boulanger C, Lüscher TF (1990). Release of endothelin from the porcine aorta. Inhibition of endothelium-derived nitric oxide. *J Clin Invest* **85**:587–90.

Bowen V (1988). Microsurgical growth plate transfers. In: HK Uthoff, JJ Wiley (eds), *Behavior of the Growth Plate*, pp 55–9. Raven Press, New York.

Boyd JB, Mulholland RD (1993). Fixation of the vascularized bone graft in mandibular reconstruction. *Plast Reconstr Surg* **91**(2):274–82.

Brand RA (1983). Fracture healing. In: CM Evarts (ed), *Surgery of the Musculoskeletal System*, pp 76–9. Churchill Livingstone, New York.

Branemark PI (1985). Introduction to osseointegration. In: PI Branemark, GA Zarb, TA Albrektsson (eds), *Tissue Integrated Prostheses: Osseointegration in Clinical Dentistry*, pp 11–76. Quintessence Publishing Co, Chicago.

Brashear HR Jr (1963). Epiphyseal avascular necrosis and its relation to longitudinal bone growth. *J Bone Joint Surg* **45A**:1423.

Briggs PJ (1994). The effects of endothelin on the neurohumoral and metabolic control of bone blood flow. MD Thesis, University of Manchester, England.

Brighton CT (1976). Clinical problems in epiphyseal plate growth and development. Instructional course lectures. *Am Acad of Orthop Surg* **23**.

Brinker MR, Uppton HL, Cook SD, Hyman AL (1990). Pharmacological regulation of the circulation of bone. *J Bone Joint Surg* **72A**:964–75.

Brookes M (1971).*The Blood Supply of Bone*. Butterworth, London (p. 20).

Brookes M (1986). An anatomy of the osseous circulation. *Bone* **3**:32–4.

Brookes M (1987). Bone blood flow measurement: part 2. *Bone* **4**:33–6.

Brookes M, Landon DN (1964). The juxta epiphyseal vesels in the long bones of foetal rats. *J Bone Joint Surg* **46B**(2) (May).

Brough MD, Grant HR, Haria M (1993). The free fibula in mandibular reconstruction. Personal communication at the 7th Congress of the European Section of the International Confederation for Plastic, Reconstructive and Aesthetic Surgery, Berlin, June 1993.

Brown K, Marie P, Lyszakowski T, Daniel R, Cruess R (1983). Epiphyseal growth after free fibular transfer with and without anastomosis. *J Bone Joint Surg* **65B**:493.

Brunelli G, Brunelli G (1991). Free microvascular fibular transfer for idiopathic femoral head necrosis: long-term follow-up. *J Reconstr Microsurg* **7**:285–95.

Buncke HJ, Daniller AI, Schultz WP, Chase RA (1967). The fate of autogenous whole joints transplanted by microvascular anastomoses. *Plast Reconstr Surg* **39**:333–41.

Burchardt H (1983). The biology of bone graft repair. *Clin Orthop* **174**:28–42.

Burchardt H (1987). Biology of bone transplantation. *Orthop Clin North Am* **18**:187–96.

Burchardt H, Busbee GA, III, Enneking WF (1975). Repair of experimental autologous grafts of cortical bone. *J Bone Joint Surg* **57A**:814–18.

Burnstock G, Lincoln J, Fehér E, et al (1988). Serotonin is localized in endothelial cells of coronary arteries and released during hypoxia: a possible new mechanism for hypoxia-induced vasodilation of the rat heart. *Experientia* **44**:705–7.

Burwell RG (1969). The fate of bone grafts. In: AP Apley (ed), *Recent Advances in Orthopaedics*, pp 115–207. Churchill, London.

Canalis E (1985). Effects of growth factors on bone cell replication and differentiation. *Clin Orthop* **193**:246–63.

Canalis EM, Hintz RL, Dietrich JW, et al (1977). Effects of somatomedin and growth hormone on bone collagen syntheses in vitro. *Metabolism* **26**:1079.

Capanna R, Biagini R, Casadei R, Donate D, Manfrini M, Mechanie E (1991). Autograft versus allograft reconstruction: the Rizzoli Institute experience. In: K Brown (ed), *Complications of Limb Salvage: Prevention, Management and Outcome*, pp 49–52. ISOLS Publ, Montreal.

Cariou JL, LeGall R (1991). L'anatomie artérielle des lambeaux péroniers analysée par l'examen Doppler et l'artériographie. *Ann Chir Plast Esthet* **36**:405–23.

Carpenter G, Cohen S (1979). Epidermal growth factors. *Ann Rev Biochem* **48**:193.

Cernacek P, Stewart DJ (1989). Immunoreactive endothelin in human plasma: marked elevations in patients in cardiogenic shock. *Biochem Biophys Res Commun* **161**: 562–7.

Chacha PB, Ahmed M, Darvwalla JS (1981). Vascular pedicle grafts of the ipsilateral fibula for nonunion of the tibia with a large defect. *J Bone Joint Surg* **63B**:244–53.

Charkes ND (1980). Skeletal blood flow: implications for bone-scan interpretation. *J Nucl Med* **21**:91–8.

Chase SW, Herndon CH (1955). The fate of autogenous and homogenous bone grafts. A historical review. *J Bone Joint Surg* **37A**:809–15.

Chen CW, Yu ZJ, Wang Y (1979). A new method of treatment of congenital tibial pseudarthrosis using free vascularized fibular graft. *Ann Acad Med Singapore* **8**:465–73.

Chen G, Suzuki H, Weston AH (1988). Acetylcholine releases endothelium-derived hyperpolarizing factor and EDRF from rat blood vessels. *Br J Pharmacol* **95**:1165–74.

Chung MS (1976) The arterial supply of the developing proximal end of the human femur. *J Bone Joint Surg* **58A**:961–70.

Clinkscales CM, Wood MB, Sim FH (1991). Vascularized fibula transfer for salvage of failed allograft reconstruction. In: K Brown (ed), *Complications of Limb Salvage: Prevention, Management and Outcome*, pp 8–11. ISOLS Publ, Montreal.

Clohisy DR, Mankin HJ (1991). The impact of complications on the long-term results of bicondylar proximal tibial osteoarticular allografts in the management of skeletal defects after tumor resection. In: K Brown (ed), *Complications of Limb Salvage*, pp 15–16. ISOLS Publ, Montreal.

Clozel M, Loffler BM, Gloor H (1991). Relative preservation of the responsiveness to endothelin-1 during reperfusion following renal ischemia in the rat. *J Cardiovasc Pharmacol* **17** (Suppl 7):S313–S315.

Codivilla A (1906). On the care of congenital pseudarthrosis of the tibia by means of periosteal transplantation. *Am J Orthop Surg* **4**:163.

Coleman JJ, Wooden WA (1990). Mandibular reconstruction with composite microvascular tissue transfer. *Am J Surg* **160**:390–5.

Comtet JJ, Bertrand HG, Moyen B (1980). Free autogenous composite joint fragment use in multiple finger injuries. *Int Microsurg* **2**:121–4.

Coutellier L, Delloye C, De Nayer P, Vincent A (1984). Aspects microradiographiques des allogreffes osseuses massives chez l'homme. *Rev Chir Orthop* **70**:581–8.

Craigmyle MBL (1960). Studies of cartilage autografts and homografts in the rabbit. *Br J Plast Surg* **8**:93–100.

Crock HV (1967). *The Blood Supply of the Lower Limb Bones in Man*. Livingstone, London.

Crock JG, Morrison WA (1992). A vascularized periosteal flap. *Br J Plast Surg* **45**:474.

Cruess RL (1984). Healing of bone, tendon and ligament. In: Rockwood CA and Green DP (eds), *Fractures in Adults*, pp 147–67. Lippincott, Philadelphia.

Cumming JD, Nutt ME (1962). Bone marrow blood flow and cardiac output in the rabbit. *J Physiol* **162**:30–4.

Curtis BF, Morrey MD (1893). Cases of bone implantation and transplantation for cyst of tibia, osteomyelitic cavities and ununited fractures. *Am J Med Sci* **106**:30.

Daniel G, Entin MA, Kahn DS (1971). Autogenous transplantation in the dog of a metacarpo-phalangeal joint with preserved neurovascular bundle. *Can J Surg* **14**:253–9.

David D, Tan E, Katsaros J, Sheen R (1988). Mandibular reconstruction with vascularized iliac crest: a 10 year experience. *Plast Reconstr Surg* **82**:792–801.

Davidson J, Boyd JB, Gullane P, et al (1991). A comparison of the results following oromandibular reconstruction using a radial forearm flap with either radial bone or a reconstruction plate. *Plast Reconstr Surg* **88**:201–8.

Davis JB, Taylor AN (1952). Muscle pedicle bone grafts. *Arch Surg* **65**:330–6.

Davis TRC, Wood MB (1992). Endothelial control of long bone vascular resistance. *J Orthop Res* **10**:344–9.

Davis TRC, Wood MB (1993). The direct effects of acidosis and alkalosis on long bone vascular resistance. *J Orthop Res* **11**:834–9.

Davis PK, Mazur JM, Coleman GN (1982). A torsional strength comparison of vascularized and nonvascularized bone grafts. *J Biomechanics* **15**:875–80.

Dean MT, Wood MB, Vanhoutte PM (1992). Antagonist drugs and bone vascular smooth muscle. *J Orthop Res* **10**:104–11.

DeBoer HH (1988). Vascularized fibular transfer. Thesis, Leiden, The Netherlands.

DeBoer HH, Wood MB (1989). Bone changes in the vascularized fibular graft. *J Bone Joint Surg* **71B**:374–8.

DeBoer HH, Wood MB, Hermans J (1990). Reconstruction of large skeletal defects by vascularized fibula transfer. *Int Orthop* **14**:121–8.

DeBruyn PPH, Breen PC, Thomas TB (1970). The microcirculation of the bone marrow. *Anat Rec* **168**:55–68.

DeHeyde A (1684). *Anatomia mytuli, subjecta centuriae observatorium*. Janssonio Waesbergios, Amsterdam.

Dell PC, Burchardt H, Glowczewskie FP Jr (1985). A roentgenographic, biomechanial and histological evaluation of vascularized and non-vascularized segmental fibular canine autografts. *J Bone Joint Surg* **67A**:105–12.

DeMey JG, Vanhoutte PM (1982). Hetergeneous behavior of the canine arterial and venous wall: importance of the endothelium. *Circ Res* **51**:439.

DeMey JG, Vanhoutte PM (1983). Anoxia and endothelium dependent reactivity of the canine femoral artery. *J Physiol* **335**:65–74.

D'Ercole AJ, Applewhite GT, Underwood LE (1980). Evidence that somatomedin is synthesized in multiple tissues in the fetus. *Dev Biol* **75**:315.

Doi K, Tominaga S, Shibata T (1977). Bone grafts with microvascular anastomosis of vascular pedicles. An experimental study. *J Bone Joint Surg* **59A**:809–15.

Donski PK, O'Brien MMcC (1980). Free microvascular epiphyseal transplantation. An experimental study in dogs. *Br J Plast Surg* **33**:169–78.

Driessens M, Vanhoutte PM (1979). Vascular reactivity of the isolated tibia of the dog. *Am J Physiol* **236**:H904–H908.

Driessens M, Vanhoutte PM (1981). Effect of calcitonin, hydrocortisone, and parathyroid hormone on canine bone blood vessels. *Am J Physiol* **241**:H91–H94.

Drinker CK, Drinker KR (1916). A method for maintaining an artificial circulation through the tibia of the dog, with a demonstration of the vasomotor control of the marrow vessels. *Am J Physiol* **40**:514–21.

Duncan CP, Shim SS (1977). The autonomic nerve supply of bone. An experimental study of the intraosseous adrenergic nervi vasorum in the rabbit. *J Bone Joint Surg* **59B**:323–30.

Eglen RM, Michel AD, Sharif NA, Swank SR, Whiting RL (1989). The pharmacological properties of the peptide, endothelin. *Br J Pharmacol* **97**:1297–1307.

Ehrlich MG, Lorenz J, Tomford W, Mankin HJ (1983). Collagenase activity in banked bone. *Trans Orthop Res Soc* **8**:166.

Elliott JS, FInn HA, Simon MA (1991). Late complications of cylindrical allografts following resection of malignant tumours in the femur and proximal tibia. In: K Brown (ed), *Complications of Limb Salvage: Prevention, Management and Outcome*, pp 33–4. ISOLS Publ, Montreal.

Enneking WF, Mindell ER (1991). Observations on massive retrieved human allografts. *J Bone Joint Surg* **73A**:1123–42.

Enneking WF, Eady JL, Burchardt H (1980). Autogenous cortical bone grafts in the reconstruction of segmental skeletal deficits. *J Bone Joint Surg* **62A**:1039–57.

Farmer AW (1952). The use of a composite pedicle graft for pseudarthrosis of the tibia. *J Bone Joint Surg* **34A**:591–600.

Feletou M, Vanhoutte PM (1988). Endothelium-dependent hyperpolarization of canine coronary smooth muscle. *Br J Pharmacol* **93**:515–24.

Felix R, Cecchini MG, Fleisch H (1990). Macrophage colony stimulating factor restores in vivo bone resorption in the op/op osteopetrotic mouse. *Endocrinology* **127**:2592.

Finley JM, Acland RD, Wood MB (1978). Revascularized periosteal graft: a new method to produce functional new bone without bone grafting. *Plast Reconstr Surg* **61**:1.

Finseth F, May JW, Smith RJ (1976). Composite groin flap with iliac bone flap for primary thumb reconstruction. *J Bone Joint Surg* **58A**:130–2.

Fisher DH, Klein AH (1981). Thyroid development and disorders of thyroid function in the newborn. *New Engl J Med* **304**:702.

Flye MW (1989). Immunosuppressive therapy. In: MW Flye (ed), *Principles of Organ Transplantation*, pp 155–75. Saunders, Philadelphia.

Foster LN, Kelly RP, Watts WM (1951). Experimental infarction of bone and bone marrow. *J Bone Joint Surg* **33A**:396–401.

Foucher G (1988). Vascularized joint transfer. In: DP Green (ed), *Operative Hand Surgery*, 2nd edn, pp 1271–93. Churchill Livingstone, New York.

Foucher G, Citron N, Merle M, Dury M (1987). Free compound transfer of the distal interphalangeal joint. A case report. *J Reconstr Microsurg* **3**:297–300.

Foucher G, Sammut D, Citron N (1990). Free vascularized toe joint transfer in hand reconstruction. *J Reconstr Microsurg* **6**:201–7.

Foucher G, Citron E, Sammut D (1991). Compound vascularized island joint transfer in hand surgery. A report of 16 cases. *French J Orthop Surg* **5**:32–9.

Friedlander F von (1904). Beitrag zur Kenntnis der Architektur spongioser Knochen. *Anat Hefte Add 1, 23:* **35**:282.

Friedlaender GE (1983). Immune response to osteochondral allografts: current knowledge and future directions. *Clin Orthop* **174**:58–68.

Friedlaender GE (1987). Bone grafts: the basic science rationale for clinical applications. *J Bone Joint Surg* **69A**:786–90.

Friedlaender GE (1991). Bone allografts: the biological consequences of immunological events. *J Bone Joint Surg* **73A**:1119–22.

Friedlaender GE, Strong GM, Sell KW (1984). Studies on the antigenicity of bone. II. Donor specific anti-HLA antibodies in human recipients of freeze-dried allografts. *J Bone Joint Surg* **66A**:107–22.

Frodel JL, Funk GF, Capper DT, et al (1993). Osseointegrated implants: a comparative study of bone thickness in four vascularized bone flaps. *Plast Reconstr Surg* **92**:449–55.

Fukuroda T, Nishikibe M, Ohta Y, et al (1992). Analysis of responses to endothelins in isolated porcine blood vessels by using a novel endothelin anatogonist, BQ-153. *Life Sci* **50**:PL107–PL112.

Furchgott RF (1983). Role of the endothelium in reponses of vascular smooth muscles. *Circ Res* **53**:557.

Furchgott RF (1988). Studies on relaxation of rabbit aorta by sodium nitrite: the basis for the proposal that the acid-activatable inhibitory factor from bovine retractor penis is inorganic nitrite and the endothelium-derived relaxing factor is nitric oxide. In: PM Vanhoutte (ed), *Vasodilatation, Vascular Smooth Muscle, Peptides, Autonomic Nerves and Endothelium*, pp 401–14. Raven Press, New York.

Furchgott RF, Zawadzki JV (1980). The obligatory role of endothelial cells in the relaxation of arterial smooth muscle by acetylcholine. *Nature* **288**:373–6.

Ganong WF (1989). Cardiovascular regulatory mechanisms. In: Ganong WF (ed) *Review of Medical Physiology*, 14th edn, pp 503–13. Appleton and Lange, Norwalk, Connecticut.

Garnet MF, Randolph MA, Schofield BH, Yaremchuk MJ, Weiland AJ (1991). Immunologic and ultrastructural changes during early rejection of vascularized bone allografts. *Plast Reconstr Surg* **88**:860–8.

Gerritsen ME, Cheli CD (1983). Arachidonic acid and prostaglandin endoperoxide metabolism in isolated rabbit and coronary microvessels and isolated and cultivated coronary microvessel endothelial cells. *J Clin Invest* **72**:1658–71.

Gibson T, Davis WG, Curran RC (1958). The long term survival of cartilage homografts in Man. *Br J Plast Surg* **11**:177.

Gilbert A (1976). Composite tissue transfers from the foot: anatomic basis and surgical technique. In: AL Daniller, B Strauch (eds), *Symposium on Microsurgery*, pp 230–42. Mosby, St Louis.

Gilbert A (1979). Surgical technique: vascularized transfer of the fibular shaft. *Intl J Microsurg* **1**:100–2.

Gilbert A (1980). Essai de révascularisation de la tête fémorale, en collaboration avec J. Judet, H. Judet. *Rev Chir Orthop* **66**:65.

Gilbert A (1981). Free vascularized bone grafts. *Intern Surg* **66**:27–31.

Gilbert A (1982a). Les transferts osseux libres vascularisés dans le traitement de la pseudarthrose congénitale. Presented at the Conference Enseignement. SOFCOT 30–31, Expansion Scientifique Française, Paris, France.

Gilbert A (1982b). Toe transfer for congenital hand defects. *J Hand Surg* **7**:118.

Gilbert A, Mathoulin C, Brunelli F, et al (in press). Reconstruction fémorale par transfert libre de péroné vascularisé. Publication pending.

Glimcher MJ (1968). A basic architectural principle in the organization of mineralized tissues. *Clin Orthop* **61**:16–36.

Gluckman PD, Grumbach MM, Kaplan SL (1981). The neuroendocrine regulation and function of growth hormone and prolactin in the mammalian fetus. *Endocrine Rev* **2**:363.

Goldberg VM, Porter BB, Lance EM (1980). Transplantation of the canine knee joint on a vascular pedicle. *J Bone Joint Surg* **62A**:414–24.

Goldberg VM, Shaffer JW, Field G, Davy DT (1987). Biology of vascularized bone grafts. *Orthop Clin North Am* **18**:197–205.

Gonzales del Pino J, Knapp K, Gómez-Castresana F, Benito M (1990). Revascularization of femoral head ischemic necrosis with vascularized bone graft: a CT scan experimental study. *Skeletal Radiol* **19**:197–202.

Gotfried Y, Yaremchuk MJ, Randolph MA, Weiland AJ (1987). Histological characteristics of acute rejection in vascularized bone allografts. *J Bone Joint Surg* **69A**:410–25.

Goto K, Kasuya K, Matski N, et al (1989). Endothelin activates the dihydropyridine-sensitive voltage-dependent CA^{2+} channel in vascular smooth muscle. *Proc Natl Acad Sci USA* **86**:3915–18.

Granick M, Newton ED, Hanna D (1986). Scapular free flap for repair of massive lower facial composite defects. *Head Neck Surg* **8**:436–41.

Greenberg BM, Jupiter JB, McKusick K, May JW Jr (1989). Correlations of postoperative bone scintigraphy with healing of vascularized fibula transfer: a clinical study. *Ann Plast Surg* **23**:147–54.

Gross PM, Heistad DD, Marcus ML (1979). Neurohumoral regulation of blood flow in bones and marrow. *Am J Physiol* **237**:H440–H448.

Guo F, Ding BF, Morrey MD (1981). Vascularized free fibula transfer in the treatment of bone tumors. Report of three cases. *Arch Orthop Trauma Surg* **98**:209–15.

Gupta A (1995). Vascularized epiphysis and hemi-joint transfer for treatment of hemifacial microsomia. In: *Transactions of the 11th Congress of the International Confederation of Plastic, Reconstructive and Aesthetic Surgery*, p 9. Kugler Publications.

Haas SL (1915). Experimental transplantation of the epiphysis with observations on the longitudinal growth of bone. *JAMA* **65**:1965.

Haas SL (1917). The localisation of the growing point in the epiphyseal cartilage plate of bones. *Am J Orthop Surg* **15**:563–86.

Haas SL (1931). Further observations on the transplantation of the epiphyseal cartilage plate. *Surg Gynecol Obstet* **52**:958–63.

Haines RW (1933). Cartilage canals. *J Anat* **68**:45–64.

Hall BK (1971). Histogenesis and morphogenesis of bone. *Clin Orthop* **74**:24.

Ham AW (1930). A histologic study of early phases of bone repair. *J Bone Joint Surg* **12**:827–44.

Ham AW, Harris WR (1956). Repair and transplantation of bone. In: GH Bourne (ed), *The Biochemistry and Physiology of Bone*, pp 475–505. Academic Press, New York.

Han CS, Wood MB, Bishop AT, Cooney WP III (1992). Vascularized bone transfer. *J Bone Joint Surg* **74A**:1441–9.

Hancox NM, Boothroyd B (1963). Structure–function relationships in osteoclasts. In: RR Sognnaes (ed), *Mechanism of Hard Tissue Destruction*, pp 497–514. American Association for the Advancement of Science, Washington.

Harmon PH (1945). A simplified surgical approach to the posterior tibia for bone grafting and fibular transference. *J Bone Joint Surg* **27**:496–8.

Harris WH (1960). A microscopic method of determining rates of bone growth (letter). *Nature* **188**:1035–9.

Haw CS, O'Brien BM, Kurata T (1978). The microsurgical revascularization of resected segments of tibia in the dog. *J Bone Joint Surg* **60B**:266–9.

Heiple KG, Chase SW, Herndon CH (1963). A comparative study of the healing process following different types of bone transplantation. *J Bone Joint Surg* **45A**:1593–1612.

Heppenstall RB (1983). Bone grafting. In: CM Evarts (ed), *Surgery of the Musculoskeletal System*, pp 89–104. Churchill Livingstone, New York.

Hertel R, Masquelet AC (1989). The reverse flow medial knee osteoperiosteal flap for skeletal reconstruction of the leg. *Surg Radiol Anat* **11**: 257.

Herzig E, Root WS (1959). Relation of sympathetic nervous system to blood pressure of the bone marrow. *Am J Physiol* **196**:1053–6.

Heslop BF, Zeiss IM, Nisbet NW (1960a). Studies on transference of bone. 1. A comparison of autologous and homologous bone implants with reference to osteocyte survival, osteogenesis and host reaction. *Br J Exp Pathol* **41**:269–87.

Heslop BF, Morrey MD, Zeiss IM, Nisbet NW (1960b). Studies on transference of bone. 1. A comparison of autologous and homologous bone implants with reference to osteocyte survival, osteogenesis and host reaction. *Br J Exp Pathol* **41**:269–87.

Heublein DM, Rodeheffer RJ, Cavero PG, et al (1989a). Relationship between plasma endothelin and atrial natriuretic factor in humans with congestive cardiac failure. *Am J Hypertens* **2**:37A.

Heublein DM, Cavero PG, Aarhus LL, Miller WL, Burnett JC (1989b). Detection of circulating endothelin in dog plasma by a sensitive radioimmunoassay. *J Vasc Med Biol* **1** (Abstr): 176.

Heyner S (1969). The significance of the intercellular matrix in the survival of cartilage allograft. *Transplantation* **8**: 666–7.

Heyner S (1973). The antigenicity of cartilage grafts. *Surg Gynecol Obstet* **136**:298–305.

Hickey KA, Rubanyi G, Paul RJ, Highsmith RF (1985). Characterization of a coronary vascoconstrictor produced by cultured endothelial cells. *Am J Physiol* **248**:C550–C556.

Hidalgo DA (1989). Fibula free flap: a new method of mandible reconstruction. *Plast Reconstr Surg* **84**:71–9.

Hidalgo DA (1991). Aesthetic improvements in free-flap mandible reconstruction. *Plast Reconstr Surg* **88**:574–85.

Hintz RL (1980). The somatomedins. *Adv Pediatr* **28**:293.

Hintz RL, Seeds JM, Johnsonbaugh RE (1977). Somatomedin and growth hormone in the newborn. *Am J Dis Childhood* **131**:1249.

Hintzsche E (1931). Uber Unbildungen in jungen menschlichen hyalin Knorpel. *Z Mikrost Anat Forsch* **25**:320–61.

Hirata Y, Yoshimi H, Takata S, et al (1988a). Cellular mechanism of action by a novel vasoconstrictor endothelin in cultured rat vascular smooth muscle cells. *Biochem Biophys Res Commun* **154**: 868–75.

Hirata Y, Yoshimi H, Takaichi S, Yanagisawa M, Masaki T (1988b). Binding and receptor down-regulation of a novel vasoconstrictor endothelin in cultured rat vascular smooth muscle cells. *FEBS Lett* **239**:13–17.

Hoffman S, Siffert RS, Simon BE (1972). Experimental and clinical experience in epiphyseal transplantation. *Plast Reconstr Surg* **50**:58–65.

Hohmann EL, Elde RP, Rysavy JA, Einzig S, Gebhard RL (1986). Innervation of periosteum and bone by sympathetic vasoactive intestinal peptide-containing nerve fibers. *Science* **232**:868–71.

Horowitz MC, Friedlaender GE (1991). Induction of T-cell responsiveness to allogenic bone. *J Bone Joint Surg* **73A**:1157–68.

Hunter W (1743). Of the structure and diseases of articulating cartilages. *Philos Trans R Soc London* **42**:514–21.

Huntington TW (1905). Case of bone transference. Use of a segment of fibula to supply a defect in the tibia. *Ann Surg* **41**:249–51.

Ihara M, Fukuroda T, Saeki T, et al (1991). An endothelin receptor (ET_A) antagonist isolated from *Streptomyces misakiensis. Biochem Biophys Res Commun* **178**:132–7.

Ihara M, Noguchi K, Saeki T, et al (1992). Biological profiles of highly potent novel endothelin antagonists selective for the ET_A receptor. *Life Sci* **50**:247–55.

Ilizarov GA, Devyatov AA, Kamerin VK (1980). Plastic reconstruction of longitudinal bone defects by means of compression and subsegment distraction. *Acta Chir Plast* **22**:32–41.

Innis PC, Randolph MA, Paskert JP, et al (1991). Vascularized bone allografts: in vitro assessment of cell-mediated and humoral responses. *Plast Reconstr Surg* **87**:315–25.

Inoue A, Yanagisawa M, Kimura S, et al (1989). The human endothelin family: three structurally and pharmacologically distinct isopeptides predicted by three separate genes. *Proc Natl Acad Sci USA* **86**:2863–7.

Jaffe EA (1985). Physiologic functions of normal endothelial cells. *Ann NY Acad Sci* **454**:279–91.

Jansen M, Schaik FMA, Ricker AT, et al (1983). Sequence of cDNA encoding human insulin-like growth factor I precursor. *Nature* **306**:609.

Jaroma HJ, Ritsila VA (1988). Behavior of cancellous bone graft with and without periosteal isolation in striated muscle: an experimental study. *Scand J Plast Reconstr Surg Hand Surg* **22**:47.

Johnson RW (1927). A physiological study of the blood supply of the diaphysis. *J Bone Joint Surg* **9**:153–94.

Jones NF, Swartz WM, Mears DC, Jupiter JB, Grossman A (1988). The "double barrel" free vascularized fibular bone graft. *Plast Reconstr Surg* **81**:378–85.

Jost A, Picon L (1970). Hormonal control of fetal development and metabolism. *Adv Metab Disord* **4**:168.

Judet H, Padovani JP (1968). Transplantation d'articulation complète avec rétablissement circulatoire immédiat par anastomoses artérielle et veineuse. *Mem Acad Chir* **94**:520–6.

Judet H, Padovani JP (1973). Transplantation d'articulation complète avec rétablissement circulatoire immédiat par anastomoses artérielle et veineuse chez le chien. *Rev Chir Orthop* **59**:125–8.

Judet H, Gilbert A, Judet J (1981). Essai de revascularization de la tête fémorale dans les nécroses primitives et post-traumatiques. *Rev Chir Orthop* **67**:261–6.

Judet PR, Patel A (1972). Muscle pedicle bone grafting of long bones by osteoperiosteal decortication. *Clin Orthop* **87**:74–9.

Jupiter JB, Bour CJ, May JW Jr (1987). The reconstruction of defects in the femoral shaft with vascularized transfer of fibula bone. *J Bone Joint Surg* **69A**:365–74.

Katusic ZS, Vanhoutte PM (1986). Anoxic contractions in isolated canine cerebral arteries. Contribution of endothelium-derived factors, metabolites of arachidonic acid and calcium entry. *J Cardiovasc Pharmacol* **8** (suppl):S97–S101.

Katusic ZS, Shepherd JT, Vanhoutte PM (1988a). Potassium-induced endothelium derived rhythmic activity in the canine basilar artery. *J Cardiovasc Pharmacol* **12**:37–41.

Katusic ZS, Shepherd JT, Vanhoutte PM (1988b). Endothelium-dependent contractions to calcium ionophore A23187, arachidonic acid and acetylcholine in canine basilar arteries. *Stroke* **19**:476–9.

Katz D, Téot L, Gilbert A (1985). Potentiel de croissance des tranferts épiphysaires vascularisés. *Ann Chir Main* **4**:249–58.

Kemp SF, Hintz RL (1980). The action of somatomedin on glycosaminoglyscan synthesis by cultured chick chondrocytes. *Endocrinology* **115**:1577.

King KF (1976). Periosteal pedicle grafting in dogs. *J Bone Joint Surg* **58B**:117.

Komori K, Vanhoutte PM (1990). Endothelium-derived hyperpolarizing factor. *Blood Vessels* **27**:238–45.

Kon V, Yoshioka T, Fogo A, Ichikawa I (1989). Endothelin may be the vasoconstrictor causing the persistent glomerular hypoperfusion in post-ischaemic kidneys. *Kidney Int* **35**:410.

Korstanje C, Mathy M-J, van Charldorp K, de Jonge A, van Zwieten PA (1985). Influence of respiratory acidosis and alkalosis on pressor responses mediated by α_1 and β_1 adrenoceptors in pithed normotensive rats. *Naunyn Schmiedebergs Arch Pharmacol* **330**:187–92.

Kort JS, Schink MM, Mitchel SN, Bassett CAL (1962). Congenital pseudarthrosis of the tibia: treatment with pulsing electromegnetic fields. *Clin Orthop Relat Res* **165**:124–37.

Kroll SS, Schusterman MA, Reece GP (1992). Cost and complications in mandibular reconstruction. *Ann Plast Surg* **29**:341–7.

Kuo ET, Ji ZL, Zhao YC, Zhang ML (1984). Reconstruction of metacarpophalangeal joint by free vascularized autogenous metatarsophalangeal joint transplant. *J Reconstr Microsurg* **1**:65–74.

Kwan CY, Grover AK, Daniel EE (1988). Cell membrane and regulation of cytoplasmic levels of Ca^{2+} in vascular smooth muscle. In: PM Vanhoutte (ed), *Vasodilatation, Vascular Smooth Muscle, Peptides, Autonomic Nerves and Endothelium*, pp 21–27. Raven Press, New York.

Lacroix P (1949). *L'organization des os* (Masson: Paris).

Langer K (1876). Uber das gefassytem der rohrenknochen, mit beitragen zur kenntnis des baues und der entwicklung des knochengewebes. *Denkschr Akad Wiss* **36**:1–40.

Langer F, Gross AE (1974). Immunogenicity of allograft articular cartilage. *J Bone Joint Surg* **56A**:297–304.

Langer SZ, Hicks PE (1984). Alpha-adrenoreceptor subtypes in blood vessels: physiology and pharmacology. *J Cardiovasc Pharmacol* **6** (suppl 4):S547–S558.

Lapierre F, Masquelet AC, Aesch B, Romaña MC (1990). Cranioplasties par lambeau libre vascularisé ostéopérioste fémoral. *Neurochirurgie* **36**:366,

Lau RS, Leung PC (1982). Bone graft viability in vascularized bone graft transfer. *Br J Radiol* **55**:325–9.

Lee EH, Goh, JCH, Helm R, Pho RWH (1990). Donor site morbidity following resection of the fibula. *J Bone Joint Surg* **72B**:129–31.

Leung PC, Chan KT (1986). Giant cell tumour of the distal end of the radius treated by resection and free vascularized iliac crest graft. *Clin Orthop* **202**:232–6.

Leung PC, Hung LK (1989). Bone reconstruction after giant cell tumor resection at the proximal end of the humerus with vascularized iliac crest graft: a report of three cases. *Clin Orthop* **247**:101–5.

Levi-Montacini RA (1982). Development neurobiology and the natural history of nerve growth factor. *Ann Rev Neurosci* **5**:341.

Lexer E, Kuliga P, Turek W (1904). Untersuchungen über Knochenarterien. Hirchwald, Berlin.

Lin HY, Kaji EH, Winkel GK, Ives HE, Lodish HF (1991). Cloning and functional expression of a vascular smooth muscle endothelin 1 receptor. *Proc Natl Acad Sci USA* **88**:3185–9.

Lincoln J, Burnstock G (1990). Neural–endothelial interactions in control of local blood flow. In: JB Warren (ed), *The Endothelium: An Introduction to Current Research*, pp 21–32. Wiley-Liss, New York.

Lindblad BE, Nielsen LB, Bjurholm, Hansen S (1993). Vasoconstrictive action of neuropeptide Y in bone. *Presented at the 39th Annual Meeting of the Orthopedic Research Society, abstr 249.*

Liu JJ, Gu XH, Casley DJ, Nayler WG (1990). Reoxygenation, but neither hypoxia nor intermittent ischemia, increaes (125I) endothelin-1 binding to rat cardiac membranes. *J Cardiovasc Pharmacol* **15**:436–43.

Loeb L (1926). Autotransplantation and homotransplantation of cartilage in the Guinea-pig. *Am J Pathol* **2**:111–22.

Lombard JH, Harder DR, Stekiel WJ (1988). Hypoxic vasodilatation and hypertension. In: PM Vanhoutte (ed), *Vasodilatation, Vascular Smooth Muscle, Peptides, Autonomic Nerves and Endothelium*, pp 61–4. Raven Press, New York.

Lopez-Curto JA, Bassingthwaighte JB, Kelly PJ (1980). Anatomy of the microvasculature of the tibial diaphysis of the adult dog. *J Bone Joint Surg* **62A**:1362–9.

Lundgaard A, Aalkjaer C, Mulvany MJ, Bjurholm A, Stender Hansen E (1993). Effects of calcitonin gene-related and vasoactive intestinal peptide on resistance vessels isolated from cancellous bone. *Presented at the 39th Annual Meeting of the Orthopedic Research Society, abstr 77.*

Lundholm L, Anderson RGG, Arnqvist HJ, Mohme-Lundholm E (1977). Glycolysis and glycogenolysis in smooth muscle. In: NL Stephens (ed), *The Biochemistry of Smooth Muscle*, pp 159–207. Universal Park Press, Baltimore.

Lüscher TF, Vanhoutte PM (1986). Endothelium-dependent contractions to acetylcholine in the aorta of the spontaneously hypertensive rat. *Hypertension* **8**:344.

Lüscher TF, Richard V, Tschudi M, Yang Z (1990). Serotonin and the endothelium. *Clin Physiol Biochem* 8 (suppl 3):108–19.

Luyten FP, Cunningham NS, Ma S, et al (1989). Purification and partial amino acid sequence of osteogenin, a protein initiating bone differentiation. *J Biol Chem* **264**:13377–80.

McBride AM, Stelling FH (1972). Infantile pseudarthrosis of the tibia. *J Bone Joint Surg* **54A**:1354–5.

McDonald DJ, McGuire MH (1991). Complications with large fragment allografts. In: K Brown (ed), *Complications of Limb Salvage: Prevention, Management and Outcome*, pp 25–8. ISOLS Publ, Montreal.

McInnis JC, Robb RA, Kelly PJ (1980). The relationship of bone blood flow, bone tracer deposition, and endosteal new bone formation. *J Lab Clin Med* **96**:511–22.

McKibbin B (1971). Immature joint cartilage and the homograft reaction. *J Bone Joint Surg* **53B**:123–35.

McKibbin B (1978). The biology of fracture healing in long bones. *J Bone Joint Surg* **60B**:150–62.

MacLeod A, Robinson D (1982). Reconstruction of defects involving the mandible and floor of the mouth by free osteo-cutaneous flaps derived from the foot. *Br J Plast Surg* **35**:239–46.

McMahon EG, Palomo MA, Moore WM, McDonald JF, Stern MK (1991). Phosphoramidon blocks the pressor activity of porcine big endothelin-1-(139) in vivo and conversion of big endothelin-1-(1-21) in vitro. *Proc Natl Acad Sci USA* **88**:703–7.

McMinn RMH, Pritchard JJ (1969). In: *Tissue Repair: Bone*, pp 148–68. Academic Press, New York.

Macquin-Mavier I, Levame M, Istin N, Harf A (1989). Mechanisms of endothelin-mediated bronchoconstriction in the guinea pig. *J Pharmacol Exp Ther* **250**:740–5.

Manaster BJ, Coleman DA, Bell DA (1990). Magnetic resonance imaging of vascular anatomy before vascularized fibular grafting. *J Bone Joint Surg* **72A**:409–14.

Mangiarua EI, Bevan RD (1986). Altered endothelium-mediated relaxation after denervation of growing rabbit ear artery. *Eur J Pharmacol* **122**:149–52.

Mangiarua EI, Joyce EH, Bevan RD (1986). Denervation increases myogenic tone in a resistance artery in the growing rabbit ear. *Am J Physiol* **250**:H889–H891.

Mankin HJ, Dappelt S, Tomford W (1983). Clinical experience with allograft implantation. The first ten years. *Clin Orthop* **174**:69–88.

Mankin HJ, Gebhardt MC, Tomford WW (1987). The use of frozen cadaveric allografts in the management of patients with bone tumors of the extremities. *Orthop Clin North Am* **18**:275–89.

Maroudas A, Bullough P, Swanson SA, Freeman MA (1968). The permeability of articular cartilage. *J Bone Joint Surg* **50B**:166–77.

Marquardt H, Hunkapillar MW, Hood LE et al (1983). Transforming growth factor produced by retrovirus transformed in rodent fibroblasts and human melanoma cells. *Proc Natl Acad Sci USA* **80**:4684.

Martin D, Mondie JM, DeBiscop J, Schott H, Peri G (1988). The osteocutaneous outer arm flap: a new concept in microsurgical mandibular reconstructions. *Rev Stomatol Chir Maxillofac* **89**:281–7.

Maruyama Y, Urita Y, Ohnishi K (1985). Rib latissimus dorsi osteomyocutaneous flap in reconstruction of a mandibular defect. *Br J Plast Surg* **38**:234–7.

Masquelet AC, Romaña MC, Penteado CV (1989). Vascularized periosteal grafts. In: M Aebi, P Regazzoni (eds), *Bone Transplantation*, pp 259–69. Springer-Verlag, Berlin.

Masquelet AC, Lapierre F, Aesch B, Romaña MC (1992). Cranioplasties by free revascularized osteoperiosteal flaps. In: VT Hinderer (ed), *Plastic Surgery*, Vol. II, pp 269–71. Elsevier Science Publishers, Amsterdam.

Mathes SJ, Buchannan R, Weeks PM (1980). Microvascular joint transplantation with epiphyseal growth. *J Hand Surg* **5**:586–9.

Mathoulin C, Gilbert A, Azze RG (1993a). Congenital pseudarthrosis of the forearm. *Microsurgery* **13**:252–9.

Mathoulin C, Gilbert A, Judet H et al (1993b). Free transfer of the vascularized fibula in pseudarthrosis and bone-loss of the femur. *J Orthop Surg* **7**:4.

Matloub H, Larson D, Kuhn J, Youssif J, Sanger J (1989). Lateral arm free flap in oral cavity reconstruction. A functional evaluation. *Head Neck Surg* **11**:205–11.

Maulik N, Liu X, Subramanian R, Das DK (1992). Release of endothelin during reperfusion of ischemic myocardium. ET-1 release from reperfused heart. *Am J Cardiovasc Pathol* **4**:133–44.

Medgyesi S (1965). Healing of muscle pedicle bone grafts. *Acta Orthop Scand* **35**:294–9.

Medgyesi S (1973). Observations on pedicle bone grafts in goats. *Scand J Plast Reconstr Surg* **7**:110–15.

Messina EJ, Weiner R, Kaley G (1976). Prostaglandins and local circulatory control. *Fed Proc* **35**:2367–75.

Metaizeau JP, Olive D, Bey P, Bordigoni P, Plenat F, Prevot J (1984). Resection followed by vacularized bone autograft in patients with possible recurrence of malignant bone tumors after conservative treatment. *J Pediatr Surg* **19**:116–20.

Meyers MH, Harvey JP Jr, Moore TM (1973). Treatment of displaced subcapital and transcervical fractures of the femoral neck by muscle pedicle bone graft and internal fixation. *J Bone Joint Surg* **55A**:257–74.

Milch RA, Rall DP, Tobie JE (1958). Fluorescence of tetracycline antibiotics in bone. *J Bone Joint Surg* **40A**:897–910.

Miller VM, Vanhoutte PM (1985). Endothelium-dependent contractions to arachidonic acid are mediated by products of cyclooxygenase. *Am J Physiol* **248**:H432.

Milner P, Ralevic V, Hopwood AM, et al (1989). Ultrastructural localization of substance P and choline acetyl transferase in endothelial cells of rat coronary artery and release of substance P and acetylcholine during hypoxia. *Experientia* **45**:121.

Minami A, Kaneda K, Itoga H, Usui M (1989). Free vascularized fibular grafts. *J Reconstr Microsurg* **5**:37–43.

Miyauchi T, Yanagisawa M, Tomizawa T, et al (1989). Increased plasma concentrations of endothelin-1 and big endothelin-1 in acute myocardial infarction. *Lancet* **ii**:53–4.

Moncada S, Herman AG, Higgs EA, Vane JR (1977). Differential formation of prostacyclin (PGX or PGI_2) by layers of the arterial wall. An explanation of the anti-thrombotic properties of the vascular endothelium. *Thrombosis Res* **11**:323–44.

Moncada S, Korbut R, Bunting S, Vane JR (1978). Prostacyclin is a circulating hormone. *Nature* **273**:767–8.

Monstrey S, Jones N (1992). The reliability of the ostecutaneous fibular free flap. Personal communication at the Annual Meeting of the American Society of Reconstructive Microsurgery, Scottsdale USA, Nov. 1992.

Montgomery RJ, Sutker BD, Bronk JT, Smith SR, Kelly PJ (1988). Interstitial fluid flow in cortical bone. *Microvasc Res* **35**:395–407.

Moore JB, Mazur JM, Zehr D, Davis PK, Zook EG (1984). A biomechanical comparison of vascularized and conventional autgenous bone grafts. *Plast Reconstr Surg* **73**:382–6.

Moran CG, Wood MB (1993). Vascularized bone autografts. A review paper. *Orthop Rev* **22**:187–97.

Moran CG, McGrory BJ, Roorda J, Wood MB (1993). Adrenergic control mechanisms of blood flow in a vascularized canine tibia allograft. *J Orthop Res* **11**:429–37.

Morris MA, Kelly PJ (1980). Use of tracer microspheres to measure bone blood flow in conscious dogs. *Calcif Tissue Int* **32**:69–76.

Morrissy RT, Riseborough EJ, Hall JE (1981). Congenital pseudarthrosis of the tibia. *J Bone Joint Surg* **63B**:367–75.

Moses AC, Nissley SP, Short PA, et al (1980). Increased levels of multiplication stimulating activity and insulin like growth factor in fetal rat serum. *Proc Natl Acad Sci USA* **77**:3649.

Moskalewski S, Kawiak J, Rymaszewska T (1966). Local cellular response evoked by cartilage formed after auto and allogenic transplantation of isolated chondrocytes. *Transplantation* **4**:572–81.

Moskovitz GW, Lukash F (1988). Evaluation of bone graft viability. *Semin Nucl Med* **18**:246–54.

Mysorekar VR (1967). Diaphyseal nutrient foramina in human long bones. *J Anat* **101**:813–22.

Nather A, Goh JSH, Lee JJ (1990). Biomechanical strength of nonvascularized and vascularized diaphyseal bone transplants. An experimental study. *J Bone Joint Surg* **72B**:1031–5.

Neild TO, Brayden JE (1991). Neural control of resistance arteries. In: JA Bevan, W Halpern, MJ Mulvanney (eds), *The Resistance Vasculature*, Chapter 13, pp 217–40. Humana Press, Totowa, NJ.

Nettelblad H, Randolph MA, Weiland AJ (1984). Free microvascular epiphyseal-plate transplantation. An experimental study in dogs. *J Bone Joint Surg* **66A**:1421–30.

Nettelblad H, Randolph MA, Weiland AJ (1986). Growth in revascularized bone grafts in young puppies. *Plast Reconstr Surg* **64**:239–43.

Neubauer S, Zimmermann S, Hirsch A, et al (1991). Effects of endothelin-1 in the isolated heart in ischemia/reperfusion and hypoxia/reoxygenation injury. *J Mol Cell Cardiol* **23**:1397–1409.

Newington DP, Sykes PJ (1991). The versatility of the free fibula flap in the management of traumatic long bone defects. *Injury* **22**:275–81.

Norman AW, Roth J, Orci L (1983). The vitamin D endocrine system. *Endocrine Rev* **4**:331.

Nove-Josserant M (1908). Pseudarthrose congénitale de la jambe guérie par la transplantation d'un lambeau ostéo-périosté cutané pris dans la jambe saine. *Soc Chirurgie Lyon:* 920–3.

O'Brien BMcC (1977). Microvascular free small joint transfer. In: *Microvascular Reconstructive Surgery*, pp 284–9. Churchill Livingstone, New York.

O'Brien RF, McMurtry IF (1984). Endothelial cell supernates contract bovine pulmonary artery rings. *Am Rev Respir Dis* **129**: abstr A337.

O'Brien BMcC, Gould JS, Morrison WA, Russel RC, MacLeod AM, Pribaz JJ (1984). Free vascularized small joint transfer to the hand. *J Hand Surg* **9A**:634–41.

Ogden JA (1974). Changing patterns of proximal femoral vascularity. *J Bone Joint Surg* **56A**:941–50.

Ok ET, Ji ZL, Zhao YC, Zhang ML (1984). Reconstruction of metacarpophalangeal joint by free vascularized autogenous metatarso-phalangeal joint transplant. *J Reconstr Microsurg* **1**:64–74.

Ollier LM (1867). *Traité expérimental et clinique de la régénération des os et de la production artificielle du tissu osseux*, Vol 1. Masson, Paris.

Östrup LT, Frederickson JM (1974). Distant transfer of a free living bone graft by microvascular anastomosis. An experimental study. *Plast Reconstr Surg* **54**:274–85.

Paley D, Catagni MA, Argnani F, Villa A, Benedette GB, Cattaneo R (1989). Ilizarov treatment of tibial nonunions with bone loss. *Clin Orthop* **241**:146–65.

Palmer RMJ, Ferrige AG, Moncada S (1987). Nitric oxide release accounts for the biological activity of endothelium-derived relaxing factor. *Nature* **327**:524–6.

Parish FF (1973). Allograft replacement of all or part of a long bone following excision of a tumor. Report of twenty-one cases. *J Bone Joint Surg* **55A**:1–22.

Parnavelas JG, Kelly W, Burnstock G (1985). Ultrastructural localization of choline acetyltransferase in vascular endothelial cells in rat brain. *Nature* **31**:724–5.

Paterson DC, Lewis GN, Cass CA (1980). Treatment of congenital pseudarthrosis of the tibia with direct current stimulation. *Clin Orthop Relat Res* **148**:129–35.

Peer LA (1939). The fate of living and dead cartilage transplanted in humans. *Surg Gynecol Obstet* **68**:603–10.

Penteado CV, Masquelet AC, Romaña MC, Chevrel JP (1990). Periosteal flaps: anatomical bases of sites of elevation. *Surg Radiol Anat* **12**:3.

Phelps AM (1891). Transplantation of tissue from lower animals to man. *Med Records* **39**:221.

Phemister DB (1914). The fate of transplanted bone and regenerative powers of its various constituents. *Surg Gynecol Obstet* **19**:303.

Phemister DB (1947). Treatment of ununited fractures by onlay bone grafts without screw or tie fixation and without breaking down of the fibrous union. *J Bone Joint Surg* **29**:946–60.

Pho RW (1981). Malignant giant cell tumor of the distal end of the radius treated by a free vascularized fibular transplant. *J Bone Joint Surg* **63A**:877–84.

Pho RW, Levack B, Satku K, et al (1985). Free vascularized fibula graft in the treatment of congenital pseudarthrosis of the tibia. *J Bone Joint Surg* **67B**:64–70.

Piotrowski G (1975). Physical and biological aspects of repair in dog cortical bone transplants. *J Bone Joint Surg* **57A**:237–46.

Pittet J-F, Morel DR, Hemsen A, et al (1991). Elevated plasma endothelin-1 concentrations are associated with the severity of illness in patients with sepsis. *Ann Surg* **213**:261–4.

Ponsetti IV (1970). Skeletal growth in achondroplasia. *J Bone Joint Surg* **52A**:701.

Puckett CL, Hurvitz JS, Metzler MH, Silver D (1979). Bone formation by revascularized periosteal and bone grafts, compared with traditional bone grafts. *Plast Reconstr Surg* **64**:361–5.

Radomski MW, Palmer RMJ, Moncada S (1987). The anti-aggregating properties of vascular endothelium: interactions between prostacyclin and nitric oxide. *Br J Pharmacol* **92**:639–46.

Ramasastry SS, Granick MS, Futrell JW (1986). Clinical anatomy of the internal oblique muscle. *J Reconstr Microsurg* **2**:117–22.

Rapoport RM, Draznin MB, Murad F (1984). Mechanisms of adenosine triphosphate-, thrombin-, and trypsin-induced relaxation of rat thoracic aorta. *Circ Res* **55**:468–79.

Ray RD (1972). Vascularization of bone grafts and implants. *Clin Orthop* **81**:43–8.

Ray RD, Sabet TY (1963). Bone grafts: cellular survival versus induction. *J Bone Joint Surg* **45A**:337–43.

Reid JJ, Wong-Dusting HK, Rand MJ (1989). The effect of endothelin on noradrenergic transmission in rat and guinea-pig atria. *Eur J Phamacol* **168**:93–6.

Restrepo J, Katz D, Gilbert A (1980). Arterial vascularization of the proximal epiphysis and the diaphysis of the fibula. *Int J Microsurg* **2**:48–51.

Reynolds EE, Mok LLS (1990). Role of thomboxane A_2/prostaglandin H_2 receptor in the vasoconstrictor response of rat aorta to endothelin. *J Pharmacol Exp Ther* **252**:915–21.

Rhinelander FW (1968). The normal microcirculation of diaphyseal cortex and its reponse to fracture. *J Bone Joint Surg* **50A**:784–800.

Rhinelander FW (1974). Tibial blood supply in relation to fracture healing. *Clin Orthop* **105**:34–81.

Richards MA, Pool MD, Godfrey AM (1985). The serratus anterior/rib composite flap in mandibular reconstruction. *Br J Plast Surg* **38**:466–77.

Ritsila V, Alhopuro S, Rintala A (1972). Bone formation with free periosteum. *Scand J Plast Renconstr Surg* **6**:51.

Robinson RA (1965). Morphology of osteoblasts, osteocytes, and osteoclasts with remarks about their function. In: *Tumors of Bone and Soft Tissues (Eighth Annual Clinical Conference on Cancer)*, pp 69–100. Yearbook Publishers, Chicago.

Rock MG, Wood MB (1991). Vascularized bone transfer for the management of post-irradiation pathologic fracture. In: K Brown (ed), *Complications of Limb Salvage: Prevention, Management, and Outcome*, pp 585–8. ISOLS Publ, Montreal.

Rock MG, Chao EYS, Shi LY, Sim FH, Sanjoy FH, Sanjoy B (1991). Osteoarticular allografts for reconstruction after tumor excision about the bone. In: K Brown (ed), *Complications of Limb Salvage: Prevention, Management, and Outcome*, pp 17–24. ISOLS Publ, Montreal.

Rock MG, Wood MB, Fleegler EJ (1993). Reconstruction for malignant tumors of the upper limb. In: GP Bogumill and EJ Fleeger (eds), *Tumours of the Hand and Upper Limb*, pp 413–34. Churchill Livingstone, New York.

Roger WM, Gladstone H (1950). Vascular foramina and arterial supply of the distal end of the femur. *J Bone Joint Surg* **32A**:867–76.

Romaña MC, Masquelet AC (1990). Vascularized periosteum associated with cancellous bone graft: an experimental study. *Plast Reconstr Surg* **85**:587.

Rubanyi GM (1988a). Endothelium-dependent pressure-induced contraction of isolated canine carotid arteries. *Am J Physiol* **255**:H783–H788.

Rubanyi GM (1988b). Endothelium-dependent vasoconstrictor factors. In: US Ryan (ed), *Endothelial Cell*, Vol. III, pp 61–70. CRC Press, Boca Raton, Florida.

Rubanyi GM, Vanhoutte PM (1985). Hypoxia releases a vasoconstrictor substance from the canine vascular endothelium. *J Physiol* **364**:45.

Rubanyi GM, Romero JC, Vanhoutte PM (1986). Flow-induced release of endothelium-derived relaxing factor. *Am J Physiol* **250**:H1145–H1149.

Ryan US (1986). The endothelial surface and responses to injury. *Fred Proc* **45**:101–8.

Sadove RC, Powell LA (1993). Simultaneous maxillary and mandibular reconstruction with one free osteocutaneous flap. *Plast Reconstr Surg* **92**:141–6.

Saijonmaa O, Ristimäka A, Fyhrquist F (1990). Atrial natriuretic peptide, nitroglycerine, and nitroprusside reduce basal and stimulated endothelin production from cultured endothelial cells. *Biochem Biophys Res Commun* **173**: 514–20.

Sakai YK, Doi K, Kawai S (1991). Free vascularized thin cortico periosteal graft. *Plast Reconstr Surg* **87**:290.

Sakurai T, Yanagisawa M, Tatuwa Y, et al (1990). Cloning of a cDNA encoding a nonisopeptide-selective subtype of the endothelin receptor. *Nature* **348**:732–5.

Sakurai T, Yanagisawa M, Masaki T (1992). Molecular characterization of endothelin receptors. *Trends Pharmacol Sci* **13**:103–8.

Sampath TK, Reddi AH (1981). Dissociative extraction and reconstitution of extracellular matrix components involved in local bone differentiation. *Proc Natl Acad Sci USA* **78**:7599–7603.

Sara VR, Hakk K, Rodeck CH, Wetterberg L (1981). Human embryonic somatomedin. *Proc Natl Acad Sci USA* **78**:3175.

Sarmiento A, Schaeffer JF, Beckerman L (1977). Fracture healing in rat femora as affected by functional weightbearing. *J Bone Joint Surg* **59A**:369–75.

Satoh T, Tsuchiya M, Harii K (1983). A vascularized iliac musculoperiosteal free flap transfer: a case report. *Br J Plast Surg* **36**:109.

Sawaizumi M, Maruyama Y, Okajima K, Motegi M (1991). Free vascularized epiphyseal transfer designed on the reverse anterior tibial artery. *Br J Plast Surg* **44**:57–9.

Schedewie HK, Fisher DA (1980). Perinatal mineral homeostasis. In: D Tulchinsky, KJ Ryan (eds), *Maternal–Fetal Endocrinology*, p 355. Saunders, Philadelphia.

Schusterman MA, Reece GP, Kroll SS, Weldon ME (1991). Use of the AO plate for immediate mandibular reconstruction in cancer patients. *Plast Reconstr Surg* **88**:588–93.

Schusterman MA, Harris SW, Raymond K, Goepfert H (1993). Immediate free flap reconstruction: significance of adequate surgical margins. *Head Neck* **15**:204–7.

Schuurman AH, Bos KE (1991). Laser Doppler bone probe: an experimental study in dogs. *Microsurgery* **12**:246–51.

Schwarzenbach O, Regazzoni P, Aebi M (1989). Segmental vascularized and nonvascularized bone allografts. In: M Aebi, P Regazzoni (eds), *Bone Transplantation*, pp 78–81. Springer-Verlag, Berlin.

Shaffer JW, Field GA, Goldberg VM, Davy DT (1985). Fate of vascularized and nonvascularized autografts. *Clin Orthop* **197**:32–43.

Shaffer JW, Field GA, Wilber RG, Goldberg VM (1987). Experimental vascularized bone grafts: histopathologic correlations with postoperative bone scan: the risk of false-positive results. *J Orthop Res* **5**:311–19.

Sherman MS (1963). The nerves of bone. *J Bone Joint Surg* **45A**:522–8.

Shim SS (1968). Physiology of blood circulation of bone. *J Bone Joint Surg* **50A**:812–24.

Shim SS, Patterson FP (1967). A direct method of qualitative study of bone blood circulation. *Surg Gynecol Obstet* **125**:261–8.

Shim SS, Hawk HE, Yu WY (1972). The relationship between blood flow and marrow cavity pressure of bone. *Surg Gynecol Obstet* **135**:353–60.

Siegert JJ, Wood MB (1987). Thrombosed vascularized bone graft: viability compared with a conventional bone graft. *J Reconstr Microsurg* **3**:99–103.

Siegert JJ, Wood MB (1990). Blood flow evaluation of vascularized bone transfers in a canine model. *J Orthop Res* **8**:291–6.

Simonis RB, Shirali HR, Mayou B (1991). Free vascularized fibular grafts for congenital pseudarthrosis of the tibia. *J Bone Joint Surg* **73B**:211–15.

Simonson MA, Dunn MJ (1992). The molecular mechanisms of cardiovascular and renal regulation by endothelin peptides. *J Lab Clin Med* **119**:622–39.

Skoog T (1967). The use of periosteum and surgicel for bone restoration in congenital clefts of maxilla: a clinical report and experimental investigation. *Scand J Plast Reconstr Surg* **1**:113.

Smith AU (1965). Survival of frozen chondrocytes isolated from cartilage of adult animals. *Nature* **207**:782–4.

Smith JW, Bellinger CG (1980) La vascularisation des tendons. In: R Tubiana, ed, *Traité de Chirurgie de la Main*. Masson, Paris: 375.

Smith PJ, Jones BM (1985). Free vascularised transfer of a metatarso-phalangeal joint to the hand. A technical modification. *J Hand Surg* **10B**:109–12.

Smith PJ, Foley B, McGregor IA, et al (1972). The anteromedial basis of the groin flap. *Plast Reconstr Surg* **49**:41–7.

Smith SR, Bronk JT, Kelly PJ (1990). Effect of fracture fixation on cortical bone blood flow. *J Orthop Res* **8**:471–8.

Snyder CC, Bateman JM, Davis CW, Warden GD (1970). Mandibular facial restoration with live osteocutaneous flaps. *Plast Reconstr Surg* **45**:14–19.

Soutar DS, McGregor IA (1986). The radial forearm flap in intraoral reconstruction: the experience of 60 consecutive cases. *Plast Reconstr Surg* **78**:1–8.

Speer D (1982). Collagenous architecture of the growth plate and the perichondrial ossification groove. *J Bone Joint Surg* **64A**: 399–407.

Spiessl B (1989). Internal fixation of the mandibule. In: Sequin F, Texhammer R (eds) *A Manual of AO/ASIF Principles*. Springer-Verlag, Berlin.

Spira E, Farin I (1967). The vascular supply of the epiphyseal plate under normal and pathological conditions. *Acta Orthop Scand* **38**:1–22.

Stein AH, Morgan HC, Porras RF (1958). The effect of pressor and depressor drugs on intramedullary bone marrow pressure. *J Bone Joint Surg* **40A**:1103–10.

Steinberg ME, Brighton CT, Steinberg DR, Tooze SE, Hayken GD (1984). Treatment of avascular necrosis of the femoral head by a combination of bone grafting, decompression, and electrical stimulation. *Clin Orthop* **186**:137–53.

Stevenson S, Horowitz M (1992). The response to bone allografts. *J Bone Joint Surg* **74A**:939–50.

Strauch B, Bloomberg AE, Lewis ML (1971). An experimental approach to mandibular replacement. Island vascular composite rib grafts, *Br J Plast Surg* **24**:334–41.

Stump CW (1925). The histogenesis of bone. *J Anat* **59**:136–54.

Sugioka Y (1978). Transtrochanteric anterior rotational osteotomy of the femoral head in the treatment of osteonecrosis affecting the hip: a new osteotomy operation. *Clin Orthop* **130**:191–201.

Sugiura M, Inagami T, Kon V (1989). Endotoxin stimulates endothelin-release in vivo and in vitro as determined by radioimmunoassay. *Biochem Biophys Res Commun* **161**: 1220–27.

Susa JB, Widness JA, Hintz RL, et al (1984). Somatomedins and insulin in diabetic pregnancies. *J Clin Endocrinol Metab* **58**:1099.

Swartz W, Banis J, Ramasastry S, Jones N, Acland R (1986). The osteocutaneous scapular flap for mandibular and maxillary reconstruction. *Plast Reconstr Surg* **77**:530–45.

Tabuchi Y, Nakamaru M, Rakugi H, Nagano M, Mikami H, Ogihara T (1989). Endothelin inhibits presynaptic adrenergic neurotransmission in rat mesenteric artery. *Biochem Biophys Res Commun* **161**: 803–8.

Takato T, Horii K, Nakatsuka T, Ueda K, Outake T (1986). Vascularized periosteal grafts: an experimental study using two different forms of tibial periosteum in rabbits. *Plast Reconstr Surg* **78**:489.

Takato T, Horii K, Nakatsuka T (1988). The segmental evaluation of bone scintigraphy: an analysis of revascularized bone grafts. *Br J Plast Surg* **41**:262–9.

Takayanagi R, Kitazumi K, Takasaki C, et al (1991). Presence of non-selective type of endothelin receptor on vascular endothelium and its linkage to vasodilation. *FEBS Lett* **282**:103–6.

Tam CS, Reed R, Cruickshank B (1974). Bone growth kinetics. I. Modifications of the tetracycline labeling technique. *J Pathol* **114**:127–33.

Tamai S, Hori Y, Fujiwara H (1987). Treatment of avascular necrosis of lunate and other bones by vascular bundle transplantation. In: JR Urbaniak (ed), *Microsurgery for Major Limb Reconstruction*, pp 209–19. Mosby, St Louis.

Taylor G (1982). Reconstruction of the mandible with free composite iliac bone grafts. *Ann Plast Surg* **9**:361–78.

Taylor GI, Daniel RK (1975). The anatomy of several free flap donor sites. *Plast Reconstr Surg* **56**:243–51.

Taylor GI, Watson N (1978). One-stage repair of compound leg defects with free vascularized flaps of groin skin and iliac bone. *Plast Reconstr Surg* **61**:494–506.

Taylor GI, Miller GDH, Ham FJ (1975). The free vascularized bone graft. A clinical extension of microvascular techniques. *Plast Reconstr Surg* **55**:533–44.

Taylor GI, Townsend P, Corlett R (1979). Superority of the deep circumflex iliac vessels as the supply for free groin flaps. *Plast Reconstr Surg* **64**:745–59.

Taylor GI, Wilson KR, Ress MD (1988). The anterior tibial vessels and their role in epiphyseal and diaphyseal transfer of fibula: an experimental study and clinical applications. *Br J Plast Surg* **41**:451–69.

Téot L (1982). Les transferts osseux libres vascularisés avec cartilage de croissance. *Rev Chir Orthop* **61**(suppl II):40–2.

Téot L (1991). Pedicled cryoconserved epiphyseal allografts. In: *Transactions of the 37th ORS*, March, p 288.

Téot L, Bossé JP, Mouffarege R, et al (1981). The scapular crest pedicled bone graft. *Int J Microsurg* **3**:257.

Téot L, Bossé JP, Dussault RG, Gilbert A (1983a). Pedicled iliac crest epiphysis transplantation. *Clin Orthop* **180**:286–93.

Téot L, Dussault RG, Bossé JP, Pous JG (1983b). Acetabuloplasty using pedicle iliac crest epiphysis transplantation in puppies. *Int Orthop* **7**:1–9.

Téot L, Charisso U, Arnal F, Pous JG (1986). Pedicled scapular crest epiphysis transplantation. *Acta Orthop Scand* **57**:163–7.

Téot L, Dussault RG, Arnal F, Blimcke B, Pfeil J, Pous JG (1987). Azetabulumplatiken durch gestielten Transfer der Beckenkammapophyse beim Hund. *Z Orthop Grenzgebiete* **2**:125, 163–9.

Téot L, Bossé JP, Pous JG (1988). Vascularized bone transfer, including epiphyseal plate. In: G Brunelli (ed), *Textbook of Microsurgery*. Masson, Milan.

Téot L, Souyris F, Bossé JP (1992). Pedicle scapular apophysis transplantation in congenital limb malformations. *Ann Plast Surg* **29**(4):332–40.

Tøndevold E, Eriksen J, Jansen E (1979a). Observations on long bone medullary pressure in relation to mean arterial blood pressure in the anesthetized dog. *Acta Orthop Scand* **50**:527–31.

Tøndevold E, Eriksen J, Jansen E (1979b). Observations on long bone medullary pressures in relation to arterial PO_2, PCO_2,and pH in the anesthetized dog. *Acta Orthop Scand* **50**:645–51.

Toynbee J (1841). Researches tending to prove the non vascularity and the peculiar uniform mode of organisation and nutrition of certain animal tissues. *Philos Trans R Soc London* **132**:132–59.

Tran MA (1980). The effect of lumbar sympathetic stimulation of the vasculature of bone. *Br J Pharmacol* **70**:363–6.

Trotman NM, Kelly WD (1963). The effect of sympathectomy on blood flow to bone. *J Am Med Assoc* **183**:123–4.

Trueta J (1957). The normal vascular anatomy of the human femoral head during growth. *J Bone Joint Surg* **39B**:358–94.

Trueta J (1961). The vascular contribution to osteogenesis. *J Bone Joint Surg* **43B**:800.

Trueta J (1963). The role of the vessels in osteogenesis, *J Bone Joint Surg* **45B**:402–18.

Trueta J, Amato VP (1960). The vascular contribution to osteogenesis, III. Changes in the growth cartilage caused by experimentally induced ischemia. *J Bone Joint Surg* **42B**: 571–87.

Trueta J, Cavadias AX (1955). Vascular changes caused by the Küntscher type of nail. An experimental study in the rabbit. *J Bone Joint Surg* **37B**:492–505.

Trueta J, Harrison MHM (1953). The normal vascular anatomy of the femoral head in adult man. *J Bone Joint Surg* **35B**:442.

Trueta J, Little K (1960). The vascular contribution to osteogenesis. II Studies with the electron microscope. *J Bone Joint Surg* **42B**:367–76.

Tsai TM, Hanna D (1988). Free vascularized joint transfers. In: G Brunelli (ed), *Textbook of Microsurgery*, pp 397–402. Masson, Milan.

Tsai TM, Jupiter JB, Kutz JE, Kleinert HE (1982). Vascularized autogenous whole joint transfer in the hand. A clinical study. *J Hand Surg* **7**:335–42.

Tsai TM, Singer R, Elliott E, Klein H (1985). Immediate free vascularized joint transfer from second toe to index finger proximal inter-phalangeal joint. A case report. *J Hand Surg* **10B**:85–9.

Tsai TM, Ludwig L, Tonkin M (1986). Vascularized fibular epiphyseal transfer. *Clin Orthop* **210**:228–34.

Uddstromer L (1978). The osteogenic capacity of tubular and membranous bone periosteum. A qualitative and quantitative study in growing rabbits. *Scand J Plast Renconstr Surg* **12**:195.

Urbaniak JR (1987). Aseptic necrosis of the femoral head treated by vascularized fibular graft. In: JR Urbaniak (ed), *Microsurgery for Major Limb Reconstruction*, pp 178–84. Mosby, St Louis.

Urbaniak JR, Aitken GSE, Nunley JA, Goldner RD (1988). Treatment of aseptic necrosis of the femoral head by free vascularized fibular graft. *Orthop Trans* **12**:191.

Urist MR, Strates BS (1971). Bone morphogenic protein. *J Dent Res* **50**:1392–1406.

Urist MR, Silverman BF, Buring K, Dubuc FL (1967). The bone induction principle. *Clin Orthop* **53**:243.

Urist MR, Iwata H, Strates BS (1972). Bone morphogenetic protein and proteinase in the guinea pig. *Clin Orthop* **85**:275–90.

Urken ML, Weinberg H, Vickery C, Buchbinder D, Lawson W, Biller HF (1989). The internal oblique-iliac crest osseocutaneous free flap in oromandibular reconstruction: report of 20 cases. *Arch Otolaryngol Head Neck Surg* **115**:339–49.

Usui Y, Kawai K, Hirohata K (1989). An electron microscopic study of the changes observed in osteocytes under ischemic conditions. *J Orthop Res* **7**:12–21.

Van den Wildenberg FA, Goris RJ, Tutein-Nolthenius-Puylaert MB (1984). Free vascularized periosteum transplantation: an experimental study. *Br J Plast Surg* **37**:226.

Vane JR, McGiff JC (1975). Possible contributions of endogenous prostaglandins to the control of blood pressure. *Circ Res* **36** (suppl I):168–175.

Vanhoutte PM (1988). The endothelium. Modulator of vascular smooth muscle tone. *New Engl J Med* **319**:512–13.

Vanhoutte PM (1991). Platelet-derived serotonin, the endothelium, and cardiovascular disease. *J Cardiovasc Pharmacol* **17** (suppl 5):S6–S12.

Van Nes CP (1966). Congenital pseudarthrosis of the leg. *J Bone Joint Surg* **48A**:1467–83.

Van Zwieten PA (1988). The role of adrenoreceptors in circulatory and metabolic regulation. *Am Heart J* **116**:1384–92.

Vemulapalli S, Rivelli M, Chiu PJ, del Prado M, Hey JA (1992). Phosphoramidon abolishes the increases in endothelin-1 release induced by ischemia-hypoxia in isolated perfused guinea pig lungs. *J Pharmacol Exp Ther* **262**:1062–9.

Von Boehmer H, Kisielow P (1990). Self–nonself discrimination by T-cells. *Science* **248**:1369–73.

Von Walter PH (1821). Wiedereinheilung der bei der Trapanation ausgebohrten Knochenscheibe. *Journal der Chirurgie und Augen Heilkunde* **2**:571.

Warner JJP, Philip JH, Brodsky GL, Thornhill TS (1987). Studies of nontraumatic osteonecrosis. The role of core decompression in the treatment of nontraumatic osteonecrosis of the femoral head. *Clin Orthop* **225**:104–27.

Warner TD, DeNucci G, Vane JR (1989). Rat endothelin as a vasodilator in the isolated perfused mesentery of the rat. *Eur J Pharmacol* **159**:325–6.

Watanabe M, Katsumi M, Yoshizu T, Tajima T (1980). Experimental study and clinical application of free toe-joint transplantation with vascular pedicle. *Orthop Surg* **31**:1411–16.

Watanabe T, Suzuki N, Shimamoto N, Fujino M, Imada A (1991). Contribution of endogenous endothelin to the excision of myocardial infarct size in rats. *Circ Res* **69**:370–7.

Watari S, Ikuta Y, Adachi N, Murase M, Tsuge K (1978). Vascular pedicle fibular transplantation as treatment for bone tumor. *Clin Orthop* **133**:158–64.

Watermann R (1965). Vascular beds in growth symphyses and calluses in the knee joint region. *Verh Anat Ges* **115**:137–52.

Watermann R (1966). On the blood supply of the distal femoral epiphysis. *Z Orthop* **101**:247–57.

Watts JA, Chapat S, Johnson DE, Janis R (1992). Effects of nisoldipine upon vasoconstrictor responses and binding of endothelin-1 in ischemic and reperfused rat hearts. *J Cardiovasc Pharmacol* **19**:929–36.

Wei FC, Chen HC, Chuang CC, Noordhoff MA (1986). Fibular osteoseptocutaneous flap: anatomical study and clinical application. *Plast Reconstr Surg* **78**:191–9.

Weiland AJ (1981). Vascularized free bone transplants. *J Bone Joint Surg* **63A**:166–9.

Weiland AJ (1991). Clinical applications of vascularized bone grafts. In: GE Friedlaender, VM Goldberg (eds), *Bone and Cartilage Allografts*, pp 239–45. American Academy of Orthopedic Surgeons, Park Ridge, IL.

Weiland AJ, Daniel RK (1979). Microvascular anastomosis for bone grafts in the treatment of massive defects in bone. *J Bone Joint Surg* **61A**:98–104.

Weiland AJ, Daniel RK (1980). Congenital pseudarthrosis of the tibia: treatment with vascularized autogenous fibular grafts. *Johns Hopkins Med J* **147**:89–95.

Weiland AJ, Moore JR, Daniel RK (1983). Vascularized bone autografts. Experience with 41 cases. *Clin Orthop* **174**:87–95.

Weiland AJ, Moore JR, Daniel RK (1984a). The efficacy of free tissue transfer in the treatment of osteomyelitis. *J Bone Joint Surg* **66A**:181–93.

Weiland AJ, Phillips TW, Randolph MA (1984b). Bone grafts: a radiologic, histologic, and biomechanical model comparing autografts, allografts, and free vascularized bone grafts. *Plast Reconstr Surg* **74**:368–79.

Weksler BB, Marcus AJ, Jaffe EA (1977). Synthesis of prostaglandin I_2 (prostacyclin) by cultured human and bovine endothelial cells. *Proc Natl Acad Sci USA* **74**:3922–6.

Weksler BB, Ley CW, Jaffe EA (1978). Stimulation of endothelial cell prostacyclin production by thrombin, trypsin, and the ionophore A23187. *J Clin Invest* **62**:923–30.

Wiklund NP, Öhlen A, Cederqvist B (1988). Inhibition of adrenergic neuroeffector transmission by endothelin in the guinea-pig femoral artery. *Acta Physiol Scand* **134**:311–12.

Wiktor-Jedrzejczak W, Bartocci A, Ferrante AW Jr, et al (1990). Total absence of colony-stimulating factor 1 in the macrophage deficient osteopetrotic (op/op) mouse. *Proc Natl Acad Sci USA* **87**:4828–32.

Wilsman NF, Van Sickle DC (1970). The relationship of cartilage canals to the initial osteogenesis of secondary centers of ossification. *Anat Rec* **168**:381–91.

Wood MB (1983). Canine vascularized bone segment transfers. Quantitation of blood flow. *Orthop Trans* **7**:354.

Wood MB (1986). Free vascularized bone transfers for nonunions, segmental gaps and following tumor resection. *Orthopaedics* **9**:810–16.

Wood MB (1990a). Free osseous tissue transfers. In: Wood MB (ed) *Atlas of Reconstructive Microsurgery*, pp 63–91. Aspen Publ, Rockville, MD.

Wood MB (1990b). Femoral reconstruction by vascularized bone transfer. *Microsurg* **11**:74–9.

Wood MB, Cooney WP III (1984). Vascularized bone segment transfers for management of chronic osteomyelitis. *Orthop Clin North Am* **15**:461–72.

Woodhouse CF (1963). Nutrient arterial circulation control problems in bone. *Am J Orthop Surg* **2**: 290–5.

Wozney JM, Rosen V, Celeste AJ, et al (1988). Novel regulators of bone formation: molecular clones and activities. *Science* **242**:1528–34.

Wray S (1988). Smooth muscle intracellular pH: measurement, regulation, and function. *Amer J Physiol*, **254**:C213–225.

Wray RC, Mathes SM, Young VL, Weeks PM (1981). Free vascularized whole joint transplants with ununited epiphyses. *Plast Reconstr Surg* **67**:519–25.

Wright CE, Fozard JR (1988). Regional vasodilation is a prominent feature of the haemodynamic response to endothelin in anesthetized, spontaneously hypertensive rats. *Eur J Pharmacol* **155**:201–3.

Yablon I, Cooperbands S, Cavall D (1982). Matrix antigens in allografts. *Clin Orthop* **168**:243–51.

Yajima H, Tamai S, Mizumoto S, Sigimura M, Horuichi K (1992). Vascularized fibular graft for reconstruction after resection of aggressive benign and malignant bone tumor. *Microsurgery* **13**:227–33.

Yajima H, Tamai S, Mizumoto S, Ono H (1993). Vascularized fibular grafts for reconstruction of the femur. *J Bone Joint Surg* **75B**:123–8.

Yamauchi T, Ohnaka K, Takayanagi R, Umeda F, Nawata H (1990). Enhanced secretion of endothelin-1 by elevated glucose levels for cultured bovine aortic cells. *FEBS Lett* **267**:16–18.

Yanagisawa M, Masaki T (1989). Endothelin, a novel endothelium derived peptide. *Biochem Pharmacol* **38**:1877–83.

Yanagisawa M, Hurihara H, Kimura S, et al (1988). A novel potent vasoconstrictor peptide produced by vascular endothelium cells. *Nature* **332**:411–15.

Yang Z, Richard V, von Segesser L, et al (1990). Threshold concentrations of endothelin-1 potentiate contractions to norepinephrine and serotonin in human arteries. *Circulation* **82**:188–95.

Yaremchuck MJ, Nettelblad H, Randolph MA, Weiland AJ (1985). Vascularised bone allograft transplantation in a genetically defined Rat model. *Plast Reconstr Surg* **75**:335–62.

Yashimura M, Shumamura K, Iwai Y, Yamauchi J, Ueno T (1983). Free vascularized fibular transplant. A new method for monitoring circulation of the grafted fibula. *J Bone Joint Surg* **65A**:1295–301.

Yoo MC (1994). Free vascularized fibular graft in treatment of osteonecrosis affecting the hip. In: R Ueno, N Akamatsu, Y Itami, H Tagawa, S Yoshino (eds), *The Hip: Clinical Studies and Basic Research: Proceedings of the 1st Western Pacific Area Conference on the Hip*, pp 189–92. Elsevier, Amsterdam.

Yoo MC, Chung DW, Hahn CS (1992). Free vascularized fibula grafting for the treatment of osteonecrosis of the femoral head. *Clin Orthop* **277**:128–38.

Yoshizu T, Watanabe M, Tajima T (1984). Transfers libres d'articulation d'orteil avec anastomoses vasculaires. In: R Tubiana (ed), *Chirurgie de la Main*, Vol. 2, pp 539–51. Masson, Paris.

Youdas JW, Wood MB, Cahalan T, Chao EYS (1988). A quantitative analysis of donor site morbidity after vascularized fibula transfer. *J Orthop Res* **6**:621–9.

Young MH (1966). Epiphyseal infarction in a growing long bone. An experimental study in the rabbit. *J Bone Joint Surg* **48B**:826–40.

Zaleske PJ, Ehrlich MG, Piliero C, May J, Mankin H (1982). Growth plate behaviour in whole joint replantation in the rabbit. *J Bone Joint Surg* **64A**:249.

Zdeblick TA, Shaffer JW, Field GA (1988). The healing of canine vascularized segmental osteotomies: the effect of retained endosteal circulation. *Clin Orthop* **236**:296–302.

Zehr RJ, Enneking WF, Heare T, Liang TS (1991). Fractures in large structural allografts. In: K Brown (ed), *Complications of Limb Salvage: Prevention, Management and Outcome*, pp 3–8. ISOLS Publ, Montreal.

Zinberg EM, Wood MB, Brown ML (1985). Vascularized bone transfer: evaluation of viability by postoperative bone scan. *J Reconstr Microsurg* **2**:13–19.

Zoja C, Orisio S, Perico N, et al (1991). Constitutive expression of endothelin gene in cultured human mesangial cells and its modulation by transforming growth factor-beta, thrombin and a thromboxane A_2 analogue. *Lab Invest* **64**:16–25.

Zuchman J, Maurer P, Berbesson C (1968). The effect of autografts of bone and periosteum in recent diaphyseal fractures. *J Bone Joint Surg* **50B**:409–22.

Index